Praise for *How to Heal Hashimoto's*

"The time is here to take back your health! Hashimoto's is a condition that can be healed and reversed—but you will need to step out of the world of conventional medicine to do so. Marc Ryan, a practitioner of Eastern Medicine and a Hashimoto's patient, shares his extensive experience from recovering his own health and helping thousands of patients do the same. Let *How to Heal Hashimoto's* be your road map to remission and start taking your health back today."

— Dr. Izabella Wentz, pharmacist and *New York Times* best-selling author of *Hashimoto's Thyroiditis* and *Hashimoto's Protocol*

"In *How to Heal Hashimoto's*, Marc takes the best parts of both Western and Eastern functional medicine to create a methodical approach that touches all aspects of the Hashimoto's journey with grace, humor, and firm encouragement. In doing so, he has empowered patients to better understand their bodies so they can engage as active participants in their own healing."

— Datis Kharrazian, D.H.Sc., D.C., M.S., author of *Why Do I Still Have Thyroid Symptoms When My Lab Tests Are Normal?* and *Why Isn't My Brain Working?*

"*How to Heal Hashimoto's* is an important new book for the autoimmune thyroid disease community, as it is the first of its kind to loop in the ancient healing practices of Traditional Chinese Medicine. Not only does Marc Ryan do an incredible job explaining the complex inner workings of the thyroid, but he shares the often overlooked emotional and spiritual side of healing as well. If you suffer from Hashimoto's, this is an incredibly actionable book that will help you get your life back!"

— Mickey Trescott, NTP, author of *The Autoimmune Paleo Cookbook* and *The Autoimmune Wellness Handbook*

"A whole person-centered look at understanding and treating Hashimoto's."

— Dr. Mike Dow, *New York Times* best-selling author of *Healing the Broken Brain*

"*How to Heal Hashimoto's* is the deepest book on the subject and a must read. If you are tired of being tired, read it twice!"

— Julie Daniluk, author of *The Hot Detox Plan, Slimming Meals That Heal,* and *Meals That Heal Inflammation*

HOW TO heal

HASHIMOTO'S

Hay House Titles of Related Interest

YOU CAN HEAL YOUR LIFE, the movie,
starring Louise Hay & Friends
(available as a 1-DVD program and an expanded 2-DVD set)
Watch the trailer at: www.LouiseHayMovie.com

THE SHIFT, the movie,
starring Dr. Wayne W. Dyer
(available as a 1-DVD program and an expanded 2-DVD set)
Watch the trailer at: www.DyerMovie.com

❧

YOUNG AND SLIM FOR LIFE:
10 Essential Steps to Achieve Total Vitality and Kick-Start Weight Loss That Lasts,
by Frank Lipman, M.D.

THE TRUTH ABOUT CANCER:
What You Need to Know about Cancer's History, Treatment, and Prevention,
by Ty Bollinger

MEDICAL MEDIUM LIFE-CHANGING FOODS:
Save Yourself and the Ones You Love with the Hidden Healing Powers of Fruits & Vegetables,
by Anthony William

LOVING YOURSELF TO GREAT HEALTH:
Thoughts & Food—the Ultimate Diet,
by Louise Hay, Ahlea Khadro, and Heather Dane

All of the above are available at your local bookstore, or may be ordered by visiting:

Hay House USA: www.hayhouse.com®
Hay House Australia: www.hayhouse.com.au
Hay House UK: www.hayhouse.co.uk
Hay House South Africa: www.hayhouse.co.za
Hay House India: www.hayhouse.co.in

Marc Ryan, L.AC.

HOW TO heal

HASHIMOTO'S

AN INTEGRATIVE
ROAD MAP TO REMISSION

HAY HOUSE, INC.
Carlsbad, California • New York City
London • Sydney • Johannesburg
Vancouver • New Delhi

Published and distributed in the United States by: Hay House, Inc.: www.hayhouse.com® • *Published and distributed in Australia by:* Hay House Australia Pty. Ltd.: www.hayhouse.com.au • *Published and distributed in the United Kingdom by:* Hay House UK, Ltd.: www.hayhouse.co.uk • *Published and distributed in the Republic of South Africa by:* Hay House SA (Pty), Ltd.: www.hayhouse.co.za • *Distributed in Canada by:* Raincoast Books: www.raincoast.com • *Published in India by:* Hay House Publishers India: www.hayhouse.co.in

Indexer: Jay Kreider • *Cover design:* Karla Baker • *Interior design:* Riann Bender
Illustrations: Maklin Ryan • Photography on pages 56, 115, 166, 219, 285, and 324 by Olesia Farberov • Images on pages 5, 14, 15, 65, 66, 68, 92, 140, 197, 203, and 335 licensed from depositphotos.com • Images on pages 27, 84, 94, 134, 193, 269, and 304; Five Element logo; and A.P.A.R.T. System logo courtesy of the author • Image on page 275 Zhuangzi Butterfly Dream: Ike no Taiga, Japan, 1723–1776 • Image on page 20: Hyperthyroidism Before/After: *The Practitioner,* January 1915, vol. XCIV, No. 1

A previous edition of this book was published under the title *Roadmap to Remission* (ISBN: 978-1515022879).

Library of Congress Cataloging-in-Publication Data

Names: Ryan, Marc,
Title: How to heal Hashimoto's : an integrative road map to remission / Marc
   Ryan, L.AC.
Description: Carlsbad, California : Hay House, Inc., [2017]
Identifiers: LCCN 2017001069 | ISBN 9781401953607 (paperback)
Subjects: LCSH: Thyroid gland--Diseases. | Thyroid gland--Diseases--Alternative treatment. | Self-care, Health. | BISAC: HEALTH & FITNESS / Diseases / Immune System. | HEALTH & FITNESS / Alternative Therapies. | HEALTH & FITNESS / Healing.
Classification: LCC RC655 .R93 2017 | DDC 616.4/4--dc23 LC record available at https://lccn.loc.gov/2017001069

Tradepaper ISBN: 978-1-4019-5360-7

10 9 8 7 6 5 4 3 2 1
1st Hay House edition, June 2017

Printed in the United States of America

SUSTAINABLE FORESTRY INITIATIVE

Certified Sourcing
www.sfiprogram.org
SFI-01268

SFI label applies to text stock only

To the three most important and influential women in my life:
My partner, Olesia, my daughter, Ava,
and my mother, Joyce.
This book would not have been possible
without your love and support.

Acknowledgments

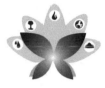

Drawings: Thank you to my son, Maklin Ryan, for his beautiful, original drawings of each of the five elements. These are true works of art, worthy of framing!

Photography: Thank you to Olesia Farberov for her photos of me doing qi gong exercises.

Editing: Thank you to Jeannie Ewing and Ava Ryan for their contributions to correcting the boatload of errors that I somehow missed the first time around.

Formatting: Thank you to Adam Timm for his help in formatting the book for print.

Thought Leaders: Thank you to my many colleagues in this movement to improve care for thyroid and Hashimoto's patients. Dr. Datis Kharrazian; Dr. Izabella Wentz and her husband, Michael Wentz; Dr. Sarah Ballantyne; Stacey Robbins; Dana Trentini; Mickey Trescott; the folks at Hashimoto's 411; and many more who toil daily to help educate and empower patients worldwide.

My Clients and Patients: Thank you for entrusting me with your care and for inspiring me to improve my craft on a daily basis to help solve the puzzle that is autoimmunity and Hashimoto's thyroiditis.

Contents

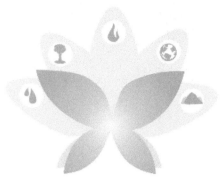

Foreword

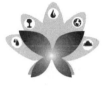

Few Chinese medicine practitioners are willing or able to explain Chinese medicine concepts in Western terms. But Marc Ryan, L.Ac., who calls Traditional Chinese Medicine (TCM) the "original functional medicine," gamely builds us a bridge between the Eastern and Western arts of healing.

If you've read my books, you'll see familiar functional medicine concepts of Hashimoto's hypothyroidism management. Not simply a problem of the thyroid, Hashimoto's is an autoimmune disease in which the immune system attacks and destroys the thyroid gland.

Thus, Hashimoto's is a problem of the immune system that involves a complex web of dysfunction and requires careful attention to the root causes of its debilitating symptoms.

What sets Marc's book apart is how he takes us on a functional medicine journey of Hashimoto's hypothyroidism through the lens of TCM.

Where Western medicine concerns itself with science and studies, Chinese medicine tells us a story about the human body, weaving in natural phenomena and earthly elements.

The Hashimoto's patient will find herself surprised by the uncanny knowing of this ancient healing art. For instance, in Chinese medicine the thyroid is seen as the place where communications and dreams are generated. When this area becomes clogged due to an inflamed and underfunctioning thyroid, the patient may feel stuck in her situation and unable to express her needs.

Marc weaves many such examples in, along with Chinese concepts of yin and yang, the five elements, Chinese herbs, and Chinese healing exercises. For the Hashimoto's patient, this book is a fascinating integration of sound functional medicine with an introduction to Chinese medicine's view of thyroid and immune function.

What's more, Marc presents the material in a conversational style that is fun to read. Hashimoto's is a complex topic that can seem overwhelming at first. Many people with Hashimoto's have difficulty with concentration, which makes it hard to read a complicated book about the topic.

In response, Marc has gone the extra mile to make his information easy to absorb with short paragraphs, clear descriptions, real-life examples, and helpful summaries. Throughout the book, his warm sense of humor, upbeat attitude, and genuine concern for helping people really shine through.

At the same time, staying true to Chinese medicine's broad-sweep approach to healing, he continually reminds us of the bigger picture—the spiritual nature of our journey, the connection of our health to that of the planet, and how facilitating the flow of energy through the organs is reflected in our flow through life's journey.

I have taught thousands of practitioners over the years and I know Marc to be a passionate and dedicated practitioner with clear integrity and humility, one of the few who leaves a seminar and reads and rereads the manuals in order to master the material. This, combined with his innate ability to incorporate larger life meanings of the Hashimoto's journey, has moved him beyond the role of practitioner into that of healer.

This passion was born out of Marc's personal experience as someone with Hashimoto's and the parent to a child with the disease. Knowing he was sick long before he knew why, his experiences were like that of many Hashimoto's patients.

These include: being told he'd have to wait until he was much worse before getting any treatment; being offered immunosuppressant therapy that would disable his body further; being dismissed by doctors; and, most important, his doctors not getting to the root of the problem.

It was when he decided to step outside of outdated, traditional modes of treatment that he made progress.

He went on to become an experienced acupuncturist and herbalist whose entire medical practice is now devoted to Hashimoto's. He truly cares that patients have the opportunity to understand how their bodies work, what is out of balance, and what steps they must take to live in a state of vitality and wellness again.

With the disconnect between conventional hypothyroidism care and the realities of Hashimoto's, the medical world clearly needs a renewed approach.

In *How to Heal Hashimoto's*, Marc takes the best parts of both Western and Eastern functional medicine to create a methodical approach that touches all aspects of the Hashimoto's journey with grace, humor, and firm encouragement.

In doing so, he has empowered patients to better understand their bodies so they can engage as active participants in their own healing.

Datis Kharrazian, D.H.Sc., D.C., M.S., author of *Why Do I Still Have Thyroid Symptoms When My Lab Tests Are Normal?* and *Why Isn't My Brain Working?*

Preface

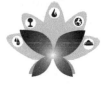

I wrote this book to help people who are suffering from the debilitating effects of Hashimoto's thyroiditis. Therefore, I have set a personal goal to help 100,000 people and I hope that you will be one of them.

I sincerely hope that you will experience at least some small victories along your journey and then build on those victories to gain some positive healing momentum and, eventually, reach remission.

MY STORY

Like many of the people I have worked with, I also have Hashimoto's and have lived with it for many years. Overcoming the struggles that it has presented has been a major motivator for me and is the reason why I'm so passionate about helping others.

For several years, I had no idea what was happening to me. I knew something was wrong, but I couldn't put my finger on it.

I was tired all the time, I couldn't sleep, I was in pain, I couldn't concentrate, my memory was shot, I couldn't focus, my digestion was horrible, my joints hurt, I had gained about 20 pounds of bloating and inflammation, and the worst thing was I had this really bad eye pain that just wouldn't stop.

Finally I went to a couple of eye doctors, and one of them did a battery of tests. At that point they discovered that I had a marker called HLA-B27, which is seen in people with Crohn's disease, and something called ankylosing spondylitis, which can cause the vertebrae in your spine to fuse.

I had some chronic back pain, but I didn't really have any other symptoms. Doctors told me that we'd wait and see and when it got bad enough, they'd put me on immunosuppressant therapy and pain-relieving drugs to completely disable my immune system and, they hoped, keep me out of pain.

As a functional medicine practitioner, that made no sense to me. Wait until my spine is severely damaged and then do something to disable another part of my body?

The truth is if a person has to live through that, it evolves into a gradual, or sometimes not-so-gradual, loss of function and quality of life. It's miserable. I've worked with people who had gotten to that point.

I'M NOT GOING THAT ROUTE

Well . . . no! No, no. I didn't want to go that route.

In response, I started treating myself using what I knew from functional medicine. I began a strict autoimmune diet and took some supplements. Through that, I was able to start to get my life back.

Then something interesting happened: I lost those extra 20 pounds, and because I could actually see my body differently, I discovered some nodules on my thyroid.

I went to see a physician friend, and he sent me for an ultrasound and some blood tests. Thank God, the nodules were not cancerous, but my antibodies were really high, and I was diagnosed with Hashimoto's.

And the funny thing was, I was in the same place all over again. My doctor said, "Yeah, you have elevated antibodies [at the time, my thyroid peroxidase (TPO) antibodies were 1,200], but all your thyroid numbers are in the normal range."

He continued, "So we're going to keep an eye on it and when it gets bad enough, we'll put you on Synthroid, and that will take care of it."

So, once again, do nothing until my thyroid is sufficiently destroyed and then act. It was then that the light went on in my head and I realized . . .

"There is nothing for us!"

Holy crap, I thought to myself, most emphatically, *there is nothing for those of us who are in this in-between stage of discovering we have autoimmune disease and major destruction of the tissue that's being attacked. Nothing.*

This doctor was well-intentioned; he was a personal friend. I know he had my best interest at heart, yet that was all he had to offer.

It was then that I decided to devote my life to finding other ways of solving this problem that could turn people's lives around *before* it was too late.

I had to really step up what I was doing and study a lot to try and figure out how to heal this disease, because I was determined not to let it ruin my life.

After many years of personal and clinical experience, I have found that to achieve remission from Hashimoto's, you must:

- First, understand, at least somewhat, what's happening to your body.

- Second, identify the problem areas and prioritize which are the worst.

- Third, acquire the necessary tools for fixing those problem areas and start initiating the healing process.

- And, last, follow through with the healing process on all systems of the body that have been impacted and use that healing to build positive momentum.

In addition, I sincerely hope to provide you with some inspiration of what is possible, some practical knowledge, and some clinical insights that you might not have had before about this incredibly complex, mysterious, and beautiful vessel we call the human body.

If you are like many of the people with Hashimoto's whom I've worked with, then you may be easily overwhelmed and have difficulty retaining a lot of information. We've tried to design the book to minimize that discomfort and to allow you easy access to the information.

As you read, you'll notice that the paragraphs are short, headlines summarize the essential ideas, and there are many summaries and recaps of important takeaways at the end of each chapter.

In addition, you may observe that the subject matter is not strictly technical and clinical in nature. In my opinion, real life is more than physiology and science.

For example, I have included some additional commentary in the form of what I call "Hashimoments" and "Clinical Pearls."

Hashimoments are positive affirmations for people with Hashimoto's. They come from the lessons I have learned about the process of healing.

Clinical Pearls are insights into treatment that I have had after working with so many people in this patient population.

Healing requires more than a laundry list of drugs and supplements, so this book includes plenty of emotion, stories, opinions, spirit, and curiosity.

And I'll warn you, I can be irreverent, opinionated, silly, and unorthodox. It's all in the name of trying to bring life to material that can sometimes be a bit dry and boring.

That's what makes things fun and worth pursuing. I'd be bored writing a book without that. And you'd probably be bored reading it. If you're looking for a standard-grade medical text, this book is probably not for you.

Most important: Keep in mind that remission is not the magical disappearance of your Hashimoto's. Nor is it a cure or license to go back to the things that made you sick in the first place.

Remission is a *journey*.

It involves taking responsibility for your life and circumstances and doing whatever is necessary to change that life and those circumstances.

The road to your remission should be ever-evolving and growing, and it should be a process that you continue to improve upon and refine.

So it is not a destination. Getting there is just half the battle. Staying there is the other half. And the only way you can stay there is to be committed for the long haul.

Measurable goals should be:

- normal thyroid lab tests;

- antibodies within the normal range;

- a healthy range for a number of other key indicators (which we will explore in upcoming chapters of the book).

These goals are just that. They are meant to be targets. You may not reach them 100 percent. And that's okay. Not reaching them 100 percent does not mean that you failed or that you should give up and quit trying. These are just numbers, and numbers in isolation are never a complete measure of success or failure.

One important thing to remember about laboratory tests is that they are not meaningful outside the context of what you are experiencing in your own body.

So you must always be aware of what is happening in your body, of how you feel, and also of what factors led up to that. Try to pay attention to both the good and the bad.

What you feel is clinically relevant and diagnostically important. And really, everything you do and try is just a test. What happens as a result is data that we can use; it provides us with clues and valuable information.

In addition, one should never keep forcing a solution when the evidence before you plainly shows that it isn't working.

You must change your plan when that happens.

This can be tricky, but it is possible to do it if you have a system.

Unfortunately, this is usually not part of the mainstream approach. With conventional medicine, medication is often the first treatment option, diet and lifestyle changes are ignored or dismissed, and the experiences that you have within your body are not given the importance that they deserve.

To address this problem and offer an alternative way of approaching healing that does take important factors like diet, lifestyle, physical, emotional, and spiritual experiences into account, I've created a simple system for you to use.

THE A.P.A.R.T. SYSTEM

It's called **The A.P.A.R.T. System** because this approach stands apart—and so will your results if you use it.

This is a simple, easy-to-remember acronym for getting better results that aren't based on protocols, dogma, or preconceived ideas.

It goes like this:

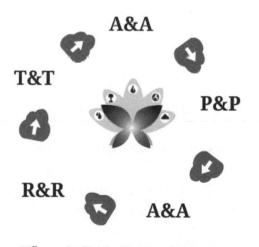

The A.P.A.R.T. System

Each letter has two ideas that are associated with it.

1. A = Ask and Assess

Data has healing power, *if* you know what data to collect and analyze, and *if* you know what to do with that information. (Both are big ifs.)

You need to ask what the symptoms are and assess the different systems of the body to find out where these symptoms are coming from.

Every bodily system and lifestyle practice needs to be a suspect. Don't exclude something because you're attached to it, feel like you can't do without it, or have decided that it isn't a problem.

Everything in your life should be evaluated with equal scrutiny, and if it isn't working to make you better, it may have to be eliminated.

This includes people, places, and things (like your favorite foods and drinks).

2. P = Prioritize and Plan

Not everything has the same level of importance. This is what 80/20 teaches us, that 20 percent of your issues cause 80 percent of your symptoms. I'll go into this in more detail in the Introduction.

Some things have more of an impact than others. Figure out which they are (the positive feedback loops, or the things that are repeated and reinforced in your body and mind) and focus on those first. Then make a plan to fix them.

I have created a Cheat Sheet in the back of the book that contains what I believe are the most common 20 percent issues that cause 80 percent of our problems.

3. A = Act and Adapt

Act and put your plan into motion. Then observe what the results are. Double down on what works and change what doesn't. Results should be apparent relatively quickly. If they aren't, you need to make changes.

The common practice of a doctor or practitioner prescribing something and then telling the patient to come back in three to six months is not the best approach, in my opinion. That's way too long, especially if it isn't working.

4. R = Reassess and Readjust

Retest, reassess, and ask all over again. Figure out what worked and what didn't. Double down on what worked and either eliminate or re-create a plan for what didn't.

It sounds obvious, but it is often overlooked or forgotten. Testing and reevaluating what you have done to see the result of your treatment is essential for good care.

Quick side note here: What I have learned over many years of practice is that you need to trust what the data is telling you. In most cases, when you make the right choice, you start feeling better.

Things like a "healing crisis," a "die-off," or a "detox reaction" sometimes occur, but they can also be a cover for incompetence. The right decision should result in a positive result relatively quickly.

If you are doing something and you aren't getting better, or you continue to feel worse, or it causes more discomfort, pain, and adverse symptoms, then you need to question whether that is the best course of action.

Eliminate it, reduce variables, and find out which part of what you are doing is causing that reaction or set of symptoms.

And all of this should not be done on the basis of lab tests alone. With Hashimoto's, assessments must also include a thorough examination of signs and symptoms.

Remember: What you feel is diagnostically important and clinically relevant.

5. T = Try and Try Again

Keep doing it, keep refining, keep building on the positive results, and keep looking for the remaining positive feedback loops that are causing vicious cycles.

People sometimes give up before giving a certain approach a chance, or they get some good results and then slide back to their old ways of doing things. When you find something that works, keep doing it. Don't quit and don't give up.

> **Our main goal is the transformation of vicious cycles into positive healing momentum. This means you start to feel better and then you build on that success.**

Lab work and symptoms should all confirm that this has taken place.

Again, lab tests must always be viewed in context to how you feel. It is the combination of these two factors that determine success or failure.

In addition, you must create realistic goals that are small enough to achieve and then build upon them. Acknowledge and celebrate your small victories. You can't go from sick to perfect in a couple of weeks.

As I said, remission is a journey. It is measured by how you feel, by your lab tests, and by your quality of life.

In other words, this journey is all about creating a lifestyle that will sustain and foster ongoing success.

Introduction

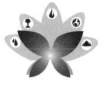

Over the past four years, I've had more than 2,000 conversations with people who suffer from this disease. And one of the most common questions I am asked is, "Why doesn't my doctor understand what is happening with Hashimoto's?"

People often share with me that they feel like they're being dismissed and that their symptoms are not being taken seriously by their doctors.

They want to know, "Why do doctors say things like, 'Hashimoto's isn't a real disease' or 'People just want to blame everything on this disease'?"

I don't know exact reasons or circumstances, but one possible explanation is the popularity of the drug Synthroid. This drug is a synthetic form of the thyroid hormone T4.

It is also the number-one branded synthetic hormone therapy for thyroid disease and the most widely prescribed medication in the United States.

According to Drugs.com, total sales of Synthroid in 2013 exceeded $800 million.[1]

Because of the drug's popularity and market share, the manufacturers have influenced the research and treatment of hypothyroidism and Hashimoto's.

And, of course, doctors know how important thyroid hormone is in the body, so there are good reasons for prescribing this drug. But, there are also consequences to the dogma of this approach.

The problem with a dogmatic approach to these principles is that they aren't always true when you're dealing with autoimmune diseases like Hashimoto's. And when this treatment doesn't work, it can have a big impact on people's lives.

---

1   "Synthroid Sales Data," Drugs.com. Retrieved February 1, 2014, from www.drugs.com/stats/synthroid

TWO THEORIES THAT LEAD TO DECLINES IN QUALITY OF LIFE

As a result, the following two theories have become common practice:

1: Synthetic T4 has been deemed the only treatment that is necessary and it is the standard of care for the majority of patients with Hashimoto's and hypothyroidism.

Results are considered confirmed by testing TSH (thyroid-stimulating hormone) and total T4.

As long as TSH is within the normal range, the patient is considered healthy.

For all intents and purposes, this practice is nothing more than TSH management with synthetic T4.

2: The thyroid can be lost and simply replaced by thyroid hormone medication. Letting the thyroid be destroyed by autoimmunity or having it surgically removed are both presented as viable, and sometimes preferred, treatment options.

This may seem like an exaggeration, but I have heard from many patients that this was the advice they received from their physicians. And they were told that supplementation with synthetic T4 would be all that is necessary once the thyroid is removed or destroyed.

This is supported by research as well. In a study published in 2011 in the *American Journal of Surgery*,[2] researchers found that the percentage of patients having total thyroidectomy increased from 17.6 percent (from 1993 to 1997) to 39.4 percent (from 2003 to 2007) for benign, noncancerous, thyroid disease.

Both of these theories have widespread consequences that affect the lives of millions worldwide, sometimes dramatically. The problem is that this approach doesn't always work and often doesn't address the underlying cause, which is the autoimmune process.

To date, I have found only one evidence-based study that supports the idea that removing the target tissue (that part of the body being attacked—in this case, the thyroid) improves symptoms of Hashimoto's in some cases, but there is no evidence that surgery completely removes autoimmunity from the body.[3]

---

2   "Utilization of thyroidectomy for benign disease in the United States: A 15-year population based study," by T. W. T. Ho et al, 2011, *The American Journal of Surgery*, 201, pp. 570–574.

3   "Total thyroidectomy in patients with Hashimoto's disease leads to elimination of anti-thyroid peroxidase (anti-TPO) levels and to elimination of severe accompanying ailments," by I. Guldvog et al, Poster 136, International Thyroid Congress 2015.

Furthermore, that theory makes no sense physiologically. The more we learn about autoimmune disease, the more we understand it to be systemic, and it often attacks multiple body parts.

These two theories are also responsible for the decline in quality of life for some people, which can mean loss of employment due to inability to work and function. It may also result in painful alienation and isolation from friends, family, and loved ones.

This is not a quality of life that any sane person would feel is acceptable or desirable, yet this is often the accepted quality of care in today's conventional medical system.

When these two approaches don't work, patients are sometimes advised to get psychiatric evaluations and prescribed antidepressants and antianxiety medications.

It doesn't have to be this way. There are other options for approaching this problem.

In upcoming chapters we will explore alternatives to this methodology and seek to understand, first, what is happening in the bodies of people who suffer from Hashimoto's. Second, we will examine the solutions that are effective for treating this disease.

I've already shared my personal story. Now here's a little about me professionally, so that you can get a sense of how I have worked to transform my personal struggles into helping others.

MY WORK

I have Hashimoto's, one of my children has Hashimoto's, and my entire practice is devoted to studying, researching, treating, and helping people recover from this disease.

I'm also a graduate of Cornell University and a licensed acupuncturist and herbalist who practices functional medicine. If you don't know what this means, it is a marriage of Western diagnostic testing and natural medicine.

I've been in practice for about 13 years. My life isn't perfect, but I have an amazing life today. I'm able to be present for my family, spend time with my kids, and walk my crazy dog twice a day.

I have the energy to do all this and to work with lots of people with Hashimoto's. I'm excited about jumping out of bed in the morning.

TREATING HASHIMOTO'S IS ALL I DO

I love what I do, and all I do is treat Hashimoto's. It's all I *want* to do. And there's no end to the challenges, believe me!

My passion has enabled me to work with people all over the world. I am fortunate to have the clinical and personal experience to really help my Hashimoto's patients—something that mainstream medicine, as we have seen, sometimes struggles to do.

But I didn't really plan it this way. I didn't wake up one day and decide to become "The Hashimoto's Guy." There was a time when I was suffering from the debilitating effects of this disease just like many other people.

I started my website, www.hashimotoshealing.com, and our Facebook support group, Hashimoto's Healing, so that I could share information and support my patients.

My hope was to reach a few hundred people and share some things that I had learned. Since then, this endeavor has absolutely exploded.

My site and others that are devoted to helping people heal from Hashimoto's and other autoimmune diseases have become popular, and I've come to realize that there are millions of people worldwide who are suffering from this disease.

HASHIMOTO'S IS *EVERYWHERE*

It's an epidemic, and many are starting to take notice as they seek alternatives to the treatment and care that is currently being offered. For a lot of us, the current treatment approach is inadequate at best, and at worst, just plain worthless.

To give you a sense of the sheer numbers, I have worked with more than 1,000 people (and spoken to more than 2,000) with Hashimoto's in the past four years.

Here's what I've learned: The average age of those people was 46; 96 percent were female, and 55 percent were on thyroid hormone (the most common brand was Synthroid, followed by levothyroxine, Armour Thyroid and Nature-Throid). The most common symptoms were (in order) fatigue, brain fog, weight gain, depression, anxiety, hair loss/thinning, constipation, and insomnia.[4]

The majority of these conversations have been free consultations that I offer for two reasons: First, I genuinely want to help these people and, second, I want to learn

---

4   I interviewed 904 individuals who were diagnosed with Hashimoto's. These interviews took place from April 2013 to June 2015. See Commentary in the back of the book for more information.

everything I can. And what better way than to actually speak to the people who are living with Hashimoto's?

It's crazy. These are people who reached out to me who know they have this disease. Imagine how many more are out there who have *not* been diagnosed.

The majority of the people I've talked to, including myself, went a number of years before anyone figured out what was going on with them. Even though Hashimoto's is so widespread, it is commonly misdiagnosed or ignored.

So I really think we're seeing the tip of the iceberg.

MY MISSION IN LIFE

Since this profound revelation, I have had the good fortune to study with some of the best teachers and practitioners in the world, like Dr. Datis Kharrazian, D.C. and Matt Van Benschoten, O.M.D.

I am indebted to them and many others who have devoted countless hours in study and research and have generously shared their knowledge, understanding, personal stories, and experience with those of us who are hungry to find another way.

While it was not easy, I was gradually able to find my way. Today I have plenty of energy and very little pain; I've figured out how to effectively treat and reverse the brain fog that really made it hard for me to function; and I have decided to commit my life to helping other people with Hashimoto's turn their lives around.

And it doesn't have to be so hard for you. Today we are very fortunate to live in a time when there is a lot of great information at our disposal. The tricky part is sorting out which information is best for you and your unique set of circumstances.

THE 80/20 PRINCIPLE

I'd like to share something with you that I believe is a really valuable mind-set for healing.

Earlier this year, I had an epiphany.

As I mentioned in the preface of this book, I stumbled upon something called the 80/20 principle, and it applies here.

It's an idea that is often applied to business. It's also called the Pareto Principle; basically, it came from a discovery by an economist named Vilfredo Pareto.[5]

Okay, so what does this have to do with Hashimoto's?

Well, it turns out that this basic idea applies to just about everything in the natural world.

Look around you . . .

. . . 80 percent of the traffic travels on 20 percent of the roads in your town or city. Most people spend 80 percent of their time with 20 percent of their friends. Go look in your closet: You wear 80 percent of your clothes less than 20 percent of the time.

You can apply this to everything, including your body and your health. And it's not about the numbers.

The point is that there is an imbalance in cause and effect. Relatively few things cause the majority of results.

Why does this matter?

Well with Hashimoto's, if this is true, it means that 80 percent of our problems are caused by 20 percent of the things we need to work on.

Or let me put it another way:

If you are like many of the people I have worked with, then 80 percent of your symptoms are caused by 20 percent of the choices you made today.

Now imagine if you could fix 80 percent of your symptoms fast by figuring out what those 20 percent choices are and then make some changes, making that 20 percent really count.

This would get you feeling 80 percent BETTER. How awesome would it be:

To have 80 percent MORE ENERGY?

To have 80 percent more MENTAL CLARITY AND FOCUS?

To feel 80 percent HAPPIER?

To lose 80 percent of THAT WEIGHT YOU WANT TO LOSE?

To FEEL LIKE YOUR OLD SELF 80 percent of the time?

Who doesn't want that?

Obviously the most important thing is to figure out what that 20 percent is, right?

---

5   "Understanding the pareto principle (the 80/20 rule)," by K. Azad. Retrieved February 2014 from betterexplained.com/articles/understanding-the-pareto-principle-the-8020-rule/

After working with hundreds of people, studying for thousands of hours, and reading tons of research, I think I have a general sense of what this 20 percent encompasses for most people. This book will help you discover where it is for you.

One thing you can be sure of is that it is usually found in the things you spend the most time doing.

If we break that down to practical terms, it comes down to four areas of your life:

1. Your DIET

2. How you handle STRESS and BLOOD SUGAR—these are totally interrelated

3. EXERCISE—hugely important for your brain, for your immune system, for dealing with stress, etc.

4. And really getting good at FINDING THE 20 PERCENT in your body

Get to know your body, so you can identify where the problems are. Be conscious of what's happening on a daily basis and learn to take responsibility for the way your actions and behavior affect your health. It's remarkable how easy it is to forget that the answer is often inside of us.

And when you do become conscious, present, and aware, it can dramatically improve your chances of getting better. Championships don't happen by accident. They are the result of a huge number of small, conscious decisions.

Become a superstar in healing yourself. It is time, energy, and effort well spent. In fact, I'll go out on a limb and say there is no better use of your time, energy, and effort. When you lose your health, you often lose many of the things that make life worth living.

Metal

Fire

Earth

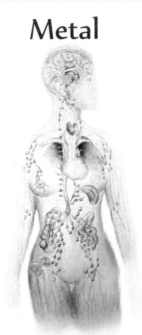

Five Elements of
Thyroid Health

Wood

Water

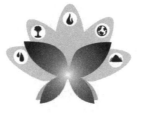

Chapter 1

FUNCTIONAL MEDICINE AND THE FIVE ELEMENTS OF THYROID HEALTH

Western medicine seeks to determine what is going on with the body and how disease affects function, but is more focused on naming and identifying that disease. Pharmaceutical treatment often alters or shuts down some physiological process, working against nature and causing long-term, unintended consequences. Then, over time, more drugs are added to shut down or alter more functions.

Functional medicine, on the other hand, seeks to understand how disease affects the body's physiology. When things go wrong and people become sick, it is caused by something in their body not working properly. Functional medicine aims to correct what is going wrong and tries to help return the body to its normal function. The goal is to work with the body to help it heal itself.

Traditional Chinese Medicine (TCM) is, in many ways, the original functional medicine. *Ancient Chinese doctors sought to figure out which parts of the body were not working properly and then tried to find ways to restore the body to balance.*

A BRIEF HISTORY OF TRADITIONAL CHINESE MEDICINE

Traditional Chinese Medicine (TCM), like Western medicine, developed in a feudal culture.[6] Hippocrates, Galen, and the other "fathers" of Western medical thought had their respective Chinese counterparts.

In China, Zhang Zhong-jing[7], Sun Si-miao, Wu You-ke, Ye Tian-shi[8] and many others were considered "fathers" of Chinese medicine, and they enjoyed the support of the Chinese court.

Indeed, the government was quite generous in fostering Chinese medical ideas and was responsible for organizing, gathering, and developing many of its theories and concepts as early as A.D. 500[9].

BASED ON OBSERVATION

Chinese medicine is based on observation, just as is Western medicine. Observations of the natural world and cosmos were used as analogies for explaining physiological function.

It was recognized that what was found in the macrocosmos was also true in the microcosmos of the human body.

In much the same way, physics now recognizes that phenomena on the microscopic level is, in many ways, similar to phenomena that takes place in the larger universe.

In fact, many of the concepts of the ancient Taoists (the philosophical fathers of TCM) have been embraced by modern quantum physicists because of their unique insights into the nature of physical phenomena.[10]

---

6   *Medicine in China: A history of ideas*, by P. Unschuld, 1985. Berkeley, CA: University of California Press.

7   *Shāng hán lùn*, by C. Mitchell et al, 1999. Brookline, MA: Paradigm Publications.

8   *Warm disease theory*, by J. M. Wen and G Siefert, 2000. Brookline, MA: Paradigm Publications.

9   *Medicine in China,* by P. Unschuld, pp. 154–188.

10   *The tao of physics*, by F. Capra, 2000. Boston, MA: Shambhala Publications.

LOOKING AT DISEASE

Diseases were recognized and described. However, the focus was not on the organization and classification of disease. Instead, Chinese medicine has chosen to organize and classify patterns of physiological dysfunction.

This was done because it was recognized that everyone who has cancer, hepatitis, Hashimoto's, or any other disease may not have the exact same symptoms.

This is true for a variety of reasons; no two people have the exact same genetic makeup, not everyone is diagnosed at the same level of progression of their particular disease, not every illness travels the same linear path of development, and not every person has the same strength of immunity (or dysfunction of the immune system).

In Chinese medicine, the study of disease was focused on how a patient's particular disorder had compromised physiological function.

This was a valuable insight because it allowed doctors to treat diseases far more effectively with the tools they had at that time.

Treatment in Chinese medicine is focused on restoring natural physiological balance, which inherently involves proper function. This concept is referred to as *zheng*.

French physiologist Claude Bernard (1813–1878) had a similar concept, believing that health was the result of maintaining a proper internal environment, *milieu interieur*. Walter Cannon, an American physiologist (1871–1945), was the first to define these same ideas; he coined the term *homeostasis*.

ANATOMY AND PHYSIOLOGY

TCM has a rather sophisticated understanding of physiology, biology, organ function, heredity, and infectious disease. *The Yellow Emperor's Classic of Medicine*, compiled between 600 and 300 B.C.E., explains the basic concepts of physiology.[11]

It provides surprisingly accurate and detailed information on the human body, with some ideas clearly equivalent to modern Western physiology.

Biochemistry was not described in Western terms, but examination of any modern *materia medica* will demonstrate that the pharmacological use of Chinese herbs is clearly done with an in-depth understanding of biochemical processes, and it is not

---

11   *Dao of Chinese medicine*: Understanding an ancient healing art, by D. E. Kendall, 2002, pp. 30–55. Oxford: Oxford University Press.

difficult to ascertain that different classes of herbs are used to treat disease in much the same way that modern pharmaceutical drugs are used.

For example, herbs that "clear heat" have broad-spectrum antiviral and antibacterial properties and were first used in the treatment of epidemic diseases; herbs that are "yang tonics" have androgen-like effects; herbs that are "qi tonics" stimulate the development of immune cells; herbs that "move blood" have pain-relieving effects,[12] and so on.

Descriptions of the organs and detailed descriptions of organ function are also found in Chinese medical literature.

In fact, all the major organs were identified by the early Chinese, including the kidneys, heart, lungs, liver, spleen, stomach, and large and small intestines.[13] The size and weight of all the internal organs were also measured and recorded by early Chinese physicians.

Measurement standards have changed over the centuries; however, relative measurements between values in the ancient texts do compare well to their modern counterparts.[14]

The early Chinese also identified heredity as *jing* (or essence), something inherited from one's mother and father.

While not fully understanding the mechanism for the transmission of heredity, they were able to describe its effects and even identified that it was responsible for birth defects.[15]

TCM theory is designed to explain patterns of dysfunction, and it has created systems that describe the relationships between the different parts of the body.

Two popular systems for explaining the relationships of different parts of the body are yin and yang and the five elements.

---

12   *Chinese medical herbology and pharmacology*, by J. K. Chen and T. T. Chen, 2004, pp. 103, 878, 835, 637. City of Industry, CA: Art of Medicine Press.

13   *Dao of Chinese medicine*, by D. E. Kendall, p. 36.

14   *Dao of Chinese medicine*, by D. E. Kendall, p. 46, Tables 3.5, 3.6.

15   *The yellow emperor's classic of medicine*, by M. Ni, 1995, p. 111. Boston, MA: Shambhala Publications.

YIN AND YANG THEORY

Chinese medical theory, though scientific in its own right, is built on a foundation of ancient philosophical thought. Many of these ideas are based on observations of the natural world and are the reason why TCM has remained a truly holistic approach to health and well-being.

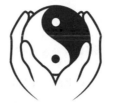

The theory of yin and yang is one such philosophy. It is said to date back nearly 6,000 years to the third or fourth millennium B.C. and is attributed to an enlightened philosopher named Fu Shi, also credited with creating *I-Ching*, or *Book of Changes*.[16]

The basic premise of yin and yang is that the only constant factor in natural events is universal change.

In other words, nothing remains the same: no disease, no condition, no emotion, no treatment or diagnosis. Absolutely everything is in a constant state of flux and, therefore, subject to the laws of change.

YIN AND YANG ARE METAPHORS FOR CONSTANT CHANGE

Yin and yang are metaphorical images used to express these constantly changing interactions. They have no fixed, precise definition.

Instead, they describe two broad categories of complementary concepts that include the relationships of positive and negative, dynamic and inert, creative and destructive, gross and subtle, and kinetic and potential.

This is quite similar to the notion of dialectics as expressed in Western philosophy. Within dialectics, the whole is the sum of its parts and, in turn, part of the sum of a greater whole.

---

16   *Tao: The subtle universal law and the integral way of life*, by H. Ni, 2014. Santa Monica, CA: Tao of Wellness.

As these various components interact, they become their opposites; e.g., variables become constants, causes become effects, and the process of creation leads to destruction.

Furthermore, this idea is demonstrated in modern physics where subatomic interactions are the result of ever-shifting polarities and constantly vacillating magnetic attractions and repulsions.

THE WHOLE UNIVERSE CAN BE SEEN AS YIN AND YANG

The entire universe may be seen as the interplay and alternation of yin and yang.

Originally the Chinese character for yin represented the moon, and the character for yang represented the sun.

Gradually these terms were broadened to include yin as night and yang as day, yin as winter and yang as summer, and yin as female and yang as male.

In fact, there is nothing that cannot be viewed from the standpoint of yin and yang.

EXAMPLES OF YIN

Yin is that which maintains and endures; it is nourishing and supports growth and development, as well as being something that contracts and moves inward. Representing yin are:

- Earth
- Autumn
- Cold, coldness
- Moisture

EXAMPLES OF YANG

Yang is that which is creative and generating; it develops and expands, and it is dynamic and full of movement. Representing Yang are:

- Heaven
- Spring, summer

- Heat, warmth

- Dryness

It is important to remember that yin and yang are not static concepts and that they are constantly influencing and determining one another. There is always some measure of yin within yang and vice versa.

In this fluid model it must be understood that neither yin nor yang can ever exist without the other.

In fact, extreme yin will become yang: An example of this can been seen in the popular expression, "The darkest hour is just before the dawn."

Naturally, the opposite is also true.

YIN AND YANG IN THE BODY

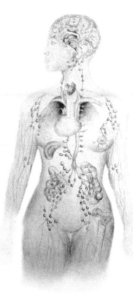

Yin and yang relationships become significant when they impact the body's anatomy and physiology, and it is precisely these designations that are used in the diagnosis of imbalances in TCM.

For a TCM practitioner, the name of the disease is of secondary importance. The primary key to a proper diagnosis of syndromes is the identification of the condition in terms of yin or yang.

EVEN LIFE IS YIN AND YANG

To understand what this means, let us examine these concepts in the context of human life.

Beginning at conception, the sperm, which is yang, unites with the ovum, yin, and a new life is formed. As that life develops and progresses, the energetic stages of youth are yang, whereas the later years, as life slows and becomes more deliberate, are yin.

Each stage is also relative to the others and contains a measure of both yin and yang. For example, the quick growth of early childhood is yang within yang, while the transition from middle age to old age is yin within yang.

YIN AND YANG ANATOMY AND PHYSIOLOGY

We can also see this philosophy expressed in the human body. In respiration, the expansion of inhalation is yang, while the emptiness, which results from exhalation, is yin.

In digestion, the yin substance of food is transformed by the metabolic activity of yang. The yin blood carries the yang hormones, which cause many physiological changes.

The physical body itself expresses this model. The lower part of the body, which connects to the earth, is yin; the upper body and extremities, which are free to move, are yang. The front, which can easily be protected, is yin; the exposed back is yang.

The internal organs, which are enclosed and protected, are yin, relative to the surface of skin and muscle, which are yang.

In addition, the internal organs can be further differentiated into *fu* (yang), the "hollow" organs that are involved with digestion and elimination, and *zang* (yin), which are involved in assimilation and storage.

Each yin organ has a corresponding yang partner, and while these connections are not recognized in Western medical terms, they are often utilized in the treatment of disease in TCM.

YIN AND YANG IN DISEASE

Finally, disease and disease progression can be viewed using this paradigm. If the body's yang (the immune system) is weak, it will be unable to ward off the invasion of a pathogen.

If the yin is weak, there will not be enough nourishment and support for the yang and the result will be the same.

Expressed in other terms, without the substance or yin the active immune system is weakened, and without activity or yang the substance (yin) becomes vulnerable.

Therefore, if yin is deficient over time, then yang also becomes deficient and vice versa. Not only do yin and yang balance each other, they mutually generate one another.

It is precisely this balance that the TCM practitioner restores using various treatment strategies. The idea is to reestablish the body's innate ability to maintain health and defend itself from disease.

The nature and progression of disease can also be understood using this pattern. When a disease develops rapidly, it is in the acute or yang stage.

As it progresses and becomes more chronic, it enters the yin stage. Usually acute diseases affect the surface or superficial aspects of the body, while chronic diseases have already overwhelmed the body's defenses and gone deeper into the interior.

Hashimoto's is a perfect example. As it progresses, it travels deeper into the body and impacts more and more systems.

When conflicting signs are present, they usually point to a more complex condition, and the TCM practitioner must evaluate all the symptoms together to determine the appropriate treatment strategy.

YIN AND YANG SUMMARY

In summary, yin and yang are universal and extend into every aspect of life.

Because of its universal nature, the theory of yin and yang is a very useful tool for understanding natural phenomena and therefore can be a helpful diagnostic aid.

While this is an ancient paradigm, it is not primitive, and though simple, it can be developed into surprising complexity.

FIVE ELEMENTS THEORY

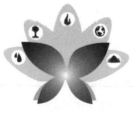

Another theory that is used to understand relationships in the body is the Five Elements Theory. The five elements really are a way of organizing functional relationships within the body.

The five elements are earth, metal, water, wood, and fire. In the upcoming chapters, I will introduce them and go into more depth about each one.

Each five-element pairing has a yin and yang organ, a sphere of influence, and specific relationships to other elements in the system.

For example, the wood element involves the liver and gallbladder. Its sphere of influence includes the nervous system, eyes, and tendons. Anger and depression are the negative emotions of the liver.

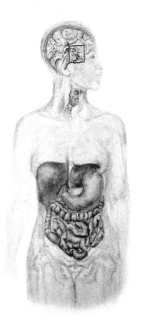

In regard to physiological function, all of these connections to the wood element can be explained. For example, the liver and gallbladder work together to metabolize fat and fat-soluble toxins.

Many studies have shown that poor detoxification in the liver can lead to neurological disorders, chemical sensitivities, adverse drug reactions, fatigue, autoimmune disease, poor conversion of thyroid hormones, and so forth.

Serotonin is also synthesized in the liver, which can explain anger and depression as being emotions of the liver.

In addition, the liver (wood element) has a unique relationship with the spleen (earth element). The physiological functions that are described as belonging to the spleen include many of the functions of the pancreas.

If you look at it in this light, then many of the problems described as liver/spleen dysfunction, such as sugar balance and fat storage in the liver, start to make a whole lot of sense.

And you can see this repeated over and over again in the five-element relationships.

The heart and small intestine represent the fire element.

What unites them? The cardiovascular system. Where is the highest concentration of fine capillaries in the body? They surround the small intestines.

The fire element has a unique relationship with the water element of the kidneys. Here we can see the role of the kidneys in managing blood pressure and its impact on the cardiovascular system.

USING THE FIVE ELEMENTS THEORY TO EXPLAIN HASHIMOTO'S

To help my own understanding and to help explain the impact of hypothyroidism and Hashimoto's on the human body, I use the Five Elements System to describe how this disease impacts the whole body.

And because TCM doesn't do a great job of explaining endocrine or neurological function, my approach is really a hybrid of TCM and functional medicine filtered through my mind from many years of clinical experience.

I don't care about being a purist; I'm looking for answers.

What really matters is, can this information and ways of looking at the body help us get better?

I believe the answer is *yes*, so let's jump in and explore this way of looking at the mind, body, and spirit effects of Hashimoto's thyroiditis.

Chapter 2

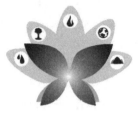

Thyroid:

UNDERSTANDING
THE TERRAIN

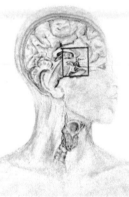

One thing I want to do is to give you a good sense of what is happening in your body so that when you have a blood test or when you have symptoms, you can start to understand it and not feel like you are at the mercy of someone else to explain what is going on.

The truth is that many medical providers have only a vague idea of what is really happening in your body.

The person who has the best understanding of that is you.

In this and in every chapter following, we are going to look at Hashimoto's from two perspectives: the Western medical model and the TCM model.

I have decided to do this because, in my view, Hashimoto's and any other disease, for that matter, is really a mind, body, and spirit condition.

And if we are really interested in healing, which I believe we all are, then we need to understand that these things are all connected. And these connections extend everywhere in our bodies.

As we go through the anatomy and the physiology, I want you to keep a couple of key ideas in mind. First, the body is not a machine with isolated parts that you can replace like a car.

The body, like our world, is a series of interconnected ecosystems that are all living and breathing, and what happens in one ecosystem influences and has consequences in others.

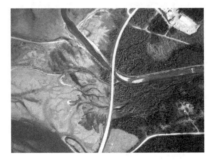

Ecosystems both inside and outside the body are connected.

For example, if you dump a bunch of chemicals in the Mississippi River in Iowa, it's going to have an impact off the coast of Louisiana.

The same thing happens in your body every day. What you eat, the chemicals you are exposed to, and the medications you take—they all have an impact.

Even a small amount of some things can have a pretty large impact on the body, such as environmental toxins and certain foods, like those containing gluten.

The second thing to understand is that the body has a natural tendency to balance itself. This is called homeostasis, and it is a very important process because a lot of what we are about to look at is the direct result of this very delicate balancing act.

A lot of symptoms from Hashimoto's are a result of this balancing act gone haywire. Somewhere in the hormones, the immune system, the digestive system, the liver, etc., things have gotten all confused.

In this confusion normal function starts to go wrong. And this is the problem when trying to heal and treat Hashimoto's. So many connections cause many systems to get out of whack.

Hashimoto's is complicated; it involves *multiple* systems.

It's not just a thyroid problem, or even a thyroid and immune system problem. It's a multisystem problem.

The best way to fix that type of problem is to make sure you keep the big picture in mind and don't get too fixated on one system alone.

YOU'RE THE SINGLE PARENT OF A LARGE DYSFUNCTIONAL FAMILY

The best analogy I have been able to come up with for describing Hashimoto's is that it is like being the single parent of a large dysfunctional family.

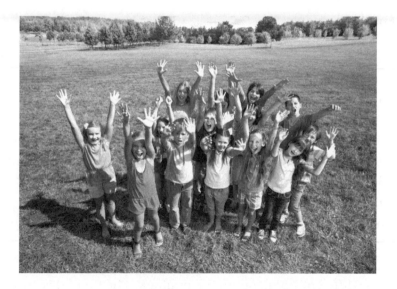

You're a single parent because, in most cases, you are on your own. The current Western medical approach to Hashimoto's treatment and management is failing. That's the simple truth. So you are on your own, like a single parent who must fend for herself.

So you are the parent, and your dysfunctional children are all the systems of your body that are being affected: the thyroid, the adrenals, the stomach, the kidneys, the liver, the gallbladder, the small intestine, the pancreas, the heart, the brain, and others.

Every one of these systems can become compromised and then can affect all the other systems, just as one sibling affects all the others in a family.

If you think about it this way, how do we heal a dysfunctional family?

Well, not by focusing treatment on only one child. To heal the family you must treat the *whole* family, not just one or two children.

That being said, let's take a look at the child that usually gets the most attention first: the thyroid.

WHAT DOES THE THYROID DO?

Simple answer? *Everything!*

It is responsible for growth, for cell differentiation (helping cells grow into different specialists), reproduction, sexual function, intelligence, and brain development. It is responsible for pretty much everything.

Thyroid function also affects every major system of the body. Its influence is literally felt everywhere.

And through lots of signals coming from all over the body, a part of the brain called the hypothalamus gets messages that say, "Hey, we need more thyroid, hit the gas."

Or, "Whoa! Slow our roll. We're getting too hyped up, less thyroid." This process happens all the time, 24/7, throughout your life.

And it's normal. When you're cold, the hypothalamus sends a signal to speed things up and increase circulation so you get warmer. When you are stressed and freaking out, it sends signals to slow things down so you can relax.

It sends nine different hormones to the pituitary. The thyroid is only one of nine systems that the pituitary is regulating.

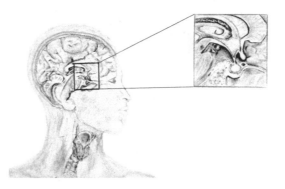

*The hypothalamus sends messages to the pituitary
to release thyroid-stimulating hormone (TSH).*

The hypothalamus sends these signals to the pituitary in the form of thyrotropin-releasing hormone (TRH). The pituitary is considered the master endocrine gland. The pituitary then releases thyroid-stimulating hormone (TSH) to the thyroid.

TSH is the test that many doctors believe is the most important test for determining thyroid function. The pituitary produces TSH.

Think about that for a second.

The test deemed most important in determining your entire care (in some cases) is measuring something that doesn't come from the thyroid. TSH is coming from your pituitary. And TSH is really a measure of pituitary function in relation to the thyroid and signals from the body.

Let me repeat that.

The test deemed most important in determining your entire care (in some cases) is measuring something that doesn't come from the thyroid. TSH is really a measure of pituitary function in relation to the thyroid and signals from the body.

So what happens next?

TSH stimulates an enzyme called thyroid peroxidase (TPO). One of the tests used to diagnose Hashimoto's includes checking for the presence of TPO antibodies. Results can mean that your immune system is attacking this enzyme and destroying it.

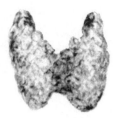

TSH causes thyroid peroxidase (TPO) to create
T4 and T3 hormones in the thyroid using iodine.

What TPO does is use iodine to create thyroid hormones T4 and T3. The majority of thyroid hormone produced is T4 (about 93 percent); the remaining 7 percent is T3. So when the immune system destroys enough of it, your thyroid produces too little thyroid hormone.

As we have already discussed, the most common drug that is prescribed for people with Hashimoto's, and for those who are hypothyroid, is Synthroid or levothyroxine. This is synthetic T4. The rationale is that T4 is most of what your body produces, so that's all you need.

Well, the body doesn't really use T4. It has to be converted into something else that the body can use to get important stuff done like growing and making different cells, making babies, thinking, and learning. Super-important stuff!

Where is T4 converted? Sixty percent is converted in the liver to T3, which is what the body uses.

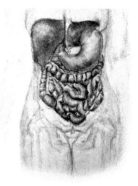

In the liver, 60 percent of T4 is converted to T3;
20 percent or more becomes reverse T3 (rT3).

The liver is a really important place for thyroid hormones to be made usable. This means that if the liver is congested or not working properly, it will have trouble making thyroid hormones work.

If the gallbladder is not functioning properly, that can have a negative effect on the process as well.

And guess what? With Hashimoto's the liver is often not working properly for a bunch of reasons.

In the chapter on the wood element we will get into this in a lot more detail. Right now, we're focusing on the big picture. The liver is really important for making thyroid hormones work.

From the liver, about 20 percent of converted T3 becomes reverse T3 (rT3), which the body can't use but which can provide a really useful test result because it tells us important information about how your body is using thyroid hormone.

Your body may actually push more T4 into rT3 when it wants to slow things down. Usually this occurs during times of extreme stress or when you have experienced physical trauma. But when you live your life in chronic stress mode, this can also happen gradually.

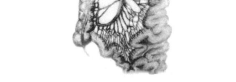

In the digestive tract, good bacteria converts 20 percent of T4 to active T3.

Next, 20 percent more of T4 is converted to T3 in the intestines. And the important thing there is your good bacteria. Remember the ecosystem?

Well, if you've taken lots of antibiotics or your diet consists mostly of processed and fast foods, or if you're taking lots of antacids or nonsteroidal anti-inflammatory drugs (NSAIDS) such as ibuprofen or acetaminophen, then your intestinal ecosystem might be totally out of whack.

This can have a big effect on whether you are able to convert and use thyroid hormone.

The liver is very important for thyroid hormone conversion.
The ecosystem of the intestines is also very important for absorbing thyroid hormone.

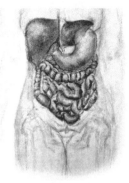

*The rest of T4 is converted in the peripheral tissues
such as the heart, fat (adipose), and skeletal muscles.*

The last bits of T4 are converted in the tissues of the body: in the heart, in fat, in the glial cells of the brain, and in skeletal muscles. If you have inflammation in your body (and autoimmune disease is, at its root, a disease of inflammation), this will make converting thyroid hormone in your tissues more difficult.

Guess how many people with Hashimoto's have inflammation all over their bodies? Almost everyone. Take a look at these classic before-and-after thyroid photos.

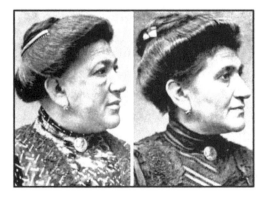

*The same woman appears in both photos;
in the photo on the left, inflammation is plain to see.*

So can you see how these systems—the liver, the intestines, and the tissues of your body—are connected? They are all responsible for making thyroid hormones work. Problems in those places mean your medication may not be working well at all.

This is one of the reasons why some people in the thyroid/Hashimoto's community advocate adding T3 to your medication regimen. You can take this in a synthetic form such as Cytomel (liothyronine sodium), or you can get it with natural desiccated hormones like WP Thyroid, Nature-Throid, or Armour Thyroid.

And this does really help some people. But again, nothing is perfect. There are so many variables here that you can still run into problems when taking natural desiccated hormones or adding T3.

For example, you may have an immune reaction to natural desiccated hormone, and too much T3 can make you really anxious, make you feel hyperthyroid symptoms, and it can have a powerful effect on heart-muscle function.

What is the best thing to do? Assess what is going on in your body and work on the other systems to improve conversion and absorption. *The importance of doing both can't be overstated.*

So let's go back to the pituitary for a second. Remember how I said it was doing nine different jobs at once?

The pituitary doesn't really have time to focus only on the thyroid. It's like, "Hey, thyroid, you good? Cool! I got other stuff to do." Just like a mother with nine children, she only has so much time.

So one important question is, how does the pituitary absorb thyroid hormone? Because it is making TSH, and TSH is the be-all and end-all of treatment. Well, it turns out that the pituitary absorbs thyroid hormone a lot differently than the rest of the cells in your body.

Perhaps because of all the demands on it, the pituitary is much more sensitive to thyroid hormone. It can sense it easily, whereas other cells in your body have to work a lot harder to get thyroid hormone into them.

This is important clinically, because it is one of the reasons why you can have all normal lab numbers but feel like crap, especially if the doctor is only testing TSH.

FUNCTIONAL HYPOTHYROIDISM

Another thing I'd like to mention is a concept that is so common it is almost a cliché. And that is the idea of "functional hypothyroidism."

As I mentioned, I have worked with more than 1,000 people with Hashimoto's, and by far the most common complaint and source of frustration is that they have normal lab tests but they still have all the classic hypothyroid symptoms.

They are tired all the time, they have terrible brain fog and memory issues, they're losing their hair, they're constipated, they have terrible digestive issues, they may have difficulty losing weight, they're in pain—they have all of these symptoms and more.

Yet their blood work is normal, so their doctor says, "You're fine; change your diet, get some exercise. I'll see you in six months."

The problem is they *aren't* fine. And the reason is simple: Parts of their body (like their pituitary and their blood) are getting enough thyroid hormone, but it's not getting absorbed, and it's not getting utilized.

There are many potential reasons for this, but the important thing to understand is that, for all intents and purposes, they are hypothyroid and their health is declining as if they weren't getting enough thyroid hormone.

The reality is that they must be treated as though they are hypothyroid, and the process of conversion and absorption has to be improved.

——Important Takeaway ——

So, what is the important takeaway here?

How you feel really matters when it comes to thyroid symptoms. It's not in your head. And your symptoms are very important when it comes to Hashimoto's because they are telling you whether your body is able to convert, absorb, and utilize thyroid hormone.

SUMMARY: FOUR COMMON MISTAKES DOCTORS AND HEALTH-CARE PRACTITIONERS MAKE

Let's summarize the four common mistakes that doctors and health-care practitioners make regarding the thyroid.

Mistake #1: They only test TSH. TSH is really more a measure of the pituitary's function with regard to the thyroid. While this is certainly an important test, it does not indicate actual thyroid hormone levels in the body.

And because the pituitary absorbs thyroid hormone differently than other cells in the body, TSH can be normal but you can still feel lousy and be functionally hypothyroid.

Mistake #2: They ignore your symptoms. Sometimes doctors will say, "All of your numbers are normal; you're doing great!" But you don't feel that way. With thyroid issues and Hashimoto's, in particular, what you feel is diagnostic and important. Do not let anyone tell you otherwise.

Mistake #3: They ignore other systems of the body and the thyroid's impact on those systems. Many symptoms can be related to poor thyroid function, low levels of thyroid hormone in your cells, or poor conversion and poor absorption of thyroid hormone by your cells.

It's important to pay attention to these other symptoms and to see the relationships of the thyroid with different parts of the body.

This observation matters because, in a number of instances, a problem in one place can create a vicious cycle of problems in other places.

For example, low thyroid function can cause the gallbladder to slow down and not do its job properly. This can cause toxins and hormones to build up in the liver, making it unable to convert thyroid hormone properly. And on and on it goes.

Mistake #4: They believe supplementing T4 is the only thing that matters. For some people, adding T3 to the mix can really help. But this approach alone ignores all the other important issues. Improving conversion, reducing inflammation, and making sure the other systems are functioning properly are all still necessary because this is much more than just a thyroid problem.

CASE STUDY

I'd like to tell you a story about a woman who had been struggling with Hashimoto's for more than four decades. She had almost given up hope, but her life-changing experience inspires everyone she knows.

This story is a perfect real-life illustration of what we have just learned about, and how things can be done differently. The wrong approach was used for many years, but once she changed to the right approach, amazing things happened.

Here's how it went down.

Diana is a 64-year-old woman who was diagnosed with Hashimoto's 45 years ago (at age 18).

She came to us on the verge of losing all hope. She didn't believe it was possible to get better.

One night Diana was surfing the Internet and discovered our website. She started reading, and it made sense to her.

She felt a small glimmer of hope that maybe, just maybe, this time it would be different than the hundreds of other times she had tried and failed.

Like many people with Hashimoto's, Diana suffered from many digestive issues—bloating, gas, constipation—and reactions to many different foods.

Diana also experienced some fatigue after meals and felt irritable and shaky if meals were missed. She had undergone antibiotic treatment for two years for an infection that would not resolve.

In addition, she had heartburn and discomfort following her meals, which she treated with antacids. She had a history of gallbladder issues and had had her gallbladder removed several years earlier.

She had trouble sleeping, was under high amounts of stress, and didn't feel rested from sleep.

Diana was taking thyroid replacement hormone but had every hypothyroid symptom you can think of: fatigue; cold hands and feet; brain fog and memory issues; weight gain; dry, thinning hair; and she needed a lot of sleep to function.

What we saw in her were numerous vicious cycles at work, compounding symptoms and causing a downward-spiral effect.

This is a perfect example of how Hashimoto's is a multisystem disorder and how other systems become impacted and lead to more hypothyroidism. This is what we call functional hypothyroidism.

Diana was taking thyroid hormone; there was enough in her system, but it was not working.

She had also tried various combinations over the years, including taking additional T3, which made her feel horrible.

We set out to first identify the various issues Diana had been dealing with so we could work on those systems and start to heal them.

With this approach, we can transform negative vicious cycles into positive healing momentum.

In Diana's case, we found ample evidence of leaky gut along with her other digestive complaints. Getting her off of gluten, dairy, and soy had immediate benefits.

We went a step further and got Diana on a special diet designed to reduce systemic inflammation and to heal her gut. While we did that, we worked to support her liver and liver detoxification.

Diana's symptoms of low stomach acid went down dramatically with this approach, and we supplemented her to help increase stomach acid production, which eliminated many of the problems she was having.

This was also a great time to work on repairing the ecosystem of Diana's gut, which had been so disrupted by all the antibiotics.

In addition, we worked to balance Diana's blood sugar, because cortisol (the so-called stress hormone) is released when blood sugar drops, and she was routinely draining her adrenals and thyroid and then binging on sugar to try and get enough energy to get through the day.

Cortisol and systemic inflammation caused by sugar is a major factor in blocking thyroid hormone conversion and absorption.

This whole process took several months and we are happy to report that Diana has an entirely new life today.

Here's an excerpt from an e-mail she sent us:

"What a fabulous program. . . . I just love it! It is the first time in my life that I have really invested the time and energy in taking care of ME!!!! . . . I love my new life! I even purchased a bicycle! I hadn't ridden a bike for about 30-plus years! Having a blast with it. Everything is more fun, and I feel like I have a new lease on life."

I spoke with Diana recently, and what she shared with me literally had me in tears. Her enthusiasm and sense of gratitude made me feel like *I* was a Debbie Downer.

I'm serious!

I'm not claiming that everyone gets these results, nor is this something that just happened miraculously overnight.

It took persistent, hard work, and it took looking in parts of the body other than the thyroid.

Diana also continues to have some work to do. Something that's been progressing for 45 years doesn't just disappear.

But she also deserves credit for sticking to this and doing the hard work that resulted in such progress. That is something to celebrate!

What happened here is that we were able to create positive healing momentum and we were able to stop all of these vicious cycles from continuing to make everything else worse.

That's key.

Vicious cycles are the result of positive feedback in the body. Positive feedback is the result of repeated reinforcement.

And with Hashimoto's, it can give you some pretty negative outcomes.

But when you work on them and reverse that negative momentum, you make the positive feedback work for you and you get healing momentum.

Does that make sense? This process involves working with nature and your body's natural tendencies.

HASHIMOMENT:
IS IT GOOD OR BAD?

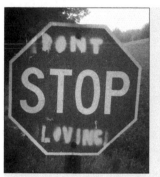

I created Hashimoments for our Facebook support group. These are positive affirmations for people with Hashimoto's.

This one tells a story that illustrates how we sometimes don't really know if something is good or bad.

It takes place in ancient China.

There was a wise farmer who toiled day in and day out in his village, doing all the work that needed to be done to run his farm and sustain his family.

One day, one of his horses ran away. His neighbor, who was a bit of a busybody, noticed.

The neighbor ran over and said, "Oh, I'm so sorry! That's such a tragedy. That's the horse you use for plowing and work. Oh, this is bad!"

The farmer shrugged and asked, "Is it?"

The very next day, the horse returned with five wild horses running after him, and the farmer and his son were able to capture all of them.

His one old horse had become six!

Seeing this, the neighbor ran over and said, "Oh my goodness! What good fortune, you are so lucky! Your one horse is now six. That's so great!"

The farmer shrugged and asked, "Is it?"

The next day, the farmer's son set to work breaking in the wild horses so they could become work horses and be sold. As he was trying to ride one of them, he was thrown to the ground violently and his leg was broken.

Hearing this, the neighbor ran over and said, "Oh, I'm so sorry. What bad luck! Now your son can't work, and you're stuck with all of these wild horses. Oh, this is bad!"

The farmer shrugged once again and asked, "Is it?"

Two weeks later, the army came to town.

They were requiring all young men in good health and of fighting age to go to the front and join the emperor's army in defending China from the invading Mongol hordes.

Many would die. But because the farmer's son had just broken his leg, he was spared. The army took just two of his new horses.

So you see, the moral of the story is that you never know what a given set of circumstances or a certain turn of events can mean.

When I was diagnosed with Hashimoto's, I thought my life was over. And for all intents and purposes, it was.

But that has turned out to be an incredible blessing, because the life I am leading now is a simpler and far more rewarding life.

It was the adversity and difficulty I went through that got me to where I am today.

So don't be so quick to judge your circumstances. It may turn out to be a really good thing for you in the long run.

Chapter 3

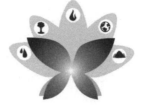

THE CHINESE MEDICINE VIEW OF THE THYROID

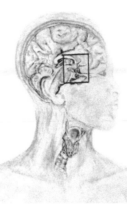

Now let's look at a different side—the energetic and emotional side of thyroid health. This isn't strictly science, but parts of real life are more than science, physiology, and lab test results.

Looking at Hashimoto's and the thyroid from this perspective gives us clues about how we can understand what we are going through and how we can heal.

In TCM, the endocrine system is thought to come from the yang energy of the kidneys. In an energetic way, the kidneys are responsible for our individual power, or will.

The yang energy is the way the ancient Chinese understood hormones. And there is something to learn in their take on this. (For a review of yin and yang philosophy, see chapter 1.)

The ancient Chinese believed that we have all been given a certain reserve or fund of yang energy at birth, and we use it throughout our lives. Sometimes we use it well, and sometimes we use it foolishly. There are whole practices devoted to helping people use this reserve in a better way.

I studied with a Taoist master named Mantak Chia many years ago in New York City. I remember going to his apartment in Chinatown and learning a special tai chi form he had adapted for small apartments. You can basically do the form right where you are standing.

One of the things he did when I worked with him was to project energy into my eyeballs with his thumb. That was really intense and gave me a blast of yang energy! The reason he did this was to quickly fill up my reserves.

Here is a drawing that illustrates a Taoist practice called the "microcosmic orbit" that I learned from Mantak Chia. It depicts an entirely different viewpoint.

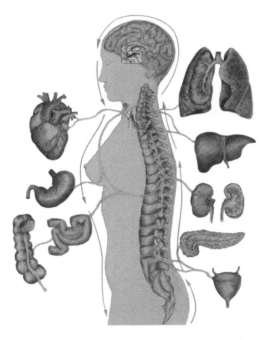

The microcosmic orbit: Energy circulates up the spine and down the front of the body.

Here we can see the process of transforming yang energy into other types of energy. For example, the ancient Taoists believed we could transform sexual energy into spiritual energy. They also believed this energy could be used to heal the internal organs and balance the nervous system.

Throughout history, Taoism has had a profound influence on Chinese medicine, and a number of Taoist ideas and practices are reflected in it.

I ask that you be open-minded, because some of this material is a bit "out there." But it also offers major insight into the emotional and spiritual aspects of the Hashimoto's journey.

LIFE IS A JOURNEY

In my opinion, life itself is a journey. We are here together taking this journey regardless of our religious beliefs. And we are all having mind, body, and spirit experiences on a daily basis.

To this point we've already established that we aren't just lab test results, and that what we feel and experience does matter.

So let's look at this from a real experiential point of view and assume that we are part of this living universe that is made up of an infinite number of ecosystems.

Let's retrace the path we took previously and look at these processes from a Chinese medicine–Taoist point of view.

First, the hypothalamus released what? Thyrotropin-releasing hormone (TRH). And sent it where? To the pituitary.

The hypothalamus is a magical place for Taoists. It represents an "on" switch to the universal force. The force is strong, Luke Skywalker . . . when your spirit awakens. This is where it is thought to happen.

This is also what connects us to the larger universe—the Big Dipper constellation, which contains the North Star and has a special meaning in Taoist cosmology. And this is where we can connect to it. (We are not alone!)

Second, the pituitary is an important energy center. It is where yang energy is thought to be transformed to spiritual energy. When opened, the pituitary is a place of wisdom and direction.

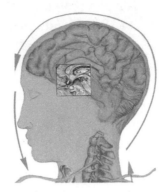

The pituitary is where yang energy is transformed into spiritual energy.

When it is open, you have a strong sense of purpose and a direct and simple knowing. When it is closed, you may be indecisive; your mind may wander and be directionless.

Meditation can really benefit the pituitary. It can create that balanced sense of purpose.

With Hashimoto's, hypothyroidism and inflammation of the brain can create some real cognitive problems. This happens because these processes can hamper neurotransmitter production and cause the immune cells of the brain to react, which then causes inflammation all over your brain (more on this in an upcoming chapter about the brain). Well, all of that affects the pituitary.

As we have seen, the pituitary sends information to the thyroid. The thyroid is considered an important energy center, too. It is the place where communication and dreams are generated.

Of course, this is where your voice comes from, both physically and emotionally. When this center is open, your expression flows, and you have greater lucidity in dreams. When it is closed, you may feel choked up and unwilling to change.

Third, we looked at how important the liver is for converting and transforming thyroid hormone. The liver is important for so many processes.

In Chinese medicine, the human eye is the sense organ connected to the liver. Eye issues are a big part of thyroid problems! Both Graves' disease and Hashimoto's have their own category of eye issues!

We can use the eyes in meditation to calm the nervous system and to send energy inward in what is a practice called the "inner smile," where you smile into your organs and systems of your body and direct healing energy there.

In terms of energy and emotion, the nature of the liver is kindness, which is maintained by the calmness and integrity of the heart. When the liver is out of balance, the negative emotion is anger, or anger turned inward—depression.

It is interesting to note that one of the most common next steps for physicians treating Hashimoto's patients is a referral for a psychological evaluation or a prescription for antidepressant medication.

When treatment with T4 doesn't result in the patient feeling better, this is sometimes the next logical step.

You see? Ancient masters really understood this stuff on a deep level.

Finally, we went to the digestive tract. This is thought to be controlled by the spleen in Chinese medicine (although the intestines also belong to other organ systems).

In Chinese medicine, Hashimoto's treatments often address the spleen and kidneys, because the yang energy is thought to be depleted and weak.

When your spleen is weak, you worry and obsess about things a lot. When it is healthy, you have a quality of fairness. You can see the big picture and be open.

The life issues of those of us with problems involving yang energy revolve around the general theme of utilizing our resources appropriately.

HASHIMOTO'S CAN BE SEEN AS A DEFICIENCY OF YANG

Hashimoto's involves a deficiency of yang. We see this in various endocrine glands: the adrenals, the pancreas, the thyroid, and the pituitary.

Chinese treatment for hypothyroidism and Hashimoto's uses therapies that *tonify* or strengthen yang. It also addresses two other issues: what the Chinese call liver depression—interesting in light of what we saw about the liver and spleen deficiency, as well as digestive and blood sugar issues. (We will explore this in more detail in the chapters on the earth and wood elements.)

With acupuncture, we treat this energy by using points like Stomach 36 (located on the lateral part of the leg just below the kneecap) and the Japanese point Large Intestine 10½ (located on the forearm, just below the elbow; they are both important *tonification* and energy-generating points.

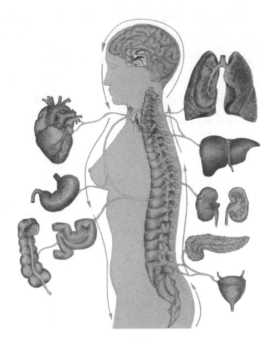

The Ren and Du channels go up the spine and down the center of the torso.

Liver acupuncture points are really helpful for anger and depression. I always recommend trying a course of acupuncture before going on antidepressants, especially for mild to moderate depression.

On the back, points for hypothyroidism often involve treating this energy pathway. The microcosmic orbit works with the energy of two main meridians, the Ren and Du channels. These run down the center of the front of the body and up the spine on the back.

These are our most primal channels and are thought to be formed at fertilization when the first cell comes into being. These channels tap into the autonomic nervous system that is so overtaxed in our society and culture.

Treating the middle of the back area and back of the neck can also be very beneficial for patients with Hashimoto's. Points in these areas have a potent effect on calming and balancing the thyroid.

In tandem with what you learned earlier, let's now look at some Hashimoto's and thyroid issues from a more energetic, emotional/spiritual perspective.

WISDOM IS A YANG VIRTUE

Wisdom is the virtue associated with the yang energy of the kidneys that empowers us to be in contact with our destiny from birth to death. This energy of the kidneys teaches us to use our wisdom to utilize the resources we have by listening to our inner voice rather than reacting to our fears.

Fear can make you impulsive and burn up your reserves. Meditation and prayer are good tools to develop that wisdom, and they enable you to get in touch with your inner voice so that you can use your energy in a more sustainable way.

You must learn to be like a boxer going 12 rounds. You always need to keep some energy in reserve, but you also need to go with the flow of the fight and use some of that energy at key times. Remain unattached to the outcome of the fight and focus instead on cultivating wisdom by listening to your inner voice.

That's an important part of this journey for treating Hashimoto's: We have to learn not to overdo it.

RECAP

In this chapter, we looked at the thyroid and how it works in your body.

We also looked at four common mistakes that many practitioners and doctors make. And we learned how what you are feeling really matters, because it can absolutely be important diagnostically. In addition, we learned:

1. **A number of spiritual and emotional pieces are attached to this entire process.** Being connected to the universe, your higher power—however you want to look at it—is traditionally related to the hypothalamus.

2. **The pituitary is a place of spiritual transformation,** a place to find wisdom and direction and one of the parts of the body that really benefits from meditation practices. Meditation can benefit the thyroid as well.

3. **The thyroid is a center for communication and dreams.** Journaling your dreams and keeping track of them can be a way to tap into this energy.

4. **The liver is, again, hugely important.** It is connected to your eyes, and to emotions of anger and depression (which can be anger turned inward).

5. **The yang of the spleen and kidney is the energetic root of the endocrine system.** This energy is responsible for many processes in the body, but has within it the seed of spiritual growth and development.

I don't know about you, but I find this way of looking at the body to be inspiring. I like it because I believe we're more than just science and physiology. It's also interesting to think about spirit, energy, and emotion, because therein lie the seeds of healing.

Chapter 4

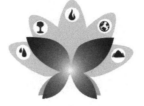

UNDERSTANDING COMMON THYROID TESTS

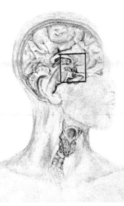

Up to this point, we've touched on some of the physiology and some of the spiritual and emotional aspects of Hashimoto's thyroiditis.

We've also looked at the more esoteric energetic side of things and examined the life challenges that might be part of this whole journey we are going through.

*That being said, I'm reminded of how important it is to **keep a journal**.*

Make a habit of paying attention to what is going on with your body, mind, and spirit. Keep track of your symptoms. Keep track of the foods you eat and of other things that you interact with for clues on what might make your condition better or worse. This is valuable data.

In this chapter I want to get to some practical information: Let's look more closely at which thyroid tests are important to order and why.

THYROID TESTING

TSH—THE STANDARD THAT NO ONE CAN AGREE ON

Thyroid-stimulating hormone (TSH), also called thyrotropin, is released by the pituitary gland after the hypothalamus releases thyrotropin-releasing hormone (TRH). TSH is the most common marker used to assess thyroid function.

Many laboratories have begun offering a test called a "thyroid cascade" in order to save themselves and insurance companies money.

Basically, if the TSH is deemed to be in the normal range, they will not order any other tests. This saves money, because they aren't paying for additional testing, but it doesn't always serve people who are trying to get better.

The problem is that there isn't a lot of agreement about what the "normal range" is.

Since 2003, the American Association of Clinical Endocrinologists has recommended that the normal range be 0.3–3.0, versus the older range of 0.5–5.5. So, according to the new standards, levels above 3.0 are evidence of possible hypothyroidism, while levels below 0.3 are evidence of possible hyperthyroidism.[17]

However, there is disagreement among doctors: Some continue to follow the older range, while others use the newer range.

TSH IS AN INVERSE MARKER

An important thing to understand about TSH is that it is an inverse number when thinking about thyroid function. Generally, the higher your TSH levels are, the more sluggish and slow (hypoactive) your thyroid is. Also generally, the lower your TSH levels, the more high-energy and fast (hyperactive) your thyroid is.

Put another way:

High TSH = hypothyroid; low TSH = hyperthyroid.

TSH levels increase as T4 levels drop, and TSH levels decrease as T4 levels rise. The reason this is the most popular test in today's medical model is because the

---

17   "Clinical practice guidelines for hypothyroidism in adults," by J. R. Garber et al, 2012, *Endocrine Practice, 18*(6). Retrieved from https://www.aace.com/files/hypothyroidism_guidelines.pdf

only treatment offered for thyroid dysfunction is thyroid hormone replacement (usually in the form of synthetic T4), and that's what doctors are checking when they test your TSH.

A TSH test alone doesn't give you information about thyroid–pituitary communication, about T4-to-T3 conversion in other parts of the body, or about whether your immune system is attacking your thyroid.

An important thing for Hashimoto's people to understand is that some antibodies can inhibit thyroid function by turning off, instead of stimulating, TSH receptors on cells. In this case, you will see high TSH levels and high antibodies.

BOTTOM LINE ON TSH

The laboratory range is somewhere between 0.3–3.0 and 0.5–5.5. That is a huge range that borders on the ridiculous. The lab range values are made based on the general population that goes to the lab.

Most people who go to the lab are taking thyroid hormones and are poorly managed or are completely undiagnosed (or both), so this is not really a good measure of optimal thyroid health. Practitioners of functional medicine (like yours truly) look at a narrower range that we, and some endocrinologists, believe is much better for assessing a healthy thyroid.

This range is 1.8–3.0. Notice that our range is higher on the low end and equal to or lower on the high end. Other people believe there's a "Goldilocks" zone, where a "just right" TSH level is somewhere between 0.5 and 2.0.

Regardless of the range, it is important to understand that these numbers mean nothing in isolation. They must be viewed in the context of your signs and symptoms, *how you feel*. You have to find your own ideal zone where you feel your best.

T4

The T4 test measures both bound and unbound thyroxine levels and is not a good marker for T4 activity when measured alone. Total T4 is increased with lower TSH and is decreased with higher TSH. It is decreased with low TSH when the pituitary gland is not functioning properly (pituitary hypofunction).

This begs the question: Are we measuring the pituitary or the thyroid?

LET'S LOOK AT SOME RESEARCH

In 2005 there was an interesting study published in *The Journal of Clinical Endocrinology & Metabolism* titled "Thyroid Hormone Concentrations, Disease, Physical Function, and Mortality in Elderly Men."

This study of 403 men investigated the association between TSH, T4, free T4, T3, thyroid-binding globulin (TBG), and reverse T3 (rT3), as well as parameters of physical functioning.

The study showed that TSH and/or T4 levels are poor indicators of thyroid hormone levels in the tissues of the body. Thus, in a large percentage of patients, those levels cannot be used to determine whether a person is euthyroid (has normal thyroid function) at the tissue level.

In fact, T4 levels had a negative correlation with thyroid hormone levels in body tissues (higher T4 levels were associated with decreased peripheral conversion of T4, low T3 levels, and high rT3).

Additionally, the study showed that rT3 inversely correlates with physical performance scores and that the T3/rT3 ratio is currently the best indicator of thyroid hormone levels in body tissues.

Furthermore, the study indicated that increased T4 and rT3 levels and decreased T3 levels are associated with hypothyroidism at the tissue level, resulting in diminished physical function and the presence of a catabolic state (breakdown of the body).

Here's what this means:

- T4 is not a good test of thyroid hormone levels in the tissues of your body (where you need it to work). T3/rT3 ratio is a much better way to determine how much thyroid hormone is getting absorbed.

- Also, the combination of increased T4 and rT3 with decreased T3 levels correlated with the study participants feeling worse physically.

- This is the state of functional hypothyroidism that I described earlier. This is also important for figuring out if you are functionally hypothyroid.

Another interesting point from the study was that many chronic diseases can lead to further decline in tissue sensitivity to hormones; these include diabetes, heart disease, hypertension, systemic inflammation, asthma, chronic fatigue syndrome, fibromyalgia, rheumatoid arthritis, lupus, insulin resistance, obesity, chronic stress, and almost any other systemic illness.

What does that mean?

All of these chronic health conditions compromise energy (yang) in the body and cause systemic inflammation. What's more, they actually make conversion and tissue sensitivity worse.

Hashimoto's is also a systemic disease, and it often involves more than one of those other issues I just mentioned, making it the perfect recipe for functional hypothyroidism.

QUICK RECAP

What tests did this study show were most helpful for figuring out if thyroid hormone is getting into the tissues/cells of the body?
T3, reverse T3, and the T3/rT3 ratio.

Let's take a look at these tests.

T3: TOTAL TRIIODOTHYRONINE (TT3)

Total T3, or TT3, gives you the total concentration of T3 in the blood. It is the preferred test for thyrotoxicosis (a hyperthyroid condition like Graves' disease).

TT3 can also be useful for identifying T4-to-T3 conversion problems in body tissue involving the enzyme 5 alpha-deodinase.

This enzyme converts T4 to T3 and stops T4 from working in the body.

REVERSE T3 (RT3)

This test measures the amount of rT3 that is being produced. (You probably figured that out!) RT3 is usually created when someone is experiencing an extreme amount of stress, such as from a serious car accident, surgery, pregnancy, or really bad chronic anxiety.

It's no surprise that rT3 is elevated after a stress response or after the body produces high amounts of the stress hormone cortisol.

Your body, especially the liver, is constantly converting T4 to rT3 as a way to get rid of any excess or unnecessary T4. As much as 40 percent of T4 converts to T3 and 20 percent of T4 converts to rT3 on any given day.

But in any situation where your body needs to conserve energy and focus on something else, such as dealing with Hashimoto's, it may increase the conversion of rT3, and then the T3 goes down because there is less T4 to convert.

Typical stressors include trauma, illness, a toxic work environment, exposure to extreme cold, diabetes, aging, or even taking certain medications. But there's another stressor for Hashimoto's folks.

We can get caught in a state of alarm, causing our body to increase rT3 in order to decrease the amount of T3 in our cells.

And the lower your T3, the worse you feel: Your body temperature lowers, you're fatigued, you may experience anxiety, weight gain, hair loss, pain, and more. These are all common symptoms of Hashimoto's and hypothyroidism.

Sometimes your levels of rT3 can climb too high. Why would you make too much rT3?

On top of the chronic stresses in your life are three common issues. The first two are related to your adrenals (low cortisol or high cortisol); the third is related to your iron levels.

The adrenal issues can be divided into two categories:

1. When you experience too much stress, your adrenal glands produce high amounts of cortisol to help you cope with ongoing hypothyroidism and lingering symptoms and conditions.

    That alone is stressful. The extra cortisol inhibits the conversion of T4 to T3, and instead produces even larger amounts of rT3, creating an rT3 problem.

2. When that stress is ongoing, your adrenals will eventually become tired, dropping from high cortisol to a mix of high and low, or all low. Those low levels create adrenal fatigue, which can also cause problems.

We will explore this in more depth in the chapter on the water element.

When you don't make enough cortisol, thyroid hormones can build up in your blood. Your body responds by converting the T4 to excess rT3 because it has to do something with the extra T4.

The third issue involves iron deficiency anemia.

When iron levels or ferritin (iron-containing protein) levels are low, as can be seen in your serum iron and saturation (quite common in thyroid patients), your red blood cells become less plentiful and carrying thyroid hormones via your blood becomes inadequate. When this happens, thyroid hormones can build up in your blood.

The body responds by producing excessive amounts of rT3 to clear out the excess T4.

You can have either an iron problem or a cortisol problem, or *both*. Other health issues can cause you to have high rT3 as well, such as low B12, excess inflammation, and leptin resistance. (Known as the "satiety hormone," leptin is a hormone produced by fat cells that is believed to regulate fat storage in the body.)

Another interesting thing to note is that interventions like meditation, qi gong, yoga, and practices like them can be helpful in lowering rT3 levels. Don't always assume a drug or supplement is the only way to get results.

FREE T3 AND FREE T4

Other tests that are helpful are free T3 and free T4. These measure the free fractions of T3 and T4, or how much of T4 and T3 are available and active in the bloodstream.

These are important, because they are what the body uses. We want to know how much is available for the body to actually use.

The final thing to look at is the ratio of T3 or free T3 to rT3. It is generally accepted that this ratio should be 20 or more with T3 or 10 or more with free T3.

However, just like TSH, this number is just a number and means very little in isolation. You must also look at it in the context of how you feel and in the context of all the other numbers. This is the best way to figure out what it means. Again, trust how you feel.

FREE T3 OR T3/ RT3 RATIO

If free T3 or T3 is low and rT3 is high, then you may be in a state of functional hypothyroidism, which means you aren't absorbing and/or converting thyroid hormone (T4) well.

You might benefit from adding T3 to your medication, and you certainly need to address the underlying issues leading to poor conversion and utilization of hormones: things like stress, inflammation, liver function, adrenals, and intestinal issues.

Calculating this result can be difficult if you are math-challenged, because different units are sometimes used for each test.

There's a great calculator at the Stop the Thyroid Madness website: www.stop thethyroidmadness.com/rt3-ratio/.

When you use the calculator, make sure to double-check that you are using the right units of measurement for each test.

THYROID ANTIBODIES

When certain antibodies are above the normal laboratory range, it can mean that your immune system is attacking your own tissue. When your body produces thyroid autoantibodies, it could create a hypo- or hyperthyroid state.

These antibodies may also be elevated if thyroid cancer is present. Some antibodies can attach to TSH receptors but they don't usually attack thyroid tissue; other parts of the immune system are responsible for this. We will explore this in more detail in upcoming chapters.

There are three autoantibodies that are tested. The first two are the most common:

1. **Thyroid peroxidase antibody (TPOAb):** This antibody is the one that is usually high in autoimmune thyroid conditions like Hashimoto's. It is also known as microsomal antibody.

2. **Thyroglobulin antibodies (TgAb):** These aren't seen high as often as TPOAb. A test for these antibodies is usually ordered when other thyroid lab test results seem strange, because they can interfere with thyroid hormone production. TgAb is also used to monitor progress after surgery for removing cancerous thyroid tissue.

3. **Thyroid-stimulating hormone receptor antibody (TRAb or TSIAb):**
    A test for this antibody is only ordered when a patient is hyperthyroid.
    Positive results usually mean Graves' disease.

There are some people with Hashimoto's who may not have thyroid antibodies detectible in the blood. In that case, having a thyroid ultrasound will help your physician determine the state of your thyroid and how badly it has been damaged in this process. It's not a blood test; it's an imaging test using ultrasound.

Wow! We covered a lot of ground there. That should give you a basic understanding of what to look for and how to interpret those results.

Next, let's bring it all together and apply the A.P.A.R.T. System that I introduced at the beginning of the book. This will give you some tools for taking the data we have gathered so far and using it to help create an action plan for getting better.

Let's face it, all of this information does you no good if we can't use it to find solutions.

Chapter 5

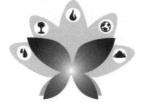

USING THE A.P.A.R.T. SYSTEM TO HEAL THE THYROID

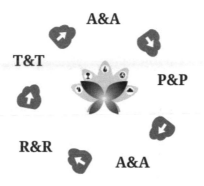

The A.P.A.R.T. System

As you may recall, I created the A.P.A.R.T System to give you a template for fixing any imbalance or disorder in the body.

First, you must take inventory and figure out what the issues are. Then, your next step is to try various treatment approaches. After that, you assess what you did and take inventory again.

Figure out what worked and what didn't. Over the long term, keep building on what works and keep eliminating what doesn't with the ultimate goal of reaching remission.

In this chapter, we look at how you can apply this approach to the thyroid.

Make sure you get a journal if you don't have one already. Make a note of your symptoms and how you feel. Create a plan for dealing with these symptoms. Experiment. Record the results of those experiments.

Double down on what worked and change what didn't. Then, lather, rinse, repeat.

1. A = Ask and Assess

Ask: Do you have any of these hypothyroid symptoms?

Hypo: tired/sluggish; feel cold—hands, feet, all over; require excessive amounts of sleep to function properly; increase in weight even with low-calorie diet; gain weight easily; difficult, infrequent bowel movements; depression/lack of motivation; morning headaches that wear off as the day progresses; thinning of outer third of eyebrow; thinning of hair on scalp, face, or genitals, or excessive hair loss; dryness of skin and/ or scalp; mental sluggishness.

Do you have any of these hyperthyroid symptoms?

Hyper: heart palpitations; inward trembling; increased pulse, even at rest; nervous and emotional; insomnia; night sweats; difficulty gaining weight.

Assess: Test thyroid levels.

Regarding testing: There are two important parts to it: One, make sure the right tests are ordered; and two, know what to do with the data that the tests reveal.

It doesn't matter what is ordered if you don't know what to do with the data.

MEDICATION AND TESTING

One really important thing to understand is the impact of your thyroid hormone medication on your blood test results. When you're tested and how you're tested matters.

In my experience, most doctors say you don't need to fast to test your thyroid. As with most things, we always need to ask whether or not that is true.

T3 has a relatively short half-life, which means it is only active in the body for a few hours. T4, both synthetic and natural, has a much longer period of activity.

A 2004 study showed that TSH results declined in 97 of the 100 people studied by an average of 23.39 percent when tested later in the day versus early in the morning, when they'd been fasting. So testing later in the day may result in lower TSH than early in the morning.[18]

Bottom line? Test your levels first thing in the morning, before taking any medication or consuming any food or beverage other than water. This will give you the most accurate reading.

Here are some tests for assessing thyroid function. This list is by no means a complete list of tests for Hashimoto's. We will discuss more tests in upcoming chapters.

Top Seven Thyroid Tests

Here is a good summary of some of the most important thyroid tests to take to your doctor if you suspect that you have Hashimoto's.

If you already know you have Hashimoto's, retesting antibodies may not be a good measure of success or failure.

This is because antibody levels are always changing and the number of the test result really represents a snapshot of that moment in time only.

They can be helpful to spot larger trends and to see if a given treatment strategy is having an effect on antibody numbers, but they should not be the primary focus of testing, in my opinion.

Make sure you request a copy of your thyroid labs so that you can see them yourself and double-check to make sure they were interpreted correctly.

1. TSH (thyroid-stimulating hormone)

2. Free T3

3. Free T4

4. Reverse T3

5. Thyroid peroxidase antibodies (TPOAb)

6. Thyroglobulin antibodies (TgAb)

7. Thyroid ultrasound

---

18   "Serum TSH variability in normal individuals: The influence of time of sample collection," by R.R. Scobbo et al, 2004, *West Virginia Medical Journal, 100*(4), pp. 138–142.

2. P = Prioritize and Plan

From the data, determine where the issues are and what areas need improvement. Are you converting properly? Is there enough thyroid hormone in the body? Is it being absorbed?

Compare symptoms to lab test results. If they are inconsistent, something may not be working. Create a plan based on the data. If you don't know how to do this, this is precisely the place to get help.

It is highly recommended that you keep things simple to limit variables, and that you keep a daily food and activity journal to identify patterns and successful results.

3. A = Act and Adapt:

There are many potential courses of action. Let's look at some foods, vitamins, and minerals that improve thyroid hormone conversion.

Important minerals and supplements for proper thyroid function include:

- **Zinc**—Needed to form TSH; too little can impair T4 to T3 conversion.

- **Selenium**—Acts as a catalyst to convert T4 to T3 and helps protect that body from oxidative damage.

- **Magnesium**—Proper thyroid function depends on a fine balance between calcium and magnesium. Magnesium is also used by the body in more than 300 enzyme reactions.

- **Iron**—Adequate amounts of iron are necessary to transport T3 to the cells of your body. Being even "a little anemic" is not acceptable.

- **Iodine**—A controversial nutrient, to say the least, iodine is important for proper thyroid function nonetheless. However, excessive iodine can cause significant problems for people with Hashimoto's.

- **Glutathione**—One of the most beneficial antioxidants in the body. See below for a more detailed explanation of all the good things it does.

FOOD SOURCES FOR NEEDED VITAMINS AND MINERALS

The following list of vitamins and minerals may, of course, also be taken in supplement form. I've gathered food sources for all of them because I'd like you to get in the habit of seeing your diet as your first choice for treatment and healing.

Note: There are foods on this list—such as nuts, seeds, and grains—that may not be appropriate for some people with Hashimoto's. We will discuss more on diet in the chapter on the earth element.

- **Zinc**—oysters, herring, liver, oatmeal, maple syrup, brewer's yeast, sunflower seeds, soybeans, mushrooms, sardines, pecans, pumpkin seeds

- **Selenium**—Brazil nuts, brown rice, brewer's yeast, eggs, garlic, liver

- **Magnesium**—kelp, almonds, cashews, brazil nuts, dulse, peanuts, walnuts, filberts, sesame seeds, lima beans, peas, millet

- **Iron**—dulse, kelp, rice bran, pumpkin seeds, beans, lentils, parsley, walnuts, apricots, almonds, raisins, Swiss chard, spinach, dates, figs, kale, cucumbers, cauliflower, cabbage

- **Iodine**—kelp, dulse, agar, Swiss chard, turnip greens, summer squash, mustard greens, watermelon, cucumbers, spinach, asparagus, kale, turnips

- **Glutathione**—Consume sulfur-rich foods such as garlic, onions, and cruciferous vegetables (broccoli, kale, collards, cabbage, cauliflower, watercress, etc.), along with a glutathione or N-acetyl-cysteine (NAC) supplement.

HYPOTHYROIDISM NUTRITION

- Beware of the "ides"! Avoid fluoride, bromide, chloride, and chlorine. Fluoride can be found in many toothpastes; bromide in fire retardants and furniture; and fluoride and chlorine in tap water. Since these elements may block the iodine receptors in the thyroid glands, leading to reduced hormone production and eventually hypothyroidism, it's important to avoid them. Drink steam-distilled water or reverse-osmosis water only.

- Avoid gluten, dairy, and soy 100 percent. All three have been found to aggravate autoimmunity, increase thyroid tissue destruction, and decrease availability of thyroid hormone in the body.

- Consume foods (or supplements) rich in vitamin B complex to promote the proper generation and utilization of energy.

HERE ARE SOME FOOD SOURCES OF B VITAMINS:

- **Vitamin B1**—rice bran, sunflower seeds, pinto beans, peas, lentils, almonds, turnip greens, collard greens, kale, asparagus

- **Vitamin B2**—salmon, trout, cod, mackerel, perch, oysters, mushrooms, almonds, hijiki

- **Vitamin B3**—rice bran, red peppers, wild rice, kelp, sesame seeds, peaches, brown rice, mushrooms, barley, almonds, apricots

- **Vitamin B5 (pantothenic acid)**—beef, chicken, salmon, mackerel, sardines, barley, rice, avocados, plums, raisins, almonds, dates

- **Vitamin B6**—bananas, barley, brewer's yeast, molasses, brown rice, liver, beef, cabbage, carrots, potatoes, yams

- **Vitamin B12**—beef liver, beef kidney, ham, sole, scallops, eggs, oats, pickles, amasake, algae, spirulina and chlorella, brewer's yeast

- **Folic acid**—liver, asparagus, lima beans, spinach, Swiss chard, kale, cabbage, sweet corn

Don't Believe the Hype

THE RESEARCH ON GOITROGENS

People with Hashimoto's and those with low thyroid function (which is commonly seen with other autoimmune diseases) are often told to avoid cruciferous vegetables, spinach, radishes, peaches, and strawberries because of their goitrogenic properties.

The word *goitrogen* was coined in the late 1940s to describe something that causes the formation of a goiter, also known as an enlarged thyroid gland.

The term has multiple meanings, from thyroid hormone suppression to changing the way thyroid hormone is produced in the body to slowing the rate of absorption of iodine.

Cruciferous vegetables have been called goitrogenic because they have the potential to block iodine absorption.

This was a problem in the 1950s when iodine deficiency was a much more common cause of hypothyroidism. Back then, lower iodine levels were much more of problem from a public health standpoint.

Well, this is 2017, and the world has changed. Today our world is awash with environmental toxins, radiation, and plastics, all of which are much more important health threats, in my opinion.

THE RESEARCH DOESN'T SUPPORT THIS

Avoiding these foods is not well-justified and is not supported by research. According to scientist and researcher Sarah Ballantyne, Ph.D., in her book *The Paleo Approach*,[19] this family of vegetables is a great source of a group of sulfur-containing compounds called glucosinolates.

When these vegetables are chewed or chopped, an enzyme called myrosinase breaks the glucosinolates apart into different compounds, many of which are potent antioxidants that prevent cancer. Two of them—isothiocyanates and thiocyanates— are also known goitrogens.

Isothiocyanates and thiocyanates seem to reduce thyroid function by inhibiting the action of the enzyme thyroid peroxidase (TPO).

As described in the previous chapter, during thyroid hormone synthesis, TPO is the enzyme that uses iodine to produce either T4 thyroid protein hormone (thyroxine) or the more active T3 thyroid hormone.

When isothiocyanates or thiocyanates are consumed in large enough quantities, they can interfere with the function of the thyroid gland.

However, there is no evidence of a link between normal human consumption of these compounds and thyroid pathogens unless you have iodine deficiency.

So if you are severely deficient in iodine or selenium, addressing that deficiency before eating tons of cruciferous vegetables is a good idea. In fact, addressing these deficiencies is a good idea, period.

The enzyme myrosinase is also deactivated by cooking, so cooked cruciferous vegetables can still be enjoyed while you're working on correcting any deficiencies.

---

19   *The paleo approach: Reverse autoimmune disease and heal your body*, by S. Ballantyne, 2013, pp. 209–210. Las Vegas, NV: Victory Belt Publishing, Inc.

Steaming and blanching are both good ways to cook and preserve important compounds and phytonutrients.

Another important point to consider is that these vegetables have potent anti-cancer effects. Researchers from Korea did a meta-analysis published in the *European Journal of Endocrinology* in December 2014.[20] The link between Hashimoto's and papillary thyroid cancer was established, but it is not fully understood whether the inflammation from Hashimoto's causes the cancer or if the inflammation is the result of the cancer.

Furthermore, in the case of papillary thyroid cancer the presence of Hashimoto's means a better prognosis and lower risk of reoccurrence if one does develop thyroid cancer.

In any case, given their known anti-cancer effects, eliminating these vegetables from our diets makes no sense. Also, in a recent clinical trial evaluating the safety of isothiocyanates isolated from broccoli sprouts, no adverse effects were reported[21] (including no reductions in thyroid function).

And finally, small amounts of these thiocyanate compounds, like what you would get from including cruciferous vegetables in your diet, stimulate T4 synthesis, meaning that vegetables labeled goitrogens actually support thyroid function.

HAVE THESE FOODS WITH SELENIUM

A strong connection exists between isothiocyanates and selenium in the formation of other important enzymes for the thyroid (thioredoxin reductase and glutathione peroxidase).

Consuming isothiocyanates with selenium gives the body antioxidants that can provide a major boost to your defenses and help prevent cancer. So I advise you to eat more rather than less of these fruits and vegetables, even if you have Hashimoto's, as long as you're not deficient in iodine and selenium.

As with anything, moderation is always recommended. Don't eat wheelbarrows full of cruciferous vegetables, and don't live in fear of them.

---

20   "The association between papillary thyroid carcinoma and histologically proven Hashimoto's thyroiditris: A meta-analysis," by J. H. Lee et al, 2012, *European Journal of Endocrinology*, *168*(3).

21   "Opposite effects of thiocyanate on tyrosine iodination and thyroid hormone synthesis," by A. Virion et al, 1980, *European Journal of Biochemistry*, *112*(1), pp. 1–7.

ADDITIONAL CONSIDERATIONS

TRADITIONAL CHINESE MEDICINE (TCM) FOOD PERSPECTIVE:

- According to TCM, vegetables are generally cold in nature and meats are usually warm in property. Since individuals with hypothyroidism often have yang deficiency and cold presentations, increased consumption of meats (especially lamb) may help warm up the body and dispel cold.

HYPERTHYROIDISM NUTRITION:

- Avoid gluten, dairy, and soy 100 percent. All three have been found to aggravate autoimmunity, increase thyroid tissue destruction, and decrease availability of thyroid hormone in the body.

- Check your dosage of thyroid replacement hormone. One cause of hyperthyroid symptoms may be too much medication. Another maybe related to the adrenals, which we will explore further in the chapter on the water element.

   Sometimes people have mixed presentations where they have both hypo and hyper symptoms. This can be the result of too much thyroid hormone in the system that isn't getting absorbed equally throughout the body.

- Consider doing more to address autoimmunity. Cutting out gluten, dairy, and soy are important first steps, but may not be enough. You may need to address autoimmunity more aggressively by adopting an elimination diet (an autoimmune paleo approach). We will explore this further in the chapter on the earth element.

QI GONG EXERCISE FOR THE THYROID

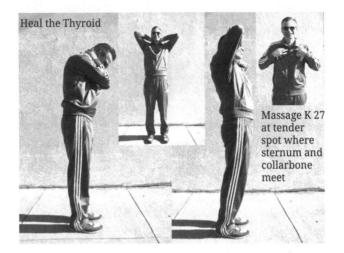

Heal the Thyroid

Massage K 27 at tender spot where sternum and collarbone meet

Here is a simple exercise that is very beneficial for the thyroid.

Neck Squeeze: You may do this exercise sitting or standing. Relax, close your eyes, and interlace your hands behind your neck. Then let your head hang forward and allow the weight of your arms to gently stretch your neck muscles. After that, bring your elbows close together in front of your face, squeezing the sides of your neck with the heels of your hands.

Inhale slowly and deeply, raising your head as you gently bring your bent elbows out to the sides. Lift your head up and let it tilt back gently. Exhale slowly and repeat the whole movement again.

Repeat this breathing exercise for two to five minutes, then continue with the next exercise, which involves the use of the K 27 acupuncture point.

K 27 Meditation: This acupuncture point is located in the tender triangle where your sternum and collarbone meet.

Close your eyes, taking slow, deep breaths as you slowly let your head turn from side to side. Visualize your entire neck region relaxing as you continue to breathe deeply, gently applying pressure or tapping on these points.

Gently let your head tilt backward and forward, slowly rotate while visualizing blood flowing peacefully into your thyroid and the area that surrounds it. Completely let go and relax.

Then sit quietly and meditate for five minutes, visualizing your thyroid healing and regenerating.

4. R = Reassess and Readjust

Execute your plan and then reevaluate in one to two weeks. If you don't feel any better, reassess. If you feel some improvement, try to determine what led to it and do more of that.

In order to do this properly, you need to establish a baseline to begin with. In your journal, note where you began, then reevaluate and compare.

CLINICAL PEARL:

One important area to reassess is your reaction to thyroid replacement hormone if you are taking it. Not everyone has the same reaction for a variety of reasons.

Also, there's no such thing as a "bad" reaction. Everything is a test, and every outcome, whether it's what we wanted or not, provides valuable information.

Here's a quick breakdown of what reactions to different types of thyroid hormone therapy may mean.

FELT BETTER WITH BIOIDENTICALS (LIKE ARMOUR, WESTHROID, ETC.)

Some people truly do feel better with bioidenticals. It's not true of everyone, but the addition of T3 can sometimes be the answer because these people:

- may need T3 due to problems with the thyroid hormone receptors on cells;

- were unable to convert T4 to T3 when using T4-only medication;

- have sensitivities to dyes or fillers in synthetic compounds that are not in bioidentical compounds;

- and/or have receptor sites on cells that simply respond better to bioidenticals than to synthetic hormones.

DID BETTER WITH T3 ONLY

Some people improve with the addition of T3, while others do their best with T3 only. And these can be synthetic or bioidentical.

This can happen for a couple of reasons:

- Their receptor sites are resistant to thyroid hormone because of high cortisol, high homocysteine, inflammation, low progesterone, vitamin A deficiency, and more.

- They have difficulty converting T4 to T3.

DIDN'T FEEL BETTER WITH T3 OR BIOIDENTICAL HORMONES

In both cases, more T3 is introduced.

- These people may not have too little T3 but instead have an active and uncontrolled autoimmune process causing the release of thyroid hormone.

- These are also the people who often vacillate from hyper to hypo. They may have an immune flare-up, more hormone is released, and then they crash; the condition calms down and they are hypo again.

- In some cases, these people can have excess adrenal hormones (e.g., epinephrine) caused by too much nicotine, caffeine, stress, or exercise.

FEEL BETTER ON SYNTHETIC HORMONES

Some people actually feel better on synthetic hormones.

- These can be people who are converting well, have an overactive metabolism, and just don't need more T3.

- They also benefit from an approach that will calm the autoimmune attacks that cause their thyroid to be revved up in the first place.

FEEL FATIGUED AND RUN-DOWN

This reaction is sometimes discounted, but it can also be meaningful.

- These people may be sensitive to the ingredients and fillers in thyroid medication.

- If they are taking bioidentical hormones and they have this reaction, they may have an autoimmune response to the replacement hormone.

5. T = Try and Try Again

Double down on what worked and change what didn't. Don't give up if at first you didn't get earth-shattering results.

This is an ongoing process; your goal should be on building long-term success.

Also, be sure to keep track of what you did that worked; take time to celebrate it and understand it, then build on those successes.

It's remarkable how often people try things without first establishing, in an organized and systematic way, where they are.

Climbing a mountain doesn't happen all at once; you get to the top one step at a time. Every step forward is a small victory that you can build on.

Make sure you stay conscious of the steps you take as best you can.

It is often these little victories that lead to more profound changes because they lead to a change of momentum.

Chapter 6

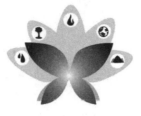

The Metal Element:
BALANCING THE IMMUNE SYSTEM

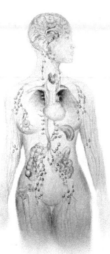

In this chapter, we're going to cover something that is fascinating but poorly understood—the immune system—which is the metal element in Chinese medicine.

You'll learn how Hashimoto's affects the immune system as well as some powerful steps for restoring balance.

You'll also discover some common triggers that can cause flare-ups and immune dysfunction.

Finally, we'll look at testing the immune system and what to do with that data.

Let's start with the big picture.

WHAT DOES THE IMMUNE SYSTEM DO?

The immune system protects the body from foreign invaders. It's like the body's military. It finds the bad guys (like bacteria, fungus, parasites, and viruses) and kills them. It also cleans things up by destroying dead and dying cells.

This is called cellular apoptosis, and if this process stops working, cancer develops. In addition, the immune system creates inflammation as part of the process of healing after an injury.[22]

The immune system is amazingly plastic and adaptive, meaning it's always changing. It continually confounds researchers, because it doesn't follow simplistic logic. It can't afford to; it must constantly defend us from so many types of invaders, literally trillions of foreign invaders in a lifetime.

Recent research in fields such as psychneuroimmunology (the study of the mind's effect on health and resistance to disease) has shown that our immune system has the ability to communicate with the nervous system, the endocrine system, and the digestive system, and that it is actively modulating and influencing the body all the time.

And it is not linear, meaning different parts of the immune system seem to do things in opposite directions at the same time. We'll look at some examples in a second.

Of course, this can get more complicated and confusing when we're trying to understand autoimmune disease, because people are also at different stages of progression, they have problems with various other systems, and they have different genetic profiles. It's no wonder that practitioners of all kinds are sometimes lost when it comes to dealing with autoimmunity.

The ancient Chinese described immunity and defense in the body as *wei qi*. This defensive *qi* (energy) was thought of as brave and fierce, which it truly is.

And where is it in the body? Much of it is found in the lymphatic system.

This is where the immune cells live and differentiate. They are born in the bone marrow and travel here to mature and do various jobs.

We have four primary barriers: the skin, the walls of the digestive tract, the lungs, and the blood-brain barrier. The lungs and the intestinal walls are heavily lined with lymph nodes, because this is where a lot of invasions (whether airborne or food-borne) happen.

22　*The immune response: Basic and clinical principles*, by T. W. Mak and M. E. Saunders, 2005, pp. 451–453. Burlington, MA: Elsevier Academic Press.

THE IMMUNE SYSTEM HAS MANY PARTS

The immune system has many different parts, but the two to remember are non-specific and specific immunity.

One theory of immune regulation involves homeostasis, or the balance between T-helper 1 (Th1) and T-helper 2 (Th2) activity. This is a very popular theory that has influenced many alternative care practitioners and treatment strategies.

As we have learned more about the immune system, the limitations of this theory have started to appear.

A LITTLE BACKGROUND ON TH1 AND TH2 THEORY

Th1 and Th2 theory traces its origins to research done on mice in 1986.[23] It was discovered that T-helper cells in mice expressed different kinds of immune proteins known as cytokines.

This theory was then applied to human immunity, and it was determined that Th1 and Th2 cells directed responses through different pathways.

Th1 cells were linked to fighting viruses and other pathogens inside cells. They also helped kill cancer cells and caused certain types of skin reactions. You can think of them as yin.

Th2 cells, on the other hand, affected antibody production and fought pathogens outside of cells. You can think of them as yang.

TH2 DOMINANCE

Th2 dominance (which means a stronger relative presence than Th1) is linked to the body's ability to tolerate transplanted tissue, for example, or a fetus during pregnancy. Normally the immune system attacks anything that is not "self."

A woman's body temporarily goes into Th2 dominance during pregnancy. This is one of the possible explanations for why some women experience the onset of Hashimoto's after pregnancy.

---

23   "Th1/Th2 balance: The hypothesis, its limitations, and implications for health and disease," by P. Kidd, 2003, *Alternative Medicine Review, 8*(3).

The temporary Th2 dominance that balances the Th1 attack on the thyroid recedes, and the immune pendulum swings back to Th1. Sometimes this happens with a vengeance. (Originally, the majority of people with Hashimoto's were thought to be Th1 dominant, but this is an oversimplification and is not always the case.)

Over time we have come to learn that Th1 and Th2 are far more nuanced than originally thought, and their proteins sometimes behave in unexpected ways. So the theory has been shown to have inconsistencies; because real life is not a textbook or a laboratory, there are rarely Th1- or Th2-exclusive patterns.

We have also learned that other immune cells, like antigen-presenting cells, can also affect the immune system in similar ways to Th1 and Th2 cells.

For example, another cytokine called interleukin-6 (IL-6) is produced by dendritic cells in the intestines, and it has been shown to promote Th2 and dampen Th1.

Why does this matter? Elevated IL-6 has been linked to lower levels of T4 and T3 in the blood. IL-6 is commonly found in the fat around the abdomen.

These different parts of the immune system can be rather confusing. The important thing to understand is that a delicate balance between the yin and yang aspects of the immune system is our ultimate goal. You can't just attack this with a heavy hand and try to shut down one side or the other or overstimulate either side.

Instead we must work to bring balance and harmony, because many diseases (like Hashimoto's) that were once considered to be exclusively Th1 or Th2 dominant have been proven otherwise when examined more closely.

Furthermore, in some experiments, Th1 dominance has actually been shown to become transformed into Th2 dominance through the depletion of glutathione.[24] So it's not always a good idea to simply push one side or the other. You might wind up with unintended consequences.

Much like real life, this theory isn't perfect, but it is a helpful framework for understanding our amazingly complex immune system. Let's take a closer look at Th1 and Th2 proteins.

---

24   "Th1/Th2 balance," by P. Kidd, p. 223.

NONSPECIFIC IMMUNITY

The nonspecific immune system—our immediate attack response—is made up of front-line soldiers that hang out in our border tissues (the mucous membranes of our lungs, digestive tract, skin, and brain) and kill invaders.

These soldiers provide our immune system's T-helper 1 (or Th1) response. These are the macrophages (the *Pac-Man* cells) and killer T cells (the elite squads) that are pathogen-killing machines.

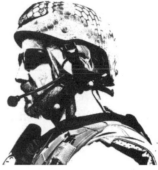

Th1 is also broken down into messenger proteins like interleukin-12 (IL-12), interleukin 2 (IL-2), interferon gamma (IFN), and tumor necrosis factor (TNF). These are the badass Navy Seals that get the job done.

IL-12 is a commander and facilitator that provokes inflammation. It's responsible for helping natural killer (NK) cells mature; it's also involved in turning on genes that result in attacks on specific organs and it stimulates the Th1 response.

An important thing to keep in mind when treating autoimmunity is that it is often the result of an overzealous immune system. IL-12 can have positive impacts in protecting the body, but in this context it can be a problem. It has been implicated as an important player in Hashimoto's attacks on the thyroid.

IL-2 is synthesized by CD4 T cells (white blood cells that help protect the body from infection), which then enables increased antibody production and improved bone marrow responses to other immune cells.

IL-15, a close relative of IL-2, has been shown to be low in people with Hashimoto's; treatment with levothyroxine can increase IL-15 levels, as do some Chinese herbs (see chapter 8).

Again, here is the contradictory nature of the immune system. Increasing IL-15, some theorize, may reduce the destruction of thyroid cells in Hashimoto's.

Yet many people thought that with Hashimoto's, Th1 was too strong. You see? Yang within yin. Yin and yang theory can help us understand contradictions in the immune system.

Tumor Necrosis Factor (TNF), also known as TNF alpha, kills tumor cells. It turns on angiogenesis (the hallmark of malignant tumors), promotes fibroblasts, and is involved in wound healing.

Drugs called biologic response modifiers (BRMs), or "biologics," block the action of TNF alpha. These have grown in popularity in recent years and are used by some rheumatologists to treat autoimmune diseases.

The downside of this type of therapy is that it makes you very vulnerable to certain kinds of life-threatening infections, like tuberculosis.

TNF beta is another commander that helps kill tumor cells, activates genes, and mediates CD8 T cells, NK cells, and helper-killer T cells to induce them to fatally injure their targets.

A TNF receptor called CD95, which is responsible for cell death, has been found to be very high in patients with Hashimoto's. It's a factor in the destruction of thyroid tissue.

SPECIFIC IMMUNITY

The specific immune system produces antibodies that label the bad guys. This part of the immune system is like the CIA: It gathers intelligence on the bad guys and labels them with an antibody.

Once an antibody labels a foreign invader, it's much easier for the killer cells to destroy it. And like the CIA, it takes a while for them to gather the intelligence, so this process is usually delayed for a period of time.

This part of the immune system is called T-helper 2 (or Th2). These cells do more than just label; they also attach themselves to certain cells like viruses to keep them from entering into our cells. This is important because once they are in our cells, they are much harder to kill, and they can replicate more quickly.

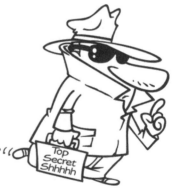

Th2 is also broken down into interleukins. IL-10 and IL-4 are two important ones.

IL-10 has been implicated in numerous autoimmune diseases, such as type 1 diabetes and multiple sclerosis. But it is a perfect example of the unpredictability of the immune system, because it turns on some immune functions and shuts off others. It can block IL-1, IL-6, and TNF alpha but turns on IL-2 and IL-4.

And to further complicate matters, research has shown that IL-10 is produced by and downregulates the function of both Th1 and Th2.[25]

IL-4 is produced by CD4 T cells and activates IgE, an immunoglobulin that's important for creating immunity to parasites; it is also involved in responding to allergens.

COMPLICATED, BUT REALLY COOL

And that's not all; we have other parts of the immune system driving the immune attack—the family of interleukins that belong to IL-1. IL-1 is released by the *Pac-Man* cells that are the front-line attackers.

IL-18 belongs in this family of cells, and a lot of it is found in Hashimoto's patients, especially those with severe symptoms that don't respond to levothyroxine treatment. IL-18 may be responsible for severe inflammation.

Both parts of the immune system are needed for certain types of invaders. For example, viruses are often microscopic and can sneak past the border security.

Next, the Th2 system uses its cellular informants to sniff out and tag viruses. This immune response can take several days to initiate and is why it takes most people a few days to recover from the common cold, which is caused by a virus.

In a general sense, the Th1 system is considered inflammatory, and the Th2 system is considered anti-inflammatory. But in reality, they are both involved in the process of inflammation.

And IL-12 and IL-18 are important drivers of inflammation in Hashimoto's.

NEW RESEARCH HAS REVEALED OTHER PARTS OF THE IMMUNE SYSTEM

Recent research has shown that there are other parts of the immune system that also play important roles in this inflammatory cascade.[26]

---

25 "Human IL-10 is produced by both type 1 helper (Th1) and type 2 helper (Th2) T cell clones and inhibits their antigen-specific proliferation and cytokine production," by G. Del Prete et al, 1993, *The Journal of Immunology, 150*(2), pp. 353–360.

26 "How do regulatory T cells work?" *by* A Corthay, 2009, *Scandinavian Journal of Immunology, 70*(4), pp. 326–336.

T-helper 3 (Th3), also known as T suppressor or T-regulatory (Treg) cells, are a part of the immune system that can calm and dampen other more aggressive cells and proteins.

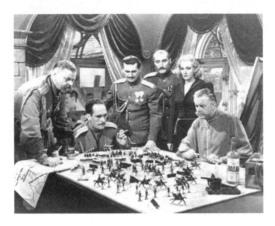

Th3 cells are like the generals of the immune system.

Th3 cells are kind of like the generals of the immune system. They call back the troops once they've attacked and keep them disciplined so they don't pillage and attack the entire body.

This part of the immune system plays an important role in autoimmune disease and must be strengthened and balanced. Both vitamin D and glutathione have been found to be quite helpful in doing this.

In addition, Th3 cells may actually have a different origin than Th1 and Th2. They seem to come from dendritic cells in the intestines.

Another type of immune cell is T-helper 17 (Th17). These cells are instigators that rev up an attack and can make the damage and the carnage much more intense. A delicate balance of all parts of the immune system is important; with an autoimmune disease like Hashimoto's, this balance is lost.

WHAT HAPPENS WITH HASHIMOTO'S?

In most cases of Hashimoto's, some combination of factors (virus, environmental toxins, genetics, gluten, breakdown of the intestinal lining) leads to a slow, gradual attack against the thyroid.

This reaction eventually causes the loss of enough thyroid cells that the condition presents as hypothyroidism (indicated on a blood test as high TSH).

TSH becomes high because, as we have learned, when the thyroid is not working properly, the pituitary gland increases production of TSH to increase thyroid gland activity. For some people with Hashimoto's, the thyroid doesn't become overactive. Rather, over time they develop symptoms of low thyroid function and are put on thyroid replacement hormone.

For others, periods of hyperactivity can occur. They may vacillate between hyper and hypo symptoms. These people may develop behavioral issues that resemble bipolar disorder.

In some cases, however, patients can develop full-blown hyperthyroidism and Graves' disease (also a thyroid-related autoimmune disease). There are even some patients who have a confirmed diagnosis of both Hashimoto's and Graves' disease.

AUTOIMMUNITY IS IGNORED WHILE TSH IS MANAGED

For many people, the issue of the autoimmune attack is never addressed. Instead, these patients are considered to be properly managed by having normalized TSH. In reality, while their TSH is being managed, the underlying problem is not being addressed.

Over time, they lose more and more thyroid cells and need more thyroid replacement hormone. The result for many people is that they continue to have hypothyroid symptoms (fatigue, hair loss, depression, constipation, and cold hands and feet), because the root cause has been largely ignored.

Since the thyroid is being destroyed, there is less thyroid hormone production. The immune system needs thyroid hormones to modulate Th1 and Th2 activity, so when thyroid hormone production decreases, the immune system can short-circuit.

This leads to a larger number of T cells and autoantibody-producing B cells, which accumulate in the thyroid and kill thyroid cells.

There are many possible scenarios that can lead to this outcome. Dr. Datis Kharrazian provides some excellent examples.

- The T suppressor (Th3) cells that regulate the immune response could be too few in number, and like a weak general who has lost control of his troops, this can lead to unchecked attacks by the immune system (and tissue like the thyroid becomes a casualty).

- Th1 has a number of different soldiers, which are the interleukins we just discussed. These all have specific jobs. For example, interleukin 2 (IL-2) is a messenger chemical that sends out orders for the killer cells to start killing.

Some people make too much IL-2, which creates a frenzy of destruction that can lead to the death of the thyroid cells. Chronic viral infections can create an excess of IL-2 and have been linked to the development of autoimmune thyroid disease. In fact, in the patient population that I have worked with, about 75 percent of the people I have seen have some history of exposure to the Epstein-Barr virus. IL-2 may be a reason why.

- Th2 also has lots of different soldiers. IL-4 deploys B cells. Like some rouge CIA agents, these cells can go crazy and tag the wrong proteins, and destruction of thyroid tissue is the result. Parasites and food allergies can cause too much IL-4 to be made.

- Too much sugar can cause the body to rapidly release insulin. Insulin spikes can stimulate the production of too many B cells, so they start tagging too many things, which leads to destruction of the thyroid.

Sugar imbalances can have a big impact on immune function.

And this is just the tip of the iceberg. There are many variables and potential reasons for the immune system to short-circuit. This is what makes treatment and management so challenging. And this is also why you must have a multipronged approach.

Initially, researchers thought Hashimoto's was a Th1 dominant disease.[27] However, this is not true for everyone and has proven to be an oversimplification.

It seems IL-18 and IL-12 also act together to cause more destruction to the thyroid. Look for the development of drugs that inhibit these two interleukins.

People with Hashimoto's also often have a weak Th3 regulatory system, and their Th2 may or may not be out of control. Th17 is also often wound up, making the attack more intense.

---

27   "Th1 and Th2 serum cytokine profiles characterize patients with Hashimoto's thyroiditis (Th1) and Graves' disease (Th2,)" by C. Phenekos et al, 2004, *Neuroimmunomodulation, 11*(4).

And none of this happens in a vacuum. This is all taking place in the context of the body where the immune system is interacting with the endocrine system, the digestive system, and the nervous system.

Talk about complicating the task of unwinding this mess; it's no wonder patients and doctors alike get frustrated and overwhelmed.

Whew! That's a lot of interleukins!

RECAP OF IMMUNE SYSTEM AND HASHIMOTO'S

1. Th1/Th2 balance is a theory that was once quite popular but is now less so, because these relationships are more nuanced than originally thought. But it is still useful and can help treatment if you can identify imbalances.

    These two parts of the immune system have a kind of yin and yang relationship, so strengthening one can sometimes help calm the other.

    Th1 cells are like the Navy Seals: They are the front-line attackers. Th2 cells are like CIA agents: They gather intelligence on the bad guys.

2. IL-18 and IL-12 are bad guys, and we want to calm them down.

3. Th17 is a troublemaker that does both good and bad stuff. But generally we want to calm it down, too.

4. Th3 cells are the command and control center, kind of like generals. They are often a weak link in Hashimoto's folks. Making the generals stronger can really be beneficial therapeutically.

We'll discuss how to influence all of these different parts of the immune system shortly.

HOW THE IMMUNE SYSTEM AND THYROID ARE CONNECTED IN HASHIMOTO'S

Before we go further, let's review a little from the last chapter and see how it relates to this chapter.

As you recall, we looked at the thyroid, so let's highlight a few of the important takeaways.

- There may be functional hypothyroidism or sufficient thyroid hormone that isn't getting into the cells of the body.

  This is a situation in which you can have normal TSH (in the pituitary) and normal T4 and still feel like crap.

  I presented this scenario to our Facebook support group and got more than 350 comments.

  The overwhelming majority of people said that they had normal TSH and T4, yet had a host of hypothyroid symptoms (fatigue, brain fog and memory issues, weight issues, constipation, anxiety and depression, hair loss, brittle hair and nails, etc.).

  Why? There are many reasons, but one is that TSH is made in the pituitary, and the pituitary absorbs and responds to thyroid hormone differently than other cells in the body.

  Add to this all the accompanying problems that are involved with Hashimoto's, like systemic inflammation, digestive issues, a poorly functioning liver, and the stress of life, and what do you get?

- The perfect recipe for diminished sensitivity and absorption of thyroid hormone into your cells.

  The best way to find out where you stand is to test your levels of T3 or free T3 and rT3, then to divide T3 by rT3. If the ratio is too low (low T3 and high rT3), then you may have a state of hypothyroidism in your cells. T4 can be elevated in these cases also.

  This is also sometimes called **low T3 syndrome**. Taking T3 may or may not help. As with everything involving Hashimoto's, there is no magic bullet. You have to evaluate everything first and then try some things.

  Inflammation, chronic stress, and autoimmune disease attacking other things (like the pituitary and other parts of the brain) can all cause low T3 syndrome and functional hypothyroidism.

  And this state of too little T3 can have a big impact on the immune system.

Thyroid hormones play a very important role in the growth, formation, and balance of immune cells. Every single immune cell has receptor sites for thyroid hormones. Immune cells need thyroid hormone to mature and to regulate Th1 and Th2 proteins and cells.

It's all connected, people.

Studies have shown that T4 may calm inflammatory proteins like IL-10 and IL-4 in mice.[28] And other researchers have found evidence of the same to be true in human subjects.

As we've discussed, when these cells get out of control, the result can mean more inflammation, more pain, and destruction of thyroid tissue.

Essentially, thyroid hormone is like the voice of reason for the angry mob of immune cells and proteins; it gets everyone to just chill out and relax.

So we clearly have the makings of a vicious cycle here. Right? One problem is reinforcing another.

Immune system imbalance can lead to more inflammation, which can prevent thyroid hormone from being absorbed properly; this leads to functional hypothyroidism and thyroid receptor issues, and back and forth they go. They create a positive feedback loop, reinforcing each other and making each other worse. And the result is definitely not positive.

To make matters worse, thyroid hormone also has a major impact on inflammation in the intestines. It is one of the things that keeps the cell walls in the intestines strong.

It also stimulates gastric cells and cells in the intestinal walls. Hypothyroidism can lead to leaky gut or intestinal permeability. This is a breakdown of the walls of the intestines. (We will explore this in detail in chapter 11.)

So, you see, we have two important factors that are constantly creating circumstances in the body that make Hashimoto's worse. These are two children with some serious issues!

---

28   "Inhibitory effects of thyroxine on cytokine production by T cells in mice," by C. Yao et al., 2007, *International Immunopharmacology, 7*(13), pp. 1747–1754.

IMPORTANT TAKEAWAY:

The most important takeaway here is that, while thyroid hormone can help auto-immune dysfunction, just throwing more thyroid hormone at the problem may not be the answer.

If you don't address the underlying autoimmunity, you'll just be spinning your wheels because the process of autoimmunity can create a state of functional hypothyroidism, which is a major factor in the downward spiral and progression of the disease.

WHY IS AUTOIMMUNITY SO OFTEN IGNORED IN HASHIMOTO'S?

It's important to understand that Hashimoto's is much more than just a thyroid disorder. It is an autoimmune disease that involves multiple systems of the body. Let's take a look now at how autoimmune disease is handled in today's health-care system.

First, we see a huge void in our health-care model for treating, managing, and even properly understanding this condition. Because so little is understood, we have basically no specialist for autoimmune disease.

Think about it. Who do you see? A rheumatologist? Maybe. And what do they do? They prescribe prednisone and other immunosuppressive agents (e.g., biologics like Enbrel).

Their goal? To completely suppress and weaken the immune system or block one aspect of the immune system from functioning properly. That's pretty much it.

I'll never forget the moment I realized that nothing was going to be done about this until things got "bad enough." Holy crap! We are on our own in the conventional medical model, especially in an early to moderate stage of tissue destruction.

DOING NOTHING IS *NOT* ACCEPTABLE

All too often, nothing is done until there is significant destruction in the body. If you're living with it, that's too late, in my opinion. This approach leads to a significant loss in quality of life, which for some means they can't work and they can't enjoy time with their family and friends.

Why isn't more attention being given to autoimmunity? When you look at the sheer number of cases, it's virtually an epidemic.

According to the American Autoimmune Related Disease Association, one out of every 12 men and one out of every nine women have an autoimmune disease.[29]

And the numbers are higher than for other major diseases: The National Institutes of Health (NIH) estimates that up to 23.5 million Americans may be afflicted with at least one autoimmune condition.[30] Just to compare, an estimated 9 million have cancer, and 22 million have heart disease.

This is especially crazy when you understand how autoimmune disease is defined. An autoimmune disease is officially recognized when about 70–90 percent of the target tissue is destroyed. You don't just go from 0–70 percent destruction overnight.

Why aren't more people talking about this? Is it because it's not life-threatening?

AUTOIMMUNE DISEASE *CAN* BE LIFE-THREATENING

No. The stakes are really high here. Actually, autoimmune disease is one of the top 10 leading causes of death in female children and women in all age groups up to 64 years of age.

I don't want to frighten you, but I want you to understand what the stakes are so that you take this part of Hashimoto's seriously. And this comes into play when you have to decide what you are going to do.

In my personal and professional experience, the most effective changes are dietary and lifestyle, some of which are major for some people.

When you see the big picture and the potential for where the disease can go and how destructive it can be, it makes not eating foods like gluten and dairy a no-brainer. It's not that big a sacrifice when your life is on the line.

I also want you to understand that these suggestions aren't some fad. They're being made because the risks of the status quo—of doing nothing or letting the disease progress unchecked—are just too high.

---

29   "Autoimmune statistics," Autoimmune disease fact sheet, American Autoimmune Related Diseases Association, Inc. Retrieved February 2014 from www.aarda.org/autoimmune-information /autoimmune-statistics

30   "Questions persist: Environmental factors in autoimmune disease," by C. W. Schmidt, 2011, *Environmental Health Perspectives*, 119, pp. a248–a253.

I'm really passionate about this for one simple reason: I've seen where the progression can lead, and I hope this information can help some of you make changes in your life to prevent that.

Now let's take a look at how Hashimoto's and autoimmunity can advance deeper into the body.

Autoimmune disease can progress in two different ways. First, it goes deeper and deeper into the body, causing more and more loss of function and the breakdown of other major systems. Second, it can progress to other autoimmune diseases.

THREE STAGES OF AUTOIMMUNE DISEASE

According to a number of researchers,[31] autoimmune disease is also a progressive disease that goes through three stages. While these are not recognized by the general medical community, they are very useful clinically.

As I stated above, autoimmune disease is not officially recognized until close to 70–90 percent of the target tissue is destroyed.

Well, wouldn't it be better to have some other way to identify these diseases before they destroy the target tissue? Before you've lost your ability to function and live and work like a normal person? For my way of thinking, the answer is YES!

Stage 1: Silent Autoimmunity

In this stage, the body has lost tolerance to its own tissue, but there are no symptoms yet and it doesn't really affect the way that the system functions. This stage can, however, be identified by lab tests that show elevated antibodies. People can stay in this stage for years.

This is the best place to begin some sort of treatment aimed at prevention, because your odds of getting good results are highest.

Physiologically, in this stage thyroid-specific antigens are presented to antigen-presenting cells (APCs) by thyroid cells, often after some kind of insult or environmental stressor(s), such as infection(s), excessive iodine, pregnancy, toxins in cigarette smoke, etc.

---

31   "Hashimoto's thyroiditis," by A. Parvathaneni et al, 2012, in *A new look at hypothyroidism*, D. Springer (Ed.) doi: 10.5772/30288.

Stage 2: Autoimmune Reactivity

In this stage, the destruction of the target tissue has begun. Elevated antibodies and some symptoms appear. However, the destruction is not significant enough to actually be labeled an autoimmune disease because 70–90 percent of the target tissue has not yet been destroyed. This stage is where a lot of Hashimoto's patients are.

They may or may not have been placed on thyroid replacement hormone, and that may or may not have normalized their thyroid lab results. However, the destructive autoimmune process is active and progressing.

This is a very important stage for treating the immune dysfunction, because you have a greater chance of slowing or stopping the destruction of tissue and likewise slowing the progression to other autoimmune diseases.

Physiologically, this is the stage when APCs differentiate into T cells and B cells and begin the process of destruction.

Stage 3: Autoimmune Disease

This stage is where Western medicine finally acknowledges the autoimmune disease. It takes this long because significant destruction of tissue has to take place before it's visible with an MRI or ultrasound.

Other findings include elevated antibodies, serious and significant symptoms, lab results, and special studies that all confirm a loss of function. Unfortunately, this is really late in the game. With Hashimoto's, the thyroid is almost completely destroyed by this stage.

Luckily, most people don't reach this stage before they have been given thyroid replacement hormone, because the symptoms have already become so serious that they will have sought out a doctor to help them before they get here.

Physiologically, at this stage positive feedback has led to massive destruction of the thyroid gland and to major loss of function in other systems of the body.

T cells have induced cytotoxicity, and B cells have produced antibodies that have led to apoptosis, or programmed cell death, of thyroid cells, and macrophages have infiltrated the thyroid and started producing the interleukin proteins we spoke about earlier.

The second type of progression is the progression to other autoimmune diseases.

COMMON AUTOIMMUNE DISEASES LINKED TO HASHIMOTO'S

According to a study from the U.K. published in *The American Journal of Medicine* in 2010, 14.3 percent of Hashimoto's patients had another autoimmune disease, with rheumatoid arthritis being the most common.[32]

This was of a group of 495 patients with confirmed Hashimoto's. I put the statistic out to our Facebook group, and we had more than 120 responses from people who had Hashimoto's and one or more additional autoimmune disease.

In my opinion, every Hashimoto's patient and every doctor who treats them should be asking the question, "Where else is it?" In an upcoming chapter, we'll look at some testing that can help you answer this question.

WHAT CAUSES AUTOIMMUNE DISEASE AND HASHIMOTO'S?

There is no single cause. In many people there is some exposure to a virus or other pathogen, such as Epstein-Barr virus (or other herpes virus), Coxsackie virus, salmonella, or bacterial pathogens such as Lyme disease and Yersenia.

One theory is that these viral fragments may resemble thyroid tissue and that may be why the immune system attacks the thyroid after fighting the virus. This is known as molecular mimicry.

There may also be exposure to environmental toxins such as mercury, bisphenol A (BPA), and others, which form what are called "neoantigens." These new antigens comprise the chemical plus our own tissue.

The formation of neoantigens initiates an immune response, which may result in antibody production against the chemical and the human tissue hybrid. Continued exposure to the chemical and the production of antibodies against various tissue antigens may result in autoimmune reactivity.

A genetic component is also a factor with Hashimoto's. We often see familial clusters affected by autoimmune disease. It is not unusual to find thyroid disease among first-degree relatives (siblings, parents, or children) of people who have confirmed Hashimoto's.

And we also know that exposure to gluten can be a factor in the formation of autoimmune disease.

---

32   "Prevalence and relative risk of other autoimmune diseases in subjects with autoimmune thyroid disease," by K. Boelaert et al, 2010, *The American Journal of Medicine, 123*(2), pp. 183.e1–183.e9.

GLUTEN SENSITIVITY, CELIAC DISEASE, AND THYROID AUTOIMMUNITY ARE RELATED

Celiac disease and autoimmune thyroid disorders share a common genetic link: the DQ2 allele.

This is a subtype of a region of cells called the human leukocyte antigen (HLA) system, located on some of our genes. Many of these are located on chromosome 6 (for those of you keeping count).

Mutations or defects of HLA have been linked to many different autoimmune diseases.

Exactly what happens is not known. There are numerous theories, but the end result is that our own tissue gets attacked and destroyed by the immune system.

With celiac disease and autoimmune thyroid diseases we see an increase in both types of antibodies that lead to attack on these tissues.

One study found that 5.4 percent of 335 adult celiac patients, of whom 83 percent complied with a gluten-free diet, had autoimmune thyroid disease (autoimmune hypothyroidism or Graves' disease).[33]

Another study found that 14 percent of celiac patients had thyroid disorders.[34] The same study noted a high prevalence of thyroglobulin antibodies (11 percent) and thyroid microsomal (TPO) antibodies (15 percent) in patients with celiac disease.

Likewise, another study found the prevalence of thyroid peroxidase antibodies to be higher in celiac patients (29.7 percent) than in healthy controls (9.6 percent).[35]

"YES, BUT I WAS TESTED FOR GLUTEN ANTIBODIES AND THE TESTS WERE NEGATIVE"

This is another area of misinformation. Most doctors test for two to four gluten antibodies.

---

33   "Autoimmune thyroid disorders and coeliac disease," by P. Collin et al, 1994, *European Journal of Endocrinology*, 130, pp. 137–140.

34   "Coeliac disease and autoimmune thyroid disease," By C. E. Counsell et al, 1994, *Gut*, 35, pp. 844–846.

35   "Thyroid and celiac disease: clinical, serological, and echographic study," by F. Velluzzi et al, 1998, *American Journal of Gastroenterology*, 93, pp. 976–979.

Current testing for gluten reactivity and celiac disease includes serum IgG and IgA against gliadin and tissue transglutaminase 2 (tTG2).

These antibodies are measured against minor components of a wheat protein called alpha-gliadin.

Here's the thing: Wheat consists of multiple proteins and peptides, including alpha-gliadin, omega-gliadin, glutenin, gluteomorphin, prodynorphin, and agglutinins.

And the important thing to understand is that *any* of these antigens can cause an immune response.

So even if you tested negative to celiac disease, you could still have gluten sensitivity or silent celiac disease (celiac disease that has caused damage to the small intestines, but has not been detected), because you may not have been tested for the right thing.

WHICH CAME FIRST, THE GLUTEN OR THE AUTOIMMUNITY?

This is a really interesting—and controversial—question. The answer is that no one really knows.

But here's what we do know.

Autoimmunity doesn't just happen for no reason. It is the result of a perfect storm of factors.

As mentioned before, genetics comes into play, as does exposure to a virus or other pathogen, and exposure to toxic chemicals—all of these cause antibodies to be produced that can result in the breakdown of the intestines.

Ground zero is the intestinal mucosa.

One theory is that gluten, which is sticky and invasive, gets into the intestines, into the spaces between the intestines (the tight junctions), and eventually into the bloodstream. Then the immune system kicks in.

Antigen-presenting cells like macrophages (those *Pac-Man* cells that munch the bad guys) start attacking and they stimulate the T-helper cells.

As we have learned, these are either Th1 or Th2 or both, and they lead to pro-inflammatory immune cells and proteins, more antibodies, cross reactions—generally, all hell breaking loose.

And finally, as this plays out and is repeated over and over again every time you eat a piece of bread, a pastry, some cake, a doughnut, or other gluten-rich food, you are unknowingly pushing your body further and further into autoimmunity.

Your immune system is so juiced it doesn't know which way is up and eventually, you lose self-tolerance.

And loss of self-tolerance means the immune system starts attacking your own tissue.

Another problem caused by gluten is that it makes thyroid hormone less effective.

CELIAC DISEASE HAS A MAJOR IMPACT ON
THYROID HORMONE ABSORPTION

An interesting study cited by the American Thyroid Association that was originally published by the Endocrine Society examined 68 patients with Hashimoto's thyroiditis alone and 35 patients with Hashimoto's thyroiditis and celiac disease. It was determined that "the average dose of levothyroxine needed to treat patients with Hashimoto's thyroiditis alone was lower than the average dose required to treat patients with Hashimoto's and celiac disease. When the patients with celiac disease went on a gluten-free diet while staying on the same dose of thyroxine, their TSH level decreased, indicating that their absorption of thyroxine had improved."[36]

The bottom line is that going gluten-free improved thyroid hormone absorption for these people. And this is not only true for people with celiac disease.

Next I'd like to share an interesting case study that someone posted on our Facebook group; it shows the remarkable effect that gluten and a strict gluten-free diet can have.

---

36   "Atypical celiac disease as cause of increased need for thyroxine: a systematic study," by C. Virili et al, 2012, *The Journal of Clinical Endocrinology & Metabolism, 97*(3).

CASE STUDY

"From December until this past Thursday, I have brought my thyroid peroxidase antibodies down from >1300 (topping out the scales) to 8. Literally, 8. My doctor is dumbfounded. I have strictly eliminated gluten (with his acknowledgment) and that is it.

However, when I say strict, I mean STRICT. He said there would be no way my numbers could change like that by elimination (he is a much older-school doctor) and he wouldn't believe it until he sees it on paper. Well, he just saw it on paper and was almost speechless.

Also, my last ultrasound, this past Wednesday, showed no enlargement of my thyroid and barely any misshape. My numbers have plummeted since February to the farthest end of hyper that the scales will show . . ."

Lori K., 4/4/15

Lori's story and outcome is quite commonplace. For some, gluten is a very serious player in the inflammation and attack on thyroid tissue. And for Lori, the change was so dramatic and the impact so great that she became hyperthyroid and had to discontinue her medication.

This is also something we see repeatedly in clinical practice. Gluten and dairy (lactose) can both block thyroid hormone absorption. In many cases, going gluten-free will improve (sometimes dramatically) the performance of thyroid replacement hormone.

In fact, sometimes it is so effective that people must lower their dosage or risk going into a hyperthyroid state.

STRESS PLAYS A MAJOR ROLE, TOO

Stress can also play a major role in the expression and proliferation of autoimmune disease and Hashimoto's. Often a large, stressful life event is the last straw.

In a 2008 study from the journal *Autoimmunity Reviews*, researchers noted that "many retrospective studies found that a high proportion (up to 80 percent) of patients reported uncommon emotional stress before disease onset. Unfortunately, not only does stress cause disease, but the disease itself also causes significant stress in the patients, creating a vicious cycle."[37]

---

37 "Stress as a trigger of autoimmune disease," by L. Stojanovich and D. Marisavljevich, 2008, *Autoimmunity Reviews*, 41(1).

This is a hugely important point that we're going to explore in an upcoming chapter. Stress and autoimmune disease go together like gamblers and con men. They just seem to bring out the worst in each other.

Stressful life events can sometimes be the final straw in a series of events and factors that lead to autoimmune disease.

RECAP OF FACTORS LEADING TO HASHIMOTO'S:

1. Exposure to a virus or other pathogen: Epstein-Barr virus, Coxsackie virus, herpes virus, Lyme disease, Yersenia or other pathogens have been linked to the initiation of thyroid autoimmunity.

2. Genetic susceptibility. Often there is a family history of thyroid disease.

3. Exposure to environmental toxins like mercury or BPA causes the body to form neoantigens or hybrids of our tissue and the toxic substance and the immune system attacks them.

4. Leaky gut or intestinal permeability. The gut is ground zero for autoimmunity; if it breaks down and your barrier systems become compromised, this can lead to the loss of self-tolerance.

5. Exposure to gluten. Gluten itself can lead to thyroid autoimmunity.

6. Stress. A major stressful event or prolonged stress can lead to thyroid (and other types of) autoimmunity.

> It's not just one thing. It's a collection of many things, and it's not your fault. You just got dealt a bad hand. What matters now is how you play that hand.

Next, let's take a look at the immune system from the Chinese medical perspective. But before we do, here's another Hashimoment.

HASHIMOMENT:
GRIEVING THE LOSS OF YOUR OLD LIFE

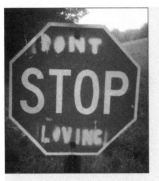

A really common theme among people who suffer from the debilitating effects of Hashimoto's is the struggle to accept the new normal.

According to Chinese medicine, one of the signs of a blocked thyroid is unwillingness to change.

Isn't that ironic? Hashimoto's forces us to change so much, sometimes!

Diet, habits, lifestyle, situations that no longer serve us.

When it starts to affect our lives, the temptation is to look at all the things we can't do anymore. And we may need to grieve the loss of that old life for a period of time.

Another irony is that in Chinese medicine, the negative emotion of the metal element is excessive grief or an inability to let go of grief.

One way to get over this is to look at it another way.

Like spring, you have an opportunity for a new life: one in which you eat a healthy diet, do the things that serve you, and let go of the stressful situations that were not good for you anyway.

Change, though difficult, can be a good thing.

Chapter 7

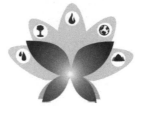

THE CHINESE MEDICINE VIEW OF THE METAL ELEMENT

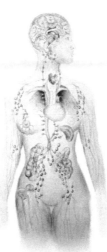

Now let's get into the Chinese medical perspective. As I said at the beginning, one important organ system that is involved with the immune response is the metal element.

Remember when I was talking about this not being linear? Well, Chinese medicine is brilliantly constructed to account for the lack of step-by-step linearity.

By observing nature and creating theories about interactions in the body, the ancient Chinese were able to describe function in the body in the way that it actually happens.

They did this by layering different theories in different directions simultaneously. You can put several of these theories on top of each other.

Right? We've already looked at yin and yang, a theme that is repeated all over the earth and throughout universe: the sun and moon, day and night, hot and cold, summer and winter, etc., *ad infinitum*. Yin, yang, yin, yang.

Then we have the five elements: Each has a yin and yang representative. In the metal element, the lungs are yin and the large intestine is yang. I was always puzzled by why. Why are these two systems connected? Well, look at the lymphatic system: That's the connection; the immune system is what unites them.

Without getting too crazy into these and other theories, I want you to see that this is exactly how the immune system and hormones and other systems in the body behave. It's a constant ebb and flow of yin and yang.

That's what a negative feedback loop is. Something gets too yin and yang intervenes, or vice versa.

HOW THE ANCIENT CHINESE UNDERSTOOD THE IMMUNE SYSTEM

The ancient Chinese described immune function as *wei qi*, a "defensive substance" that flowed into the gut, deep into lymphatic vessels, which also carry absorbed dietary fat and lymph fluid.

In the body, the lymphatic system drains into the venous blood supply at the subclavian vein—a large vein located just below the clavicle (visible in the illustration at the top of this chapter).

There is a description of this in the *Neijing Lingshu,* or *The Yellow Emperor's Classic of Medicine,* a seminal text of Chinese medicine from the 2nd century B.C. This book has two parts, the Nei Jing and the Ling Shu.

There are various translations of the Yellow Emperor's classic and in them our body's protective qi is referred to as fierce and brave and it is generated from water and grains.

"The protective qi comes out, its fierce qi is violent and quick and first moves in the four limbs, in the divisions of the flesh and the gaps of the skin and is unceasing. During the daytime it travels in the yang. At night it travels in the yin…as it moves in the five viscera and six bowels."[38]

---

38   Jing-Nuan, Wu, *The Ling Shu or Spiritual Pivot* (Honolulu: University of Hawaii Press, 1993), 226.

The "divisions of the flesh and the gaps in the skin" are a reference to the superficial lymphatics and the mesenteric system of the abdomen and chest, which are densely populated with lymph glands and vessels.

These were the first descriptions ever of the body's immune system (from 2,000 years ago). The ancient Chinese understood subtle details like the fact that *wei qi* leaves arterial circulation to mount a protective reaction and that it has both yin and yang characteristics.

In other words, they described the process of something leaving the bloodstream to protect the body. And that it was both yin and substantial (the lymph fluid) and yang and energetic (it caused an energetic reaction or triggered other events—the way the immune system causes many different changes in other systems of the body).

In addition, they spoke of immune reactions in both yin and yang terms. The inflammatory reactions of the immune response are considered yang, and the anti-inflammatory functions are yin.

This truly expresses the contradictory nature of the immune system we described earlier. It's not linear. Different parts of the immune system do different things. Sometimes the same part does things in opposite directions. Yin and yang describe this behavior quite well.

In addition to normal immune functions, *wei qi* also has a role in warming the body and controlling pores and sweating. *Wei qi* functions also include control over superficial vasodilation and the immune complement system.

UNDERSTANDING THE COMPLEMENT SYSTEM

The complement system is a group of small proteins that basically add lighter fluid to a fire. They get the killers and attackers in the immune system amped up and make the carnage much worse during an immune response. These are the guys we want to clear out because of their destructive potential.

One other interesting thing about the Chinese medical approach is that it looks at these internal organs and their connections, or spheres of influences.

It's like having friends, family, and acquaintances that you have some degree of influence over. The same is true with each element.

So the metal element has the lungs and large intestine, and it has the *wei qi* that we just described. It has the skin, the mucous membranes, and the nose. Which endocrine gland is connected to it?

The thyroid. Holy crap! Just look at all the lymph glands in the throat. The thyroid is very much connected to the immune system.

And check this out. TSH is not only produced in the pituitary. Thirty years ago, researchers discovered that immune cells actually produce TSH during times of acute infection.[39]

Where do the immune cells produce TSH? They produce it in the bone marrow where immune cells are born, by white blood cells, and also in the intestines when exposed to a virus. Remember when we were talking about IL-18 and IL-12? It turns out they also produce TSH.

HERE'S AN EXAMPLE

A female patient's lab tests showed that her TSH was too high, yet she was having many hyper symptoms such as anxiety, palpitations, mood swings, and so forth. She was going nuts.

Think about this. She had some gluten and dairy (made from cow's milk), which caused a massive immune response in her intestines. She may have been exposed to some sort of pathogen (maybe a bovine virus), and those immune cells produce TSH.

Her TSH appeared high because of these factors, but she was functionally hyperthyroid. Remember in an earlier chapter how I said what you feel is diagnostically and clinically important with Hashimoto's?

This can work both ways. A hypothyroid state creates impaired immune function. There's a lot about this that we still don't know, but one of the theories is that immune cells produce a local surge of T3, and this surge causes a systemic decline in TRH and TSH production.

One theory on this is that in times of infection and immune-induced inflammation (which autoimmune disease is in a chronic state of), the immune system shuts down thyroid function and then at some point kicks it back up again.

With Hashimoto's, this endocrine-immune communication is out of whack. The immune system may not be able to kick things up again. Or, because of chronic inflammation and tissue attack, it may not know when the "infection" is over.

---

39   "The immune system as a regulator of thyroid hormone activity," by J. R. Klein, 2006, *Experimental Biology and Medicine,* 231, pp. 229–236.

The antigen is the tissue of the body. The fight never stops. Do you understand what I'm saying?

To be honest, I just learned about this while researching this book. We are looking at some cutting-edge stuff, people! Wow. And the Chinese masters were putting it together 2,000 years ago.

Put that in your pipe and smoke it! (Not literally, though! That's not good for your lungs!)

THE EMOTIONS OF THE METAL ELEMENT

The *Neijing Suwen* (*The Yellow Emperor's Classic of Medicine*), describes the lungs as "minister and chancellor," helping the heart to regulate the body's *qi* (energy).

The lungs govern *wei qi*, which guards our outermost boundary and prevents all that doesn't match our true self from getting inside to our core. Grief is the negative emotion of the lungs, and grief can weaken them.

My father died when I was nine. The next year I got pneumonia. Maybe it was a coincidence, or maybe there is some connection.

The lungs are very vulnerable to dryness, as well. If this boundary becomes too dry, then finding our true self can become more difficult. If the lungs become too moist, then phlegm builds up and blocks our connection to the essence of life.

In health the lungs are thought to empower us to stay connected to the essence of value, even after the material things disappear. For example, after the loss of a loved one, a healthy lung can empower a connection to the spirit of that person.

But if the lung is weak, you could become fixated on the loss, become consumed by that grief, and lose appreciation of the present moment.

Grief can manifest as phlegm, a chronic cough, or a constant dripping sinus, like internal tears. Phlegm is very important in Chinese medicine. Like *qi*, it has a number of different definitions.

Good phlegm clears pathogens; it's the first line of defense. "Bad" phlegm accumulates in the joints, the kidneys, the brain, and the thyroid in the form of nodules.

The Chinese character for phlegm includes the character that means inflammation. Phlegm can also represent the antibody response to pathogens that cross-react to healthy tissues.

This kind of phlegm impairs cellular immune function, leading to chronic disease.

UNDERSTANDING THE LARGE INTESTINE'S ROLE

The large intestine is the yang partner to the lungs. According to the *The Yellow Emperor's Classic*, the large intestine is responsible for transit. All waste products go through this organ.

This is true of waste moving through the large intestine, which returns to the earth. It's also true metaphorically. The large intestine constructs a barrier between self and nonself by sorting out the things we take in and determining which acquired influences need to be kept and which need to be let go.

With autoimmune disease, so much of which begins and is perpetuated in the intestines, the barrier between self and nonself is lost. We lose self-tolerance. And a lot of this happens in the intestines.

When we fail to respond in a balanced way to a loss in life (and not just the loss of a loved one, but any loss: a job, a relationship, a pet) it is the large intestine that reacts. In an energetic way, it helps us to assimilate and process our grief.

But grief can become distorted, and it can be difficult to let go; in so doing, you hold on to things that no longer serve you. And what happens next? Diarrhea—which causes you to lose important minerals—or constipation, when you are literally holding on to things that no longer serve you.

This condition can make you pessimistic, cynical, and generally negative. It can make you judgmental of others. Leaky gut or intestinal permeability is caused by a breakdown of the intestinal lining and cell walls.

Many researchers believe that it is one of the root causes of autoimmunity and the loss of self-tolerance. (We will explore this in depth in the section on the earth element.)

Leaky gut may also have an emotional root. It can make you feel like you're not properly valued by others. You see how this is all connected?

Now let's look at some important insights that Chinese medicine offers in regard to the treatment of autoimmune disease in general and Hashimoto's in particular.

In the last chapter we talked a lot about lab tests and symptoms. Well, another thing that "bad" phlegm does is block receptor sites and impair thyroid hormone binding, which can affect lab test results and also prevent thyroid hormone from working efficiently in the body.

THREE IMPORTANT TREATMENT STRATEGIES

There are three important strategies that can be employed by using Chinese herbs to treat autoimmune disease. All three processes that these strategies address are involved in the initiation and continuation of autoimmune disease. If we want to slow or stop the progression, we may have to deal with these pathogenic processes.

1. Deal with pathogens. Chinese medicine uses the term *xie qi* to describe these pathogenic influences, one of which is wind. There is wind-cold, wind-heat, and so on.

Wind is a metaphor for airborne pathogens, such as viruses, bacteria, and so forth. Wind-cold refers to mild colds and flus; wind-heat refers to more virulent infections that cause a more intense reaction in the body and have the potential to do more damage internally.

Entire schools of Chinese medicine are devoted to the treatment of epidemic diseases caused by these pathogens. Long before the invention of antibiotics and antivirals, the ancient Chinese treated diseases with herbs.

In fact, when we look at the pharmacology of the herbs used to treat these conditions, they turn out to be broad-spectrum antibacterial, antifungal, and antiviral. As we have seen, viruses like Epstein-Barr have been linked to Hashimoto's. Sometimes these viruses can linger for years and resurface. Other bacterial and fungal infections may also be present in the body and can undermine the healing process if they aren't dealt with.

2. Limit antibody cross-reactions with healthy tissue. Cross-reactivity is an important concept. All proteins, including viral proteins, are built from amino acids. In nature there are 20 different amino acids, and they comprise the proteins of every living substance on earth. Many are very similar in structure. Since your immune system attacks these proteins, sometimes immune cells may attack the wrong things because they resemble this protein structure.

Different antibodies then attack both tissues that look alike. For example, gluten resembles cerebellar tissue. Eat gluten, and immune cells may attack your brain. This is one theory for why some autistic children may do better on a gluten-free diet. Researchers have found strong evidence that brain-reactive antibodies were increased in mothers of children with autism.[40]

---

40   "Brain-reactive IgG correlates with autoimmunity in mothers of a child with an autism spectrum disorder," By L. Brimberg et al, 2013, *Molecular Psychiatry*, *18*(11), pp. 1171–1177.

Depending upon which antibodies and which tissues we are addressing, we can choose herbs that focus on cross-reactivity. There are even herbs that can be helpful for thyroid enlargement.

Other herbs are thyroid protective.

There are still other herbs that increase or decrease thyroid hormone.

3. Slow or stop immune activation that is causing tissue destruction. It is critically important to unwind this destructive process. You can actually clear circulating immune complexes with Chinese herbs.

Nothing in Western medicine does this, except a very expensive process called plasmaphoresis, where they essentially take out all of your blood, clean it, and cycle it back in. You know, the Keith Richards treatment.

These immune complexes are amping up the attack. By clearing them you can really help calm down the immune system.

You'll find a lot more information on herbs in the next chapter. We have many of them in our herbal pharmacy.

ONE WEIRD REMEDY THAT HAS SUPERIOR HEALING PROPERTIES

One remedy, in particular, that I'd like to highlight is Cordyceps, a fungus that grows on the bodies of silkworms.

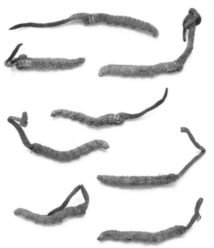

Okay, time out! How'd they find this one? I imagine the conversation going something like this.

"Hey, what's that?" "A silkworm."

"What's wrong with it?" "What do you mean?"

"What's that all over it? It looks like mold." "I don't know. Let's eat it and find out."

Seriously? God bless the brave souls who had the courage to try and test these substances. Without them, we would never have discovered their amazing healing properties.

Cordyceps actually has a kind of chocolaty taste. It also helps the body make glutathione.

The stuff is amazing. It is used traditionally to tonify kidney yang. Remember earlier we spoke about kidney yang being the source of endocrine function? It also tonifies the lungs and dissolves phlegm.

Well, since Cordyceps helps the body make and use glutathione, and glutathione has been shown to modulate immune function . . . wow and wow!

Pharmacologically, it's miraculous. Its antibiotic and anticancer, it relieves asthma, it stimulates immune function, it stimulates the adrenal glands, and it has been found to increase platelets.

All this from a fungus that grows on silkworms. Yum!

A REVIEW OF CHAPTER 7:

Okay, let's wrap up this section. So much has been covered. I mean mind-blowing stuff here, people! Let's recap.

1. **The metal element in Chinese medicine has many components of the immune system.**

   The lungs and large intestine are yin and yang pairs, and we can clearly see their connection through the lymphatic system. *Wei qi* is how the ancient Chinese explained the immune system and its activity.

2. **Emotionally, the lungs and large intestine help us deal with boundaries and loss.**

   Grief is the negative emotion of the metal element. If the lungs are weak, you can get overwhelmed by grief and loss.

   Phlegm is a by-product of this process, and in Chinese medicine phlegm is a pathogen—something that makes you sick. Bad phlegm can clog receptor sites and create nodules.

3. **Chinese herbs can clear out circulating immune complexes; Western medicine currently has no drug for that.**

   There are herbs that can help calm the immune attack. Specific herbs are also available (and can be found in our herbal pharmacy) for the various interleukins we talked about in this chapter. For more information, visit https://www.hashimotoshealing.com/contact/.

4. **Cordyceps, a fungus that grows on the bodies of silkworms, is one example.** Cordyceps helps clear out immune complexes that can increase the destructive attack by the immune system and it helps the body make glutathione.

LET'S APPRECIATE GLUTATHIONE

I would like to take this opportunity to heap praise on glutathione. The stuff is amazing.

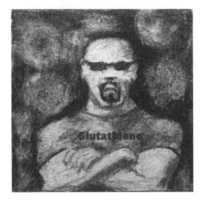

Glutathione is like the loyal bodyguard who will sacrifice his own life to save the life of the person he or she protects. There are different forms of glutathione in the body, but when we have enough of the right kind, we are protected from any number of toxic invaders.

However, when our glutathione stores start to run low, it triggers a destructive inflammatory process. Toxic chemicals and pollutants drain glutathione from the body because it is exactly what our bodies use to clean these destructive compounds out of our systems.

Glutathione is everywhere. It's in animals, microorganisms, and plants—and, because it is water soluble, it's found mainly inside cells. In fact, it is one of the most highly concentrated antioxidants inside of cells.

There are different forms of glutathione available on the market. It's important to know which kind does what. The oral form of S-acetyl-L-glutathione can be utilized by the body and is mostly absorbed by the liver.

There are liposomal creams that are absorbed by the peripheral tissue and that are effective for getting it into the bloodstream and into the thyroid itself.

And there are remedies such as Cordyceps (mentioned earlier), which helps the body recycle and reabsorb glutathione. Some doctors also offer it in IV form.

It is often depleted with Hashimoto's. It also strengthens (along with Vitamin D3) the regulatory or Th3 part of the immune system.

It does it all. I thank you, glutathione!

Chapter 8

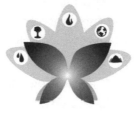

USING THE A.P.A.R.T. SYSTEM
TO HEAL
THE IMMUNE SYSTEM

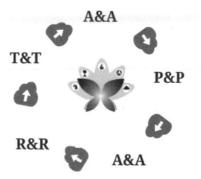

The A.P.A.R.T. System

1. A = Ask and Assess: An Overview of Immune Testing

Grab your journal and look for symptoms of problems with the metal element. Note what they are, then create a plan for addressing them. After that, you must act on your plan; follow-through is crucial.

Next, take inventory of what you did. Look at what worked and what didn't. Both will provide valuable information.

Double down on what worked and change what didn't. Keep refining your process.

Autumn is a good time of year to address issues with the metal element. Traditionally, the ancient Chinese believed that not only does the body go through daily energetic rhythms (like circadian rhythms), it also goes through annual energetic rhythms. And autumn is considered the time of the metal element.

(But don't wait to heal the intestines or lungs if something comes up at another time.)

Let's review a couple of things about testing and its availability for the immune system—particularly autoimmune-disease testing—and why it matters.

SIGNS AND SYMPTOMS OF AUTOIMMUNITY AND BARRIER SYSTEM COMPROMISE:

Ask: Do you have any of these symptoms?

- Lung deficiencies
- Common lung disorders

THE IMPACT OF HASHIMOTO'S ON THE LUNGS

The impact of Hashimoto's and hypothyroidism on the lungs and respiratory system is seldom discussed. However, there are a number of potential issues that may need to be addressed.

One thing we know is that fatigue and dyspnea (difficult or labored breathing) are common symptoms. These are some of the factors that make exercise such a challenge for Hashimoto's folks.

One explanation for an intolerance to exercise could be the effects of hypothyroidism or functional hypothyroidism on the lungs, namely: limited pulmonary reserve, limited cardiac reserve, and decreased muscle strength (especially of the diaphragm and other muscles involved in breathing).

Lower oxygen saturation has also been noted. This is interesting, because when you combine this with the various anemias that are found in Hashimoto's patients, you have a recipe for compounded fatigue.

Pleural effusion (or the buildup of fluids in the interstitial spaces between the lungs and the tissues that line the chest) has also been found to be caused by hypothyroidism. One theory is that hypothyroidism leads to capillary permeability and fewer, narrower vessels, as well.

In clinical practice, I have noted that complaints involving the upper airway are common with people with Hashimoto's. Patients frequently complain of nasal congestion, recurrent colds, voice change, sensation of swelling or a foreign object in the throat, and discomfort and dryness of the throat.

Nasal mucus may be increased, and about 20 percent of patients have tonsil enlargement. Sleep apnea is also found in this population; hypothyroidism is a well-documented cause of obstructive sleep apnea, for all of the reasons mentioned above,[41] a condition that tends to be more severe in people who are obese.

In addition to the issues that may be linked to hypothyroidism, many problems of the lungs (and large intestine) are due to a sedentary lifestyle that is also common in this day and age. Lack of activity can lead to poor respiration and elimination.

Lung and colon problems are, obviously, also made worse by a poor diet: overeating; not eating enough roughage; and consuming too much dairy, sugar, processed foods, or other congesting foods. Using recreational drugs, cigarettes, and pharmaceutical drugs can also compromise lung function.

And Hashimoto's and hypothyroidism can lead to chronic constipation.

These habits and behaviors can cause mucus to be deposited into the lungs, which blocks their proper functioning. Colds, allergies, sinus problems, bronchitis, and asthma are some of the issues that may result.

Furthermore, toxins build up in the lungs and colon and create tension, exhaustion, hair loss, and skin problems such as acne. The following syndromes give a sense of how these various conditions manifest in the lungs, and thus shed light on how to resolve them.

COMMON SYNDROMES OF THE LUNGS

Viruses most commonly cause the first lung syndrome—the onset of conditions such as the common cold and flu. As we discussed, some viruses have also been linked to the onset of Hashimoto's.

(In the patient population I have seen, the Epstein-Barr virus is the most common; I've seen the virus in the history of more than 75 percent of the people I have spoken to and worked with.)

---

41   "Association of hypothyroidism and obstructive sleep apnea," by V. Kapur et al, 1998, *American Journal of Respiratory and Critical Care Medicine, 158*(5), pp. 1379–1383.

It is important to note that the practice of prescribing antibiotics for viral respiratory infections is not only a bad strategy, it also has now been found to cause long-term damage to the immune system by killing off beneficial bacteria that are so important to healthy immune function.

Overuse of antibiotics has made our population vulnerable to superbugs (drug-resistant bacteria). Many herbal formulas are available that are quite effective for treating upper respiratory (sinus, ear, and lung) infections.

If such infections are not resolved, they can develop into what is known as "heat in the lungs."

Heat congestion in the lungs will usually produce what is known in Chinese medicine as "exterior symptoms"—fevers accompanied by chills, and a red tongue with a dry, yellow coating.

In addition, dry cough, shortness of breath, and a painful sore throat may be present; there may also be thick, yellow-green phlegm, or in even more severe cases, blood-streaked phlegm; and yellow nasal discharge.

It's important to have alternative approaches to healing, because when people with Hashimoto's become sick, it can be very debilitating.

Prescribing more and more antibiotics can further damage the ecosystem of the intestines. In some cases antibiotics may be necessary, but they should not be the first course of action—especially if the issue is caused by a virus.

Phlegm in the lungs is most often brought about by weak digestion (weak spleen/pancreas) that causes mucus. It can also result from too much mucus-forming food.

In either case, mucus accumulates in the lungs; symptoms include cough, shortness of breath, wheezing, or asthma accompanied by sticky phlegm. The tongue coating may be greasy and white if the phlegm is cold; a greasy-yellow coating indicates hot phlegm.

LARGE INTESTINE/IMMUNE ISSUES

Large intestine issues: feeling that bowels do not empty completely; constipation; hard, dry, or small stool; frequent laxative use.

Intestinal permeability issues: increased frequency of food reactions; unpredictable food reactions; aches, pains, and swelling throughout the body; unpredictable abdominal swelling; frequent bloating and distention after eating; abdominal intolerance to sugars and starches.

Chemical intolerance: multiple smell and chemical sensitivities; intolerance to smells; intolerance to jewelry, intolerance to shampoos, lotions, and detergents; and constant skin outbreaks. (This is related to the metal element because multiple sensitivities could be an indicator of a breakdown of the barrier systems. The lungs and intestines are two important barriers in the body.)

TOP THREE FOODS THAT CAN LEAD TO AUTOIMMUNE FLARE-UPS

From both my personal and clinical experience, I have found that the top three foods that may overstimulate your immune system are gluten, dairy, and soy.

1. **Gluten:** Gluten is rich in lectins (nature's own insecticides). It can bind to your intestinal walls, cause them to break down, and once through, can cause a massive immune response.

    Research also suggests that the proteins in gluten resemble certain tissues in our body. For example, there is evidence to suggest that antibodies for gluten also attack Purkinje cells (large, branched nerve cells) in the cerebellum. Therefore, when you eat gluten, your body attacks and attacks that tissue.

    (We discussed in chapter 6 what a massive impact being on a strict, gluten-free diet can have.) More dietary information concerning Hashimoto's and celiac disease is found in later in this book.

2. **Dairy:** Dairy products are some of the most immunoreactive substances in our diet. Commercial dairy is full of antibiotics and hormones, and the process of pasteurization leaves billions of dead bacteria and viruses in these products. Raw dairy products may contain live bacteria and viruses. Raw, organic dairy from grass-fed animals may be tolerated but is still a big risk.

    And the issue with dairy is not what animal it comes from or whether or not it is raw or pasteurized. It is the problems caused by dairy proteins like casein and dairy sugars like lactose.

3. **Soy:** Soy is heavily genetically modified, is also rich in lectins, and is very difficult to digest. It is also estrogenic (it acts like estrogen) in large quantities. Soy can be anti-inflammatory, but it can also be goitrogenic

and it suppresses thyroid peroxidase (TPO) enzymes (not TPO antibodies). It's okay in small quantities if you can tolerate it, but many Hashimoto's people cannot.

In some people, these foods can cause massive broad-spectrum immune responses.

Assess: Here are some tests you can do to find out more.

LOW-TECH TESTS AND LAB TESTS

Low-tech tests can be done at home. Lab tests, obviously, we order from the lab. Both can be helpful diagnostically.

Low-tech tests are basically challenge tests. They involve stimulating the immune system and seeing what happens. They can be risky, and certain people should not do them.

For example, if someone is very weak and depleted, stimulating the immune system could potentially wipe them out. So be cautious. That being said, such tests can also be really helpful.

Conceptually, whenever you consume something, whether it's medication, herbs, vitamins, or food, it has an impact on your immune system.

And if parts of your immune system are overactive and you take or eat something that stimulates that part of your system, then you can put gasoline on the fire and end up feeling like utter crap.

Does that make sense?

TH1 AND TH2 CHALLENGE TEST

Natural remedies like herbs can cause more specific responses in the Th1 or Th2 systems. This can be helpful diagnostically, because it can help you identify things that may make you feel worse.

Basically, what you do is take a mixture of herbs (listed below) that stimulate Th1 or Th2 and you do this for three days. Then you record your symptoms in your journal. You only take one of these at a time and you make sure that you limit other things that may be immune stimulating during this time. By minimizing the variables you can get a better sense of whether you are having a reaction.

This same methodology can be applied to everything in your life: Simplify, minimize the variables, and test that particular herb, food, or behavior and see how you react. And if it causes an immune response, it may be something you need to pay attention to and eliminate or avoid.

When testing Th1 and Th2, lots of things can happen. You can get a reaction from one, from both, or from neither. As I've said, it's so important to keep a journal and note anything that is out of the ordinary.

If you get a reaction, that could mean a flare-up of your symptoms like pain, fatigue, brain fog, diarrhea, digestive complaints, and neurological symptoms like mood changes, anxiety or depression, and so on.

And that is important because it can help you identify what to avoid. Sometimes these reactions are subtle, so try and note anything out of the ordinary.

Here's a good list of Th1- and Th2-stimulating compounds that comes from Mickey Trescott, author of the *The Autoimmune Paleo Cookbook*.[42]

TH1-STIMULATING COMPOUNDS:

Astragalus

Chlorella

Echinacea

Glycyrrhiza (found in licorice)

Grape seed extract

Medicinal mushrooms (Maitake and beta-glucan are common)

Melissa officinalis (lemon balm)

Panax ginseng

---

42 "How do you balance TH1 and TH2 in autoimmune disease?" by M. Trescott, 2013. Retrieved from autoimmune-paleo.com/how-do-you-balance-th1-and-th2-in-autoimmune-disease/

TH2-STIMULATING COMPOUNDS:

Caffeine

Curcumin (found in turmeric)

Genistin (found in soybeans)

Green tea extract

Lycopene (found in tomatoes and other red fruits, excluding strawberries and cherries)

Pine bark extract

Pycnogenol (found in the extract of French maritime pine bark and apples)

Quercitin (a flavanoid found in many fruits and vegetables, such as onions, berries, and kale)

Resveratrol (found in grape skin, sprouted peanuts, and cocoa)

White willow bark

DON'T CONTINUE ONCE YOU GET A REACTION

And just to be clear: Once you get a reaction, stop taking whatever caused it. You don't need to keep causing a reaction and risk potentially hurting yourself. Note the reaction and stop.

Also: This type of test is *not* for everyone. For people who are very weak or people who have certain types of autoimmunity where a flare-up can be life-threatening, or for people who are very compromised, this test can cause more harm than good.

You have to be careful. If you are in doubt about whether or not this is appropriate for you, consult a physician who has experience using these herbs (a functional medicine practitioner would be a good choice).

GABA CHALLENGE FOR TESTING THE BLOOD-BRAIN BARRIER

Another interesting test is the GABA (gamma-aminobutyric acid) challenge. It can be used to test the blood-brain barrier.

Why do we want to test this? Well, all the barriers in our body—the intestinal barrier, the lung barrier, and the blood-brain barrier—are made of the same proteins.

So if we find one to be compromised, there's a very good chance that the others are also damaged. We know that the gut and the brain have a very close connection.

For example, if we find a weakened blood-brain barrier, we know we have to intensify our efforts to heal the gut as well. It's just a good, basic rule of thumb.

Because of the blood-brain barrier (and for other reasons), the immune system in the brain is much less specialized. It doesn't have all the different immune cells and proteins and other forms of help we've been talking about.

Your brain has the microglia. And they are super hypervigilant. They're like paranoid Chihuahuas with automatic rifles. They just start firing at the slightest sign of invasion.

This is why your brain reacts so strongly to immune stimulation; it gets inflamed. And brain fog, memory issues, or concentration issues can also come from brain inflammation. One of the worst offenders? Gluten.

Regarding the GABA challenge, you simply take a large dose of GABA (1,000 milligrams), then you wait and see. Don't plan to do anything important afterward, like operating heavy machinery or using a chain saw, because you can end up with quite a buzz.

GABA is an inhibitory neurotransmitter: It calms things down. It can make you very mellow. But it's also a very big molecule and shouldn't be able to cross the blood-brain barrier.

If you get buzzed, then you may have a breach. If you do have a breach, do not, under any circumstances, get chelation therapy until you've worked to heal that barrier.

(In an upcoming chapter, we're going to delve more into the barriers and how to fix them.)

Chelation therapy draws heavy metals out of your tissues, and if you have a breach of the blood-brain barrier, it could dump mercury, lead, cadmium, and other fun stuff right into your brain and other vital organs.

This is very, very bad. I've seen some patients who were never the same after chelation therapy. Seriously. There are consequences to trying different therapies.

This is another reason to be humbled and sensitive to the complexity and stakes involved with the body in general, and blood-brain barrier specifically.

THE BEST TEST IS YOUR OWN BODY

All of these tests and the tests mentioned below can be very helpful, but the gold standard is an elimination diet, which is the initial phase of an autoimmune paleo diet.

With food-sensitivity tests you may get a false negative if you have avoided these foods for a period of time. Reintroducing foods after eliminating them for 30–60 days is often a more definitive test for determining whether or not you still have the sensitivity.

Once again, the best way to test your body is to ask your body. First eliminate the food, herb, or substance in question, and then reintroduce it after a period of time (30–60 days). Make this food, herb, or substance the only variable; take note of the response(s) it gives you.

Responses can vary from digestive upset, pain, cramping, gas, diarrhea, and/or constipation to neurological symptoms such as moodiness, anxiety, depression, brain fog, memory loss, headaches, or other cognitive problems.

LABORATORY TESTING

The best lab by far that I have found for testing autoimmune-related issues is called Cyrex Laboratories.

Their tests are called arrays, and they are extremely well-designed and supported by an enormous amount of research. They are great tools for identifying triggers and for identifying what additional autoimmunity you may have.

This data allows us to make changes early and to stop or slow the progression of autoimmune disease to other parts of your body (where it can be very destructive and, in some cases, life-threatening).

I think it's important to go over the available arrays here to give you a sense of how you or the practitioner you are working with can use them and the data they provide to better design your treatment. They are listed in order of importance.

1. Array 2: Intestinal Antigenic Permeability Screen

This array tests intestinal permeability (also known as leaky gut). So many Hashimoto's folks have leaky gut, which can contribute to flare-ups, because so much of the immune system is in the gut.

If this barrier is compromised, bacteria, viruses, protein fragments, yeast, and other things that shouldn't be in the bloodstream may get through and your immune system will never have a chance to calm down.

This becomes a constant source of immune flare-ups, which can drive the destruction of tissues in your body.

This blood test:

- Measures intestinal permeability to large molecules, which can inflame the immune system.

- Identifies the damaging route through the intestinal barrier (between cells or through the cell itself).

2. Array 3: Wheat/Gluten Proteome Reactivity and Autoimmunity

Most doctors test two or three antibodies for gluten. This test looks at 24 different gluten antibodies so that you can:

- Accurately identify gluten reactivity

- Measure antibody production against nine wheat proteins and peptides and three essential structure enzymes.

This is the preferred test for celiac disease and gluten sensitivity. This also may be a good test if you have a lot of neurological symptoms, such as brain fog, numbness, balance, or speech issues of unknown origin.

3. Array 4: Gluten-Associated Cross-Reactive Foods and Food Sensitivities

This is a great test if going gluten-, dairy-, and soy free isn't yielding results. As many as 25 other foods are known to behave like gluten and can cause an immune response. This test makes it possible to identify them quickly.

You could also do an elimination diet and then reintroduce these foods to challenge each of them.

- This test can help identify dietary proteins other than gluten that you may be reacting to.

- If a gluten-free diet isn't getting you the results you had hoped for, this test may help explain why by identifying cross-reactive foods.

4. Array 11: Chemical Immune Reactivity Screen

This test is used to identify antibodies to environmental toxins. Here's the theory about what happens in your body with these toxins.

In today's world we are exposed to chemicals, heavy metals, pesticides, and other toxic substances on a daily basis. When they enter your body, your immune system and your liver must try and get rid of them by neutralizing and excreting them.

During this process, they may bind with your own proteins and create what's called a neoantigen, which is a hybrid of your own tissue and the environmental toxin—and that is what your immune system may attack.

This attack may cause a massive immune windup that results in flare-up symptoms. These can have a big impact on the progression of Hashimoto's.

This test can tell you which chemicals are causing flare-ups in you so that they can be avoided. For some people this is an important piece of the puzzle.

5. Array 5: Multiple Autoimmune Reactivity Screen

This is the test that helps answer the question, "Where else is it?"

This test is expensive, but the information is incredibly valuable as an early warning sign for where your disease may be progressing.

It looks at 24 different antibodies for autoimmune disease in places you never thought of, such as the pancreas, brain, joints, cell walls, and stomach.

This can be an amazing tool for seeing the big picture and for understanding why certain treatments and strategies aren't working.

We know antibodies are predictive, so even if you don't have any symptoms related to a particular antibody, this information can be valuable for prevention and being proactive.

Array 5 is an incredible tool that may be recommended for those who need a little extra incentive to take the progression of autoimmunity more seriously. And fair warning, it can be a little scary because this may reveal potential problems in the future.

Discovering you have antibodies in your brain or other vital organs doesn't mean that you will automatically develop autoimmunity in these places, but it does tell you what you are at risk for.

It would also be a good idea to test the intestinal ecosystem for a variety of issues as well. You can read more about that in the next chapter.

6. Array 10: Multiple Food Immune Reactivity Screen

This is an innovative test developed by Cyrex, and it is a definite game changer.

It tests for 180 different real-world antigens, including cooked foods (because cooking changes their chemistry), raw foods, and food additives. By "real world" they mean actual chemicals and substances found in the food you are really eating.

These aren't antigens developed in a laboratory. This test and Array 4 provide a complete overview of the problem foods in your diet.

Note: These arrays must be ordered by a practitioner. And it's important that this practitioner has experience with interpreting them.

These are not common laboratory tests, and many people are not sure what to do with the data. If you're interested, you can always contact our office through our website, and we can discuss the proper steps for ordering these tests.

THE LARGE INTESTINE AND FODMAP

FODMAP stands for a list of things that you would probably never say during a normal conversation: fermentable oligosaccharides, disaccharides, monosaccharides, and polyols. These substances weren't connected before researchers found a common link among them (see below).

They are made from different kinds of sugars, such as fructose, lactose, fructo- and galacto-oligosaccharides (fructans and galactans), and sugar alcohols like sorbitol, mannitol, xylitol, and maltitol.

All of the above share three things in common:

1. They don't get absorbed very well in the small intestine. This can happen for many reasons, like a breakdown of the intestinal lining and a breakdown in the mechanisms that carry these particles across the intestinal barrier.

   Also, brush border enzymes like amylase, cellulase, and invertase may be depleted and other enzymes like hydrolases may be lacking as well. Sometimes, it's just simply that these molecules are too big to cross the barrier and get absorbed.

2. They can also be small and "osmotically active," meaning they kind of grease the wheels and get things moving. One example is lactulose, a synthetic sugar that isn't digestible. In large enough doses it works like a laxative, making the stool looser and promoting faster movement through the bowels.

3. These substances tend to be fermented quickly by bacteria. The chain length of the carbohydrate determines how fast these sugars are fermented. The shorter the chain, the faster the fermentation.

LOTS OF GAS

All of this translates into lots of farting.

Yes, I said it—bad and often really stinky gas. Treating this condition involves removing high-FODMAP foods from the diet. Google "FODMAP diet" and you will find a list of foods to avoid.

2. P = Prioritize and Plan

Examine which issues are the most severe. Obviously, this is complicated and involves the intersection of the immune system and the digestive system—where most of the immune system lives.

In my personal and professional experience, diet is the single most important thing in getting the immune system under control and in slowing and/or stopping the progression of autoimmune disease.

The diet we advocate is an autoimmune paleo approach (also known as the autoimmune diet). We will explore this diet in depth in upcoming chapters.

3. A = Act and Adapt

Act and put your plan into motion. Then observe the results. Double down on what works and change what doesn't. And results should be apparent relatively quickly. If they aren't, you need to make changes.

CLINICAL PEARL:

Another important thing to be conscious of when addressing the metal element and working with the immune system is that stimulating immune function can have some serious adverse effects.

As we have seen, stimulating parts of the immune system that are already over-excited can make things significantly worse, particularly if that part of your immune system is already attacking your own tissues (like your thyroid or your brain).

This is why the Th1/Th2 challenge test mentioned earlier can be helpful. But it's also important to remember this when you are treating other things like colds and flu. During these times you may forget and focus on trying to get better.

Common immune stimulants like echinacea, goldenseal, and astragalus are all examples of herbs that might be recommended to treat a common cold but may not be such a good idea if you have Hashimoto's.

A better approach may be to use antiviral herbs. One remedy I have used with success is a popular patent formula of Chinese herbs called Gan Mao Ling.

This contains ilex root, evodia, chrysanthemum flower, vitex, isatis root, and honeysuckle flower. It is useful as both a preventative to illness and after you've already become sick to resolve the illness more quickly.

METAL: DIETARY SOLUTIONS FOR THE LUNGS AND LARGE INTESTINE

FOODS FOR COMMON METAL ELEMENT ISSUES

Common cold: Chinese medicine has categorized two types of cold-related issues, wind-cold and wind-heat. They are considered two different conditions and have two different treatment approaches.

Wind-cold: This often occurs when there's a change in the weather and if you have a weak immune system. Symptoms include chills, fever, no sweating, headache, body aches, and clear nasal discharge.

The best way to treat this is to try and sweat the pathogen out.

Foods to help aid sweating are: ginger, garlic, mustard greens, grapefruit peel, cilantro, parsnips, scallions, cinnamon, and basil.

Wind-heat: This is usually a more serious condition; it has often progressed deeper into the body and may involve a more serious infection. Symptoms include high fever, some chills, sweating, sore throat, cough, headache, body aches, and yellow or green nasal discharge.

Foods recommended are: mint, cabbage, chrysanthemum flowers, burdock root, cilantro, dandelion, apples, pears, and bitter melon. In addition, drink plenty of water and get lots of rest.

Foods to relieve constipation: bananas, apples, figs, spinach, peaches, pears, pine nuts, sesame seeds, mulberries, grapefruit, yams, honey, apricot kernels, alfalfa sprouts, beets, cabbage, bok choy, cauliflower, Chinese cabbage, and salt water. (Epsom salts are commonly used as a laxative. Be very careful with this, as it can have a pretty dramatic effect.)

CLINICAL PEARL:

Magnesium is also very helpful for treating constipation. There are a lot of different kinds on the market. Here's a brief breakdown of those best used for constipation and other purposes.

Magnesium carbonate, which has antacid properties, contains about 45 percent magnesium.

Magnesium chloride/magnesium lactate contains only 12 percent magnesium, but has better absorption than others, such as magnesium oxide, which contains five times more magnesium.

Magnesium citrate is magnesium with citric acid, which has laxative properties.

Magnesium glycinate is a chelated form of magnesium that has some of the highest levels of absorption and it is an excellent choice for those who are trying to correct a deficiency.

Magnesium oxide is a nonchelated type of magnesium, bound to a fatty or organic acid. It has stool-softening properties.

Magnesium sulfate/magnesium hydroxide (milk of magnesia) is typically used as a laxative. Be aware that it's easy to take too much of either one of these, so be cautious and use only as directed.

Magnesium taurate contains a combination of magnesium and taurine, an amino acid. Together they tend to provide a calming effect on your body and mind.

Magnesium threonate is a newer type of magnesium supplement that has shown promise due to its ability to get past the mitochondrial membrane inside of cells.

GREAT EXERCISE FOR CONSTIPATION:

A simple exercise for stimulating peristalsis (movement through the intestines) is to rub your belly clockwise 100 times.

Transit through the intestines moves in a clockwise direction; by rubbing your stomach in this way you are stimulating that natural activity and encouraging movement through them.

OTHER LUNG-RELATED ISSUES

- **Treating heat congestion in lungs:** watercress, cantaloupe, apple, persimmon, peach, pear, strawberry, citrus, seaweeds, mushroom, daikon radish, radish, carrot, pumpkin, kuzu, cabbage, bok choy, cauliflower, chard, papaya, and white fungus

- **Treating phlegm in lungs:** fennel, fenugreek, watercress, garlic, other members of the onion family, horseradish, turnip, fresh ginger, daikon radish, mushroom, cereal grass, and seaweeds

- **Foods that specifically affect lungs and large intestine:** pungent foods—onion family, radish, turnip, ginger, horseradish, cabbage, daikon radish, white peppercorn, and especially garlic

- **Mucilaginous (create natural mucus) foods:** seaweeds, chia seeds, and okra

- **Beta-carotene foods:** carrot, winter squash, pumpkin, broccoli, parsley, kale, turnip, mustard greens, watercress, wheat or barley grass, and common green, blue green, and golden micro algae

HERBS FOR MODULATING IMMUNE FUNCTION

I. Here's a quick review of herbs that are Th1 and Th2 stimulants.

It is important to note that while there is a kind of yin and yang relationship that exists between Th1 and Th2, it's not always as simple as taking one to reduce the other.

If someone is especially inflamed or reactive, it may be best to avoid both Th1 and Th2 stimulants to allow the immune system to calm down.

TH1–STIMULATING COMPOUNDS:

Astragalus
Chlorella
Echinacea
Glycyrrhiza (found in licorice)
Grape seed extract
Medicinal mushrooms (Maitake and beta-glucan are common)
Melissa officinalis (lemon balm)
Panax ginseng

TH2-STIMULATING COMPOUNDS:

Caffeine

Curcumin (found in turmeric)

Genistin (found in soybeans)

Green tea extract

Lycopene (found in tomatoes and other red fruits, excluding strawberries and cherries)

Pine bark extract

Pycnogenol (found in the extract of the French maritime pine bark and apples)

Quercitin (a flavanoid found in many fruits and vegetables, such as onions, berries, and kale)

Resveratrol (found in grape skin, sprouted peanuts, and cocoa)

White willow bark

II. Here's an overview of herbs that can increase or decrease various interleukins that we discussed above. These come from lecture notes of Matt Van Benschoten, O.M.D., who was a brilliant herbalist and practitioner of Chinese medicine.[43]

It is not recommended to take these herbs without the supervision of a skilled physician.

Due to the unpredictable nature of immune function, some herbs that may seem like a good idea may not be and those that may seem like a bad idea may actually be beneficial.

Some herbs may also exert apparently contradictory effects and impact both Th1 and Th2 pathways. Welcome to the immune system!

As we stated earlier, test something as a single variable before you start taking lots of it. And don't just assume that it will have the same effect in your body as it has in someone else's body.

1. Th1 family cytokines
A. IL-12 increasing: celosia, ginseng, lentinus, herbal formula Xiao Chai Hu Tang
B. IL-12 decreasing: eleutherococcus, garlic, inula, salvia, herbal formula Ba Wei Di Huang Wan

---

43 *Autoimmune disease and Chinese herbal medicine,* by M. M. Van Benschoten, 2003. Santa Monica, CA: Emperor's College of Oriental Medicine.

C. IL-15 increasing: Herbal formula Si Jun Zi Tang (containing bai zhu, fu ling, ginseng, and licorice)

TNF alpha decreasing: acorus, asparagus root, camellia, capillaris, cordyceps, fagopyrum, polygala, cooked rehmannia, smilax

TNF alpha increasing: achyranthes, aloe, coix, cordyceps, reishi mushroom, ginseng, pseudostellaria

2. Th2 family cytokines

A. IL-4 increasing: agaricus mushroom, celosia, eleutherococcus, fagopyrum, inula, perilla leaf, tripterygium

B. IL-4 decreasing: angelica sinensis, epimedium, garlic, polygala, pseudostellaria, herbal formula Liu Wei Di Huang Wan

C. IL-10 increasing: coix, garlic, hoelen, inula, lentinus, Liu Wei Di Huang Wan

D. IL-10 decreasing: cordyceps, perilla leaf, Xiao Qing Long Tang

3. IL-1 family cytokines. It is recommended to avoid herbs that stimulate IL-1 and instead to take herbs and supplements that decrease IL-1.

A. IL-1 decreasing: asparagus, lentinus, picrorhiza, polygala, cooked rehmannia, rhubarb, siegesbeckia, smilax, tinospora, turmeric, quercetin, boswellia, ClearVite formula

B. IL-1 increasing: achyranthes, reishi mushroom, lentinus, American ginseng, tremella, typhonium

C. IL-18 increasing: lentinus, Ba Wei Di Huang Wan

III. Supplements for increasing Th3, regulatory T cells: vitamin D, EPA, DHA, glutathione, superoxide dismutase

IV. Supplements that decrease Th17: According to Dr. Kharrazian, the following substances reduce Th17, largely due to their ability to increase healthy nitric oxide levels in the blood: adenosine, huperzine A, vinpocetine, alpha glycerylphosphorylcholine (alpha GPC), xanthinol niacinate, L-acetyl-L-carnitine.[44]

V. Herbs for clearing pathogens: These herbs have broad-spectrum antibiotic, antifungal and antiviral properties: chrysanthemum, cinnamon twig, coptis, dandelion, forsythia, houttuynia, lonicera, magnolia bark, rhubarb, scute, siler, stemona, dermatrol

---

44 *Mastering the thyroid*, by D. Kharrazian, 2011.

VI. Herbs for clearing circulating immune complexes: angelica sinensis, atracylodes, bupleurum, cordyceps, persica, rehmannia, rhubarb, schizandra, Si Jun Zi Tang and Tao Hong Si Wu Tang herbal formulas

QI GONG EXERCISE FOR THE METAL ELEMENT

REACH FOR HAPPINESS

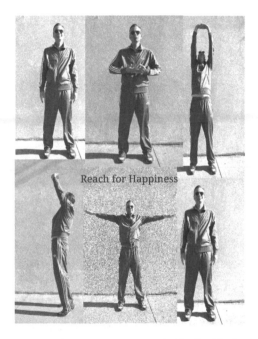

Reach for Happiness

This exercise focuses on bringing more energy and blood flow to the lungs. In Chinese medicine, the lungs are among the most important organ systems for creating energy and sustaining health and well-being.

This exercise has its origin in a famous statue of Buddha, in which he is portrayed with his hands above his head just like the photo above.

As we learned in the chapters on the metal element, the lungs and large intestine are united by the immune system. And as you can see in this drawing . . .

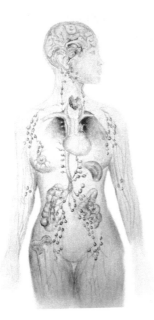

. . . they both have an enormous number of lymph glands in and around them.

So focusing on healing these areas can have a very positive effect on calming, regulating, and balancing the immune system—all valuable for people with Hashimoto's.

The qi gong exercise pictured is also good for digestive problems; heart, lung, spine, or back problems; a stiff neck; and eye problems. It helps bring more blood flow to the brain, increases lung volume, and increases blood flow back to the heart.

How to do it: Begin with a natural standing posture. Feet shoulder-width apart, hands relaxed at your side.

Inhale and gently sweep your hands out to your sides, then bring them together to meet at your abdomen, just below your navel.

Your palms should be facing up toward the sky, with your fingertips pointing up toward each other. As you sweep your hands up, imagine that you are holding a ball of energy; keep your arms rounded and your armpits open.

Next, raise your hands, lifting the energy ball slowly and steadily up to your chest. Keep your arms about six to eight inches from your body to keep the movement open. Gently hold the energy ball and imagine that you must balance it or it will fall.

Next, turn the palms down and rotate your thumbs underneath, pushing your hands out above your head. Keep your fingers interlocked and again imagine that you are balancing an energy ball, pushing it up toward the sky.

At the end of this movement, stand on your tiptoes as far as your balance allows. Push up for one or two seconds as you exhale completely. Then, inhale as deeply as you can while staying relaxed.

Finally, exhale again, unlock your fingers, and return your head and eyes to a neutral, forward position. Let your arms float outward as if gently pushing down a couple of big balloons.

Repeat the entire exercise three times, once or twice per day. When you are finished, try to maintain the posture and height that you got from doing the exercise.[45]

4. R= Reassess and Readjust

Retest, reassess, and ask all over again. Figure out what worked and what didn't. Double down on what worked and either eliminate or re-create a plan for what didn't.

If you ordered diagnostic tests, reordering them will help you figure out if what you did changed anything. This can also get expensive.

By now you should also be keeping track of your symptoms and actions in a journal. If you are doing this, you can often see patterns emerge. This can be very helpful for determining what's working and what isn't.

Journaling and keeping track of your reaction to various foods, chemicals, and other foreign substances can be really important when it comes to balancing and regulating the immune system.

If you continue to be exposed to things that your immune system reacts to and this is the same part of your immune system that is attacking your tissue, then this can become a problem that is never resolved.

5. T = Try and Try Again

Keep doing it, keep refining, keep building on the positive results, and keep looking for the remaining positive feedback loops that are causing vicious cycles.

This is a long-term project. Play the long game. Keep at it and don't quit before the miracle happens.

In my experience, this is where some people lose the will to keep going and they quit too soon.

Keep the faith; it will be rewarded.

---

45 *The healing art of qi gong*, by H. Liu, 1997. New York, NY: Warner Books.

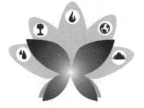

Chapter 9

The Earth Element:
GROUND ZERO FOR AUTOIMMUNITY

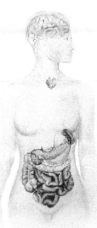

I am so excited to get into this chapter's topic, the earth system, because this is really where it all happens with Hashimoto's.

The earth system in Chinese medicine represents the digestive system.

The ancient Chinese identified this as being so important that there is an entire school of medical practice built around it called, appropriately, the Earth School.

Basically, they believe that almost every ailment comes from some problem in the digestive tract. And my experience with treating Hashimoto's folks has been the same. This is ground zero.

As you know, Hashimoto's is an autoimmune disease and a thyroid disorder.

And as we explored in the first two chapters of this book, the digestive tract is a very important place for all aspects of this condition.

It impacts thyroid hormone, and it is where most of the immune system lives. A healthy ecosystem in the gut is essential for converting and absorbing thyroid hormone and for balancing and calming immune function.

It's also hugely important for healthy brain function (which we'll cover in the chapters on the brain). What goes on in the digestive tract affects the whole family of ecosystems in your body.

Diet is the foundation of success

This is where it all happens, people. And if you don't work on your diet and healing the earth element, you won't have success treating Hashimoto's.

It's just that simple.

If you doubt that this is true, check out the results of a survey of 2,232 people with Hashimoto's conducted recently by Dr. Izabella Wentz, a colleague and friend of mine.[46]

On the question of diet, these are the results Dr. Wentz observed:

> In addition to the gluten-free diet, the other most helpful dietary interventions were going on a sugar-free diet and a paleo diet (81 percent of those who tried these diets felt better), grain-free diet (81 percent felt better), dairy-free diet (79 percent felt better), autoimmune paleo diet (75 percent felt better), and the low glycemic index diet (76 percent felt better).

In this chapter we will discuss the reasons why these types of diets yield such good results.

However, before we jump into that, let's recap the important takeaways from what we've covered so far:

---

46   "Top 10 takeaways from 2,232 people with Hashimoto's," e-mail from I. Wentz, received June 21, 2015.

- We looked at thyroid hormone conversion and the role of good bacteria in converting T4 to T3, which the body can use. We're going to explore that a bit more in this chapter.

- We also looked at the metal element, which is the immune system. The lungs, the large intestine, the lymphatic system and, amazingly, the thyroid are all part of this.

- The lung and the large intestine are linked via the lymphatic system and represent our physical, emotional, and spiritual borders with the outside world and the boundary between self and nonself.

Remember, autoimmune disease is the loss of self-tolerance and recovery, and healing of those borders and boundaries is essential.

THE EARTH ELEMENT: CENTER OF HEALING

In some diagrams of the five elements, the earth element is pictured in the center, and all the other organ systems surround it. In many ways, it is the center of healing.

The earth element includes the spleen, stomach, pancreas, and the whole digestive tract. As we explore it in more depth, you will discover that it is also the center of autoimmunity.

As we look at the earth system, try to be open to the fact that we don't know everything, and only through observation and questioning the status quo can we hope to learn.

There's something in psychology known as confirmation bias, which is the unconscious act of referencing only those theories and ideas that agree with our pre-existing views. This leads to ignoring other theories and ideas that may actually lead to breakthroughs and progress.

THE APPENDIX IS A PERFECT EXAMPLE

Did you hear the news that scientists think they have finally figured out what the appendix was for?

For many years the established dogma was that the appendix was an artifact, a useless piece of flesh that evolution somehow forgot, and therefore could simply be removed, without the slightest repercussions.

The truth is that nature is infinitely more clever than man and infinitely better at using everything that exists for some purpose. Nature does not forget things. If they have no purpose, they almost never survive evolution.

Well, so it is for the appendix. It turns out it has a purpose. What is it?

The appendix is actually a bank of good bacteria, so that when there is a die-off, or a full frontal assault for whatever reason, it acts to replenish your intestines with the species that are beneficial.[47]

The right bacteria are hugely important for many things. And one important thing with regard to Hashimoto's is the role of gut bacteria to assist in converting inactive T4 into the active form of thyroid hormone, T3. As you learned in chapter 1, about 20 percent of T4 is converted to T3 in the gastrointestinal (GI) tract.

Good bacteria helps convert thyroid hormone

HOW GOOD BACTERIA AIDS THYROID HORMONE CONVERSION

It is converted in the forms of T3 sulfate (T3S) and triiodothyroacetic acid (T3AC). The conversion of T3S and T3AC into active T3 requires an enzyme called intestinal sulfatase.

Where does intestinal sulfatase come from?

Drum roll . . .

Yup, you guessed it, a healthy balance of bacteria in the ecosystem of the gut. When this ecosystem is out of balance and there are fewer beneficial bacteria than other species, the rate of conversion of T3S and T3AC to T3 can be affected.

Here's where we see how events outside the thyroid can cause problems with thyroid hormone in the body. This is another factor that can lead to functional hypothyroidism (having hypothyroid symptoms despite normal lab test results).

---

47   "Microbial composition of human appendices from patients following appendectomy," by C. M. Guinane et al, 2013, *mBio 4*(1), pp. e00366–12.

Established dogma said the appendix was an artifact and it had no purpose. Yet we now know that the appendix is a bank of good bacteria and that good bacteria is essential for proper thyroid hormone conversion.

Do you see how it's all connected?

This is why observation and trying to figure out the mechanics are helpful practices. When you can see what's going on and find the mechanism behind it, much becomes clear.

Nature always has a method to her madness. Man has dogma. Dogma says, "What I say is the absolute truth. Don't question it." Obviously, this can stop us from learning what the real truth might be.

LET'S TALK STOMACH

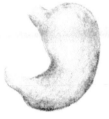

What does the stomach do and what is its relationship to the thyroid?

The stomach's role is to take food that has been chewed (hopefully well) and mix it with saliva to break it down.

Okay, what breaks all this down?

HYDROCHLORIC ACID

Hydrochloric acid (HCL) is vitally important for breaking down vitamins, minerals (like iron), and vital nutrients so that they can be absorbed by your small intestine.

A lot of people, misled by dogma, believe that stomach acid is bad. Two of the top 10 drugs prescribed in the U.S. are Nexium and Prevacid. These medications, called proton pump inhibitors, are designed to block the production of stomach acid.

Proton pump inhibitors block the production of stomach acid by inhibiting (shutting down) a system in the stomach known as the proton pump.

This is another perfect example of sales and marketing trumping good clinical decisions. According to Medscape, in 2013, Nexium alone totaled $6.1 billion dollars in sales.[48] The popularity of such medications has led to the false theory that it's okay to suppress stomach acid, in some cases indefinitely.

There's only one problem: Having sufficient stomach acid prevents food poisoning, parasites, and other critters from taking over your digestive tract. Enough hydrochloric acid also stimulates gallbladder and pancreas function to complete digestion and keep the entire digestive tract working properly.

Proton pump inhibitors also affect thyroid hormone absorption, and a study from *Endocrine Practice*, the official journal of the American Association of Clinical Endocrinologists, found their impact to be so significant that patients taking these drugs and thyroid hormone may need to adjust their dosage.[49]

So you actually do need HCL, and its production depends on the hormone gastrin. And guess what has an impact on gastrin? Thyroid hormone.

So hypothyroidism causes less gastrin to be produced, which leads to lower amounts of hydrochloric acid, which in turn leads to heartburn, bloating, gas, and . . . wait!

"Did you say heartburn?" Why yes, I did.

"But didn't you also say too little hydrochloric acid?" Why yes, I did.

Let me explain . . . mechanisms, people.

It turns out that having enough stomach acid actually prevents heartburn by thoroughly digesting your food. The burning sensation that people feel from heartburn is actually from the poorly digested food rotting in their gut and pushing up into their esophagus. This creates a kind of traffic jam.

And the esophagus has no protection from acid. Even a small amount can cause problems and irritation there.

In a 2009 editorial published in *Gastroenterology*, the authors remarked:

---

48   "Top 100 selling drugs of 2013," by M. Brooks, Retrieved January 30, 2014, from http://www.medscape.com/viewarticle/820011#vp_1

49   "Effect of proton pump inhibitors on serum hyroid-stimulating hormone level in euthyroid patients treated with levothyroxine for hypothyroidism," by I. Sachmechi et al, 2007, *Endocrine Practice, 13*(4), pp. 345–349.

"Treating gastroesophageal reflux disease with profound acid inhibition [which is exactly what proton pump inhibitors do] will never be ideal because acid secretion is not the primary underlying defect."[50]

This is true.

For decades the medical establishment has been focusing on how to reduce stomach acid secretion in people suffering from heartburn and gastroesophageal reflux disease (GERD).

Even though it's common knowledge that these conditions are not caused by too much stomach acid.

In fact, the real problem is too little stomach acid. So these drugs are ensuring that the people who use them must continue to use them indefinitely.

HOW ELSE IS HCL BENEFICIAL?

Another thing that HCL is important for is the absorption of vital nutrients like B12, iron, and calcium, and for breaking down and absorbing protein.

Too little HCL can lead to inflammation, lesions, and infections in the intestines.

All of that leads to poor absorption of thyroid hormone, which leads to . . . (this one is a gimme) . . . *the presence of hypothyroid symptoms despite normal lab test results (i.e., functional hypothyroidism).*

Too little stomach acid can also lead to anemia, because without it you can't absorb B12 and you can't properly absorb iron.

Couple this with heavy bleeding during your menstrual cycle, which can also be caused by too little thyroid hormone, and you have a recipe for iron deficiency anemia.

Wow, dogma, mechanisms, and the rantings of an addled Hashimoto's patient (that would be me).

RECAP: SUMMARY OF THE STOMACH

The stomach is important for breaking down and digesting foods and for enabling the body to absorb important vitamins, minerals, and proteins.

---

50   "Evidence that proton-pump inhibitor therapy induces the symptoms it is used to treat," by K. E. L. McColl and D. Gillen, *Gastroenterology*, *137*(1), pp. 20–22.

Too little stomach acid can lead to a host of problems, like heartburn (counterintuitive but true), anemia, and iron and protein deficiency.

All of this creates a vicious cycle of less conversion and utilization of thyroid hormone and lower stomach acid. Not good.

In my clinical experience this is a very common but underrated finding. Fixing this problem can make a really big difference, because this affects everything downstream—the pancreas, gallbladder, intestines, etc.

Now let's look at the pancreas and blood sugar issues.

TWO DIFFERENT TYPES OF SUGAR PROBLEMS

Health is all about balance, and nowhere is this more evident than with blood sugar balance.

There are two different kinds of blood sugar problems, and many people have a mixture of both. They are hypoglycemia (too little sugar in the blood) and insulin resistance (too much sugar in the blood).

With Hashimoto's either one or both of these blood sugar problems can make your symptoms worse. And just to remind you that this goes in both directions, it's important to understand that hypothyroidism can also cause blood sugar problems all by itself.

We have the makings of a *vicious cycle*.

HYPOGLYCEMIA

For our bodies, low blood sugar is a really big deal. We are genetically programmed to react to low blood sugar, because our lives literally depend on it. If we have severely low blood sugar or it continues for a long time our body can seize up, go into a coma, or, worst-case scenario, we could die.

When blood sugar levels drop below normal, the adrenal glands answer the call by secreting cortisol. Cortisol then tells the liver to make more glucose. The liver responds by bringing blood sugar levels back to where they should be.

Hypoglycemia is a condition in which there is not enough cortisol to tell the liver to raise blood sugar to the normal range.

Repeated day after day, over time this process can end up wearing out the adrenals. In fact, we often see adrenal fatigue and hypoglycemia together. And when you add the physiological stress of having an autoimmune disease like Hashimoto's, you have a recipe for both.

LOW BLOOD SUGAR AND CORTISOL

Cortisol is the body's fixer. It increases the amount of glucose available to the brain, and it helps speed up healing and tissue repair.

It also slows down functions that we don't need when we are in the middle of a crisis and our focus is to fight or run (things like reproduction, growth, and digestion). You can't eat, have sex, and grow when you're in the middle of running for your life.

Having Hashimoto's is like living in a constant state of stress. Having autoimmunity is very stressful for your body and your brain. And this can lead to repeated cortisol release.

When you add this to low blood sugar, the result is suppressed pituitary function. And the pituitary is the master gland that instructs the thyroid.

If this function isn't working properly, then "Houston, we have a problem." And where do we have a problem? In the thyroid.

LOW BLOOD SUGAR CAUSES THYROID PROBLEMS

Cortisol directly inhibits an enzyme called 5 alpha deiodinase, which converts inactive T4 into active T3. This can lead to low T3 levels.

In addition, elevated cortisol will cause thyroid hormone receptor insensitivity, meaning that even if T3 levels are high enough, they may not be able to bind normally to receptor sites. And when this happens it doesn't get into the cells.

Cortisol will also increase the production of reverse T3 (rT3), which is inactive. (It's kind of like the anti-hormone.)

Reverse T3 can cause an increase in the production of substances known as thyronamines that can cause hypothyroid symptoms, such as low basal body temperature, fatigue, and depression, along with insulin resistance symptoms of increased blood sugar.

Cortisol can also lower the levels of protein that binds to thyroid hormone so it can circulate in a stable structure.

And finally, elevated cortisol will slow TSH production by disrupting hypothalamic-pituitary feedback leading to lower TSH production.

Well, there is also a hypothalamus-pituitary-thyroid (HPT) axis.

And much like wires going through a transformer on an electric grid, the HPT and HPA axes are very closely related, and problems in one area can affect the other.

HOW TO IDENTIFY BLOOD SUGAR PROBLEMS

Common symptoms of hypoglycemia (many of which improve when you eat) include:

- Craving sweets
- Feeling irritable when meals are missed
- Depending on coffee or other sources of caffeine for energy
- Eating relieves fatigue
- Feeling shaky or jittery
- Feeling agitated or nervous
- Getting upset easily
- Poor memory, forgetful
- Blurred vision

It's important for hypoglycemics to eat often throughout the day and not skip meals. Each meal should be a combination of protein, carbohydrates, and fats. For these people, too many carbs will often cause serious problems with blood sugar levels.

INSULIN RESISTANCE

When you eat too many carbs and too much sugar, the pancreas secretes insulin to move extra glucose from the blood into the cells where glucose is used to produce energy.

But over time, the cells lose the ability to respond to insulin. It's like insulin is a little dog barking outside the cell, but the cell won't let it in.

"I hear you barking, but you can't come in."

The pancreas responds by releasing even more insulin (barking louder) in an effort to get glucose into the cells, and this eventually causes insulin resistance.

Insulin resistance and metabolic syndrome become more prevalent after menopause, and in some women this can lead to worsening of symptoms and progression of thyroid autoimmunity.

A 2015 study showed that repeated insulin spikes that come with insulin resistance increase the destruction of the thyroid gland in people with autoimmune thyroid disease [Hashimoto's].[51]

It also resulted in higher TSH and IL-6 levels, both of which have been linked to autoimmune thyroid disease.

As the thyroid gland is destroyed in this process, what happens? Thyroid hormone production falls. And this causes hypothyroidism. Not good.

INSULIN RESISTANCE CAN LEAD TO THYROID PROBLEMS

Insulin resistance can also cause a reduced conversion of T4 to T3 hormones.

When this is addressed, the cells can once again start using glucose for energy and T3 production picks up.

So for a person who is insulin resistant, a low-carbohydrate diet may help restore better T4 to T3 conversion, and often these people lose weight in the process (a nice side effect).

For other people, factors such as long-term chronic stress may be affecting their response to low-carb diets. Chronic stress can interfere with thyroid hormones in many different ways, which we will explore in the chapters on the water element.

---

51 "Associations between metabolic syndrome, serum thyrotropin, and thyroid antibodies status in postmenopausal women, and the role of interleukin-6," by L. Siemińska et al, 2015, *Endokrynologia Polska, 66*(5), pp. 394–403.

COMMON SYMPTOMS OF INSULIN RESISTANCE (WHICH GENERALLY DO NOT IMPROVE WHEN YOU EAT):

- Fatigue after meals (this is the hallmark symptom)
- General fatigue
- Constant hunger
- Craving for sweets that isn't relieved when you eat sweets
- Must have sweets after meals
- Waist girth is equal to or larger than hip girth
- Frequent urination
- Increased appetite and thirst
- Difficulty losing weight
- Migrating aches and pains

MANY PEOPLE HAVE SYMPTOMS OF BOTH

Life is not a textbook. Many people are somewhere in the middle of this blood sugar odyssey and they have some symptoms of hypoglycemia and some symptoms of insulin resistance.

I put this question to my Facebook support group, and of the 66 respondents with Hashimoto's, 24 reported symptoms of hypoglycemia, 14 reported symptoms of insulin resistance, and 16 reported some symptoms of both.

In addition, in the patient population I have treated I have found about 80 percent have symptoms of hypoglycemia, insulin resistance, or both.

While this is hardly a scientific study, it does demonstrate how common the problem is in this population.

VIRTUALLY EVERYONE HAS SOME INSULIN RESISTANCE

One thing that's important to understand is that whether you have high or low blood sugar, you probably have some amount of insulin resistance.

I explained how high blood sugar causes insulin resistance earlier, but insulin resistance can also cause low blood sugar.

This condition, called reactive hypoglycemia, happens when the body secretes excess insulin in response to a meal high in sugar and carbohydrates.

For example: A burger on a sesame seed bun with French fries and a soda causes blood sugar levels to spike and then drop below normal. (I'm *not* lovin' it!)

HYPOTHYROIDISM CAN CAUSE BLOOD SUGAR PROBLEMS, TOO

If you eat like this and you have Hashimoto's (and hypothyroidism), you are setting yourself up for a world of hurt.

Hypofunction of the thyroid can cause everything we just talked about because:

- It slows the rate that cells take in glucose.
- It slows response of insulin to higher blood sugar levels.
- It decreases the rate that the gut absorbs glucose.
- It slows the removal of insulin from the blood by the liver.

These mechanisms all appear clinically like hypoglycemia. When you're hypothyroid, your cells aren't very sensitive to glucose. (They are resistant.)

So although you may have normal levels of glucose in your blood, you'll have the symptoms of hypoglycemia (fatigue, headache, hunger, irritability, etc.).

And since your cells aren't getting the glucose they need, your adrenals will release cortisol to increase the amount of glucose available to them.

This causes a chronic stress response that suppresses thyroid function. Does this sound familiar?

We've already discussed how some people are functionally hypothyroid. In other words, they have enough thyroid hormone but it's not getting into the cells.

Many of these people also have enough sugar in their blood but it's not getting into the cells. It's another vicious cycle.

And let me tell you this from clinical experience: It is really, really, really, really, really, really, really hard to manage a Hashimoto's patient or someone with functional hypothyroidism if he or she doesn't address their sugar issues.

In fact, I'm going to say it: It's a deal breaker.

If a high-sugar diet or hypoglycemic state isn't treated, you might as well throw in the towel, pack it in, wave the white flag, say uncle, hear the fat lady sing, and give up, because it's just an exercise in futility.

All the money you're spending on supplements and therapies won't work. This is one of those areas that can undermine everything—when 20 percent of your diet is causing 80 percent of your symptoms.

KEEPING BLOOD SUGAR IN A HEALTHY RANGE

When balancing blood sugar, there are two things to consider. The first is fasting blood glucose, which can be measured first thing in the morning before eating or drinking.

The second and more important thing to measure is postprandial blood glucose. This is measured one to two hours after a meal.

In the final chapter of this section, we apply the A.P.A.R.T. System to the earth element, and I include a detailed description on balancing blood sugar using a glucose meter.

In conclusion, if you have Hashimoto's, it's important that you take steps to make sure your thyroid is properly balanced to keep your blood sugar properly balanced.

As you have seen, this thing works in both directions.

Sugar problems can disrupt thyroid function, and thyroid disorders like Hashimoto's can cause sugar problems, putting you at greater risk for hypoglycemia, insulin resistance, and—if nothing is corrected—diabetes.

This is why so many people feel better on a low-sugar, low-carb, or paleo diet. It is an excellent approach to fixing the blood sugar dilemma.

RECAP: BLOOD SUGAR ISSUES

1. Too much sugar in the diet leads to insulin resistance, which can directly lead to more aggressive destruction of the thyroid in Hashimoto's.

2. When low blood sugar (hypoglycemia) becomes chronic, it leads to cortisol release that eventually causes pituitary problems and messes with thyroid function.

3. Hashimoto's and hypothyroidism itself can lead to either one or both of these problems, creating a vicious cycle.

4. If you don't take your blood sugar issues seriously, you will have tremendous difficulty getting your Hashimoto's under control.

HASHIMOMENT:
THE FUTILITY OF WORRY

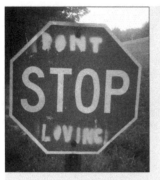

The negative emotion of the earth element is worry.

With Hashimoto's, sometimes it seems like there's a whole lot to worry about.

It can be overwhelming trying to figure everything out.

Because we have to be our own health advocates, we have a lot on our shoulders. And if you're like many people, you also have a family to take care of.

And all of these demands may make you feel like you can't get to what you need to do to feel better.

So you worry.

The problem with worry is that it doesn't help. At all. It just builds on itself and gives you more to worry about. And it can become self-fulfilling.

So a better thing to do is to stop, look around, and find things to be grateful for. Being grateful leads to acceptance.

When you achieve acceptance, things are less overwhelming.

And when you can find gratitude in adversity, you become more resilient.

So stop, take five minutes, and think about everything you are grateful for.

Don't leave anything out. You can be grateful for even the most seemingly insignificant things—the flowers, the leaves, the air you breathe, the water you drink, your clothes, the roof over your head, your dog or cat, anything and everything.

Try it and share the results with us on our Facebook page: www.facebook.com/ hashimotoshealing

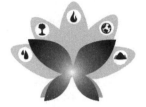

Chapter 10

THE CHINESE MEDICINE VIEW
OF THE EARTH ELEMENT

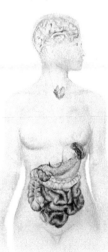

Let's take a look at the Chinese medical view of the earth element: In Chinese medicine, the yin organ of the earth element is the spleen and the yang organ is the stomach.

In previous chapters, when I discussed some of the theories of Chinese medicine, I mentioned how each of the five elements is the organ system and its sphere of influence.

The point I was making was that the emphasis of anatomy and physiology for the ancient Chinese was in determining how those organ systems function. That was the first functional medicine.

How does it differ from Western medicine?

In Western medicine, anatomy and physiology are often focused on distinct parts and their independent and distinct roles in the body. Most specialists stay in their focus area and do not leave it to look at the larger picture.

They name conditions and diseases and try to fit a patient's signs and symptoms into those conditions or diseases. Then they prescribe a drug protocol that has been designed to treat that specific condition or disease.

In Chinese medicine, the focus is on patterns of function, or dysfunction, and a lot more attention is paid to how a given disease or condition impacts the rest of the body. Additionally, there's a determination as to where it is in its progression.

Chinese medicine has theories for stages of disease. The name of the disease is far less important than the extent to which it has impacted the body and which organ system or systems have been impacted.

And the further a disease or condition has progressed, the more serious it is and, consequently, the more difficult it is to resolve.

THE LONGER YOU WAIT, THE HARDER TREATMENT BECOMES

In fact, the Chinese have an old adage that goes something like this: "Treating disease after it is formed is like digging a well after you've become thirsty." And we can add to that: "The thirstier you are, the harder it is to dig the well."

I believe that thinking this way is very important when we look at Hashimoto's, because it is precisely why I say that everyone's Hashimoto's is a little bit different.

No two people are at the same stage of development with their condition, no two people have the same level of involvement of other organ systems, and no two people have the same life factors involved, such as genetics, stress, or diet.

These considerations become incredibly important as we try to unwind the mess that Hashimoto's has created in your body.

And this is exactly why no cookie-cutter approach with a one-size-fits-all solution will work for Hashimoto's. We see this all the time: thyroid replacement hormone doesn't work for a lot of people, the (fill in the blank) protocol doesn't work for a lot of people, and so on.

In many cases, the best protocol is the one that takes into account all the different systems of your body that are impacted. And simply because this is so complex and can involve so many different parts of the body, it is virtually impossible to mass-produce an effective protocol. Often what is required is doing a whole lot more than simply treating the thyroid.

I'm sure that by now you are starting to understand the complexity of Hashimoto's and how it is a multisystem condition that requires a multisystem approach to heal it.

THE SPLEEN/PANCREAS: IT'S A HYBRID

So now let's take a look at the earth element and its sphere of influence. As I said, the yin organ is the spleen and the yang organ is the stomach.

The endocrine gland associated with the earth element is the pancreas. In fact, a lot of what the ancient Chinese ascribed to the spleen sounds, in my opinion, very much like the pancreas.

The other parts of the system that represent the earth element are the mouth, saliva, flesh, and muscles. The earth element governs the sense of taste.

The spleen governs digestion and keeps the blood circulating. We know that it is also responsible for cleaning old and dead red blood cells from the bloodstream. It also stores platelets that aid in clotting and coagulation.

The ancient Chinese recognized the spleen as an important organ for immune function. We know now that it also stores monocytes—the *Pac-Man*-like white blood cells—and that B and T cells are made and mature in the spleen.

Remember in the last chapter when we spoke about certain immune cells producing TSH? Some of those cells come from the spleen.

The sense organ associated with the spleen is the mouth; health issues involving the spleen sometimes manifest on the lips and in the corners of the mouth.

The spleen is also associated with mental and physical actions involving body movements, especially movements of the four limbs.

The negative emotion of the spleen is worry or obsessive thinking, while the energy or vitality of the earth element is intent.

This energy is linked with mental and physical activity of the body. Lack of desire or difficulty with coordination and movement of the body may reveal an issue with intent and, therefore, the spleen.

The difficulty with coordination, or a problem with moving and articulating the limbs, is associated with poor utilization of nutrients by the muscles.

What are the ancient Chinese talking about? It could be insulin utilization—the state of insulin resistance that we spoke about in the last chapter.

Almost all cells in the body have insulin receptors. So intent involves a major mental component and is also under the influence of insulin, but not always for the purpose of just utilizing glucose. Insulin can also help with the uptake of certain amino acids.

SEROTONIN IS A GREAT EXAMPLE

One interesting example of this relationship involves serotonin.

The brain's ability to absorb serotonin is enhanced by insulin. If you become insulin resistant, what happens emotionally? You lose your intent, you become depressed, and you crave carbs to try and make you feel better.

Do you see how this is all connected? These are examples of spheres of influence.

In a spiritual sense, intent affects the digestive function of thought that allows for the processing and assimilation of our life experiences in a nourishing way.

Unbalanced function leads to brooding, worry, and excessive thought patterns, such as obsessive-compulsive disorders. People who think obsessively can become stuck in a pattern of thinking for thinking's sake alone; in doing so they don't get nourished by their experiences, because they can't move on.

One of the health issues that is problematic for the spleen is dampness. Internally, this can take the form of phlegm. Phlegm is made in the spleen and then sent up to the lungs.

Metaphorically, dampness is an accumulation of everything that should be nourishing but instead has become a burden. In a psychological sense, it manifests as lethargy, boredom, mental sluggishness, obsessive thinking, and brooding.

On a physical level, phlegm dampness accumulates in the spleen, stomach, lungs, and large intestine. Sweetness is the flavor of the earth element and sugar is a common source of phlegm dampness.

From a spiritual/psychological standpoint, phlegm dampness represents the excessive need to give or receive sympathy. Therefore, it's spiritual phlegm; it is giving too much to others in lieu of taking care of yourself, or it is demanding too much so as to become a burden to others.

THE EARTH HAS ALWAYS BEEN THERE FOR US

The positive attributes of the earth element are integrity and reciprocity (giving back equally). Integrity is being faithful and truthful. The sage or enlightened being is a person who is kind to both the kind and to the unkind. He or she trusts the trustworthy and the dishonest, meaning he or she trusts nature.

The idea of reciprocity is really that of giving back appropriately what has been given to you. The earth nourishes all of us; our planet is the ultimate in faith, trustworthiness, and loyalty. The earth has always been here for us; it has sustained life for billions of years.

Well, we need to reciprocate and be good stewards of our planet or we're not going to survive as a species. Really, when it comes down to it, what's happening to our world is also happening to our bodies.

Some feel that the rise of autoimmune disease may be a direct consequence of our larger inability to care for the earth.

All the pollution, radiation, and global impact of man and industrialization are resulting in an environment that is becoming increasingly less supportive of good health.

Everything is connected—all the different ecosystems inside of our bodies and all the ecosystems in our environment.

Of course, this is more philosophy than science. But what if we all behaved with that in mind?

Healing ourselves and healing the earth would become synonymous.

QUICK RECAP

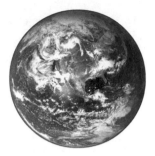

1. The earth element is the spleen, stomach, and pancreas. The spleen is yin; the stomach is yang. The pancreas is the endocrine gland associated with the earth element.

2. The negative emotion of the spleen is worry or obsessive thinking, which is linked to sugar metabolism and insulin resistance. The emotional consequences of insulin resistance can be depression and/or obsessive thinking (i.e., emotional phlegm).

3. The positive attributes of the earth element are integrity and reciprocity. They represent being faithful and truthful and giving back to the earth that has served us and given us life for billions of years.

IT'S ALL CONNECTED

Isn't it amazing how all these things are connected? These connections are the fulcrums of healing; they are the places where we can get the best results. They are also our source of hope for healing our Hashimoto's.

Now let's look at the stomach in TCM terms.

In the *Neijing* (*The Yellow Emperor's Classic*), the spleen and stomach's functions are mentioned together.

So that's interesting. And if we factor the pancreas into this equation, it makes sense. The functions of the stomach and pancreas are very much intertwined.

These two organ systems are all about acquiring and distributing the nourishment of life.

The virtues of the earth element—integrity and giving back—can be seen in the stomach, in the gathering and processing of all resources that are available in the outside world.

The spleen's job is to integrate what the stomach has acquired; it does this by adding nutrients and building our blood. Through the blood, the spleen takes this information and distributes it to all aspects of our inner being.

The spleen makes this integrity live in us by incorporating the things that are part of our lives that are sympathetic to our inner being.

Another way to think of it is that it's the process of how we integrate the energies of heaven and earth into our own beings.

When you have a separation of mind and body, this sympathy can block the stomach from looking inward to the spleen to get a true sense of what we really need in life.

Then we seek poor sources of nourishment that are ultimately unfulfilling, like junk food pumped full of salt, fat, and sugar. This leads to obsessive behavior: You reject what is good for you or you overeat in an effort to just pile it on.

A HEALTHY EARTH ELEMENT MEANS HEALTHY BOUNDARIES

The earth element impacts personal boundaries. Sometimes it's difficult to distinguish between your needs and the needs of others. The breakdown of this boundary leads you to either be too needy of other people or to take care of other people too much, at your own expense.

If someone is too needy they become like a sponge, soaking up emotional phlegm. When they do this, they can become too sweet, ingratiating themselves and sometimes manipulating others.

The other side of this earth impulse is to look for intimate relationships with other needy or sick people so that you can put your energy into nourishing them back to health instead of nourishing and healing yourself.

We all have some of this. I had to identify this in myself and completely rethink my medical practice when I realized that I was doing way too much and was losing my health as a result.

What are we trying to do in those circumstances?

Ultimately we seek to care for others in the way that we wish we were cared for. But it can leave us exhausted and depleted.

And what happens?

If you do a good job of helping that other person, they don't need you anymore. Then if you are out of balance, you can get resentful that they don't appreciate you enough. You see this with a lot of healers—they give too much and get burned out.

FIRST HEAL YOURSELF, THEN HELP OTHERS

So, to heal the earth element, we must first heal ourselves. Only then will we have the capacity to help others in a way that has integrity and balance.

It's just like being on an airplane: Put the oxygen mask on yourself first, then you can breathe and help other people around you.

How do we address these deep-seated emotional earth element challenges? Let's think about that. We have to nourish ourselves appropriately on this journey.

We have to transform the sugar burning/sugar binging mentality into one that is more integrated and ultimately more sustainable.

Does that make sense?

I'll bet you never thought that healing your Hashimoto's would mean actually healing your life, too. Well, that's the journey.

We are in this for the long haul so that we can come out the other side and not only heal ourselves but also heal our relationships with one another and with our planet.

And the truth is, if you don't address the dietary issues that are at the foundation of this process, all the herbs and supplements in the world won't give you the results you are looking for.

QUICK RECAP

1. The choices we make can have a huge impact on our lives, especially with Hashimoto's. If you don't fix your blood sugar problems, you can't heal.

2. We have to heal the earth element so that we can make appropriate decisions as to how much to give to others and how much to nourish ourselves.

3. We have to have *balance* so that we can be faithful and truthful—so that we're able to give to others without over-giving and leaving ourselves malnourished.

4. We must also learn how to get proper nourishment so we don't become burdensome to others; helping others at our own expense can leave us feeling resentful and unappreciated.

5. The foundation we use for healing involves an elimination diet (part of the autoimmune paleo protocol), which can help heal your leaky gut as well as heal and rebalance blood sugar imbalances.

If we can do these things, then we've gone a long way toward healing the earth element and getting our Hashimoto's under control.

It is by no means the only thing we have to fix, but it is sure taking some huge steps in the right direction!

CASE STUDY:
EARTH ELEMENT

Here's a real-life story about someone whose earth element was at the root of her issues.

Paula, a 45-year-old patient, suffered from a history of serious gastrointestinal problems.

A motility test revealed that her stomach wasn't emptying, that she suffered from too little stomach acid (hypochlorhydria), chronic constipation, bacterial overgrowth of the small intestine, and chronic yeast infections.

Paula could not digest fatty foods well because she had her gallbladder removed due to complications from the problems mentioned above. She also experienced fatigue after meals, which was extreme at times.

Unfortunately, and not surprisingly, she had a number of symptoms of intestinal permeability (leaky gut) and had difficulty maintaining proper iron levels along with other important nutrients. She experienced vacillations in how her thyroid medication worked.

Sometimes Paula would feel hyper, and sometimes she would feel hypo.

Clearly this was a person whose earth element needed some tender loving care. And that's just what we provided.

We got her on a strict autoimmune paleo diet, got her off of the foods that were causing problems in her gut, and worked on supporting detoxification in her liver while healing her intestinal lining using supplements like brush border enzymes.

We also worked to rebalance and repopulate the ecosystem of her intestines.

After a couple of months of faithfully following our protocol, Paula sent us this e-mail:

"By following the AIP diet very closely and taking the supplements you recommended, I was able to eliminate the fatigue I experienced from Hashimoto's and hypothyroidism. Through your program, I gained a much better understanding of what 'leaky gut' means. Doing the AIP diet and learning what foods are the most troublesome for me, plus the vitamins, for the first time in my adult life my serum iron levels are within normal ranges."

Paula L., Arizona

This was a tremendous victory for Paula. Getting her serum iron into normal range for the first time in her adult life may not seem like a big deal.

But in terms of energy, quality of life, and healing, this is a major achievement, and it allowed her to get her life back. Paula deserves the credit, because she stuck with our plan and didn't complain about not being able to eat certain foods.

She was in enough pain and discomfort where that hardly mattered anymore. Now she is enjoying life in ways she had only dreamed about before.

Chapter 11

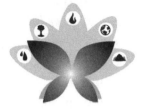

LEAKY GUT OR INTESTINAL PERMEABILITY AND OTHER ISSUES

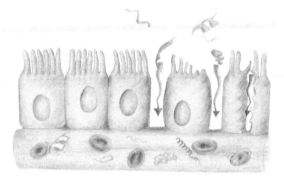

A breakdown of the intestines can happen between cells, through cells, or both.

I wanted to go into a little more detail on leaky gut in this chapter and also explore some additional obstacles you may encounter in your healing process.

First of all, what is leaky gut, and how does it lead to autoimmune disease?

Consider for a moment your digestive tract as a party: It's all the rage, lots of action, bacteria taking care of business, dancing the digestive boogie woogie . . . but it's selective—oh yes, exclusive, in fact.

Your intestinal membrane is like a big, formidable bouncer, and if someone is not on the list, they don't get in.

Now imagine that your bouncer is tired of dealing with all the stress: Damaging antibiotics are messing with the bacterial "cool kids," NSAIDs (Advil, aspirin, Tylenol, Alleve, etc.) are corroding the doors, and trigger-happy toxins are looking for a fight.

Before you know it, he's stretched too thin, leaving the doors ajar, and in walk all manner of riffraff. Now you've got a problem.

Security hustles over in the form of your immune system, and in the chaos things start getting out of control. It's a domino effect of friendly fire, toxic overload, body out of whack.

That's leaky gut syndrome—a modern ailment and a physiological indicator of the toxic world our bodies have to deal with.

Leaky gut is a malady that is not widely accepted as an official medical condition, yet a growing body of research supports the concern that practitioners of whole-body health care have been voicing for years.

Through studies and investigations it is becoming clear that when your intestinal lining becomes too permeable, the effects of the unwanted toxins and particles in your intestines have a ripple effect across your entire body.

Leaky gut is also now thought to be linked to autoimmune disease, because it causes your immune system to go into overdrive. And once your body crosses over into full-blown disease, there is often no turning back.

HOW DOES LEAKY GUT HAPPEN?

When the lining of the digestive tract is inflamed, the connections between the pieces of lining known as "tight junctions" break down and allow large, undigested compounds—toxins and bacteria—to leak into the bloodstream.

These substances all react with the intestine's immune system and cause an exaggerated immune response. This overreaction by the immune system becomes a vicious cycle that leads to more intestinal damage.

And as this problem grows, diet, lifestyle, medications, and infections may cause further intestinal inflammation that can ultimately lead to more serious problems.

In addition, after the intestinal lining becomes damaged, the damaged cells are unable to properly digest food and produce the enzymes necessary for digestion.

Such damage can lead to malnutrition, further intestinal inflammation, further permeability challenges, the development of food sensitivies, bacteria and yeast overgrowths, and an impaired immune system leading to irritable bowel syndrome (IBS), Crohn's disease, and other autoimmune diseases like Hashimoto's.

These self-destructive patterns can be very difficult to unwind.

> Leaky gut is something that must be addressed.

WHY DOES THIS MATTER?

I hope that by now you have a sense of how all of these different systems are connected and that this is way more than a thyroid problem.

In my opinion, leaky gut is a kind of fulcrum or nexus of all of these systems and it's where autoimmune disease begins and progresses. It's also the place that can make the most difference in your healing process.

Here's the thing: Leaky gut is not a static condition. It is constantly progressing, and many of the problems in other systems of your body are connected to the gut. Like any fulcrum, it's a place of maximum leverage.

Things can quickly go from bad to worse. And they can go much more quickly in the direction of healing if you focus on fixing all the factors that lead to leaky gut.

But this requires a steadfast commitment to fostering good health in the gut. In essence, you must become a farmer of your gut ecosystem. Just like a farmer must plant, seed, fertilize, and cultivate his crops and his farm, you need to do the same for your gut.

In the beginning of the book, I explained the 80/20 principle. In my opinion, leaky gut and what is happening in the ecosystem of your gut are the top 20 percent of the 20 percent.

This is arguably the most important area, and if you get nothing else from this book I want you to come away with an understanding of the factors that lead to leaky gut, because they contain the seeds of healing (and remission) in them.

So of course this begs the question: What are these factors?

Diet, insulin resistance (sugar addiction), low stomach acid, adrenal stress (which can lead directly to hypothyroidism), imbalance of healthy bacteria, poor fat digestion, constipation, and problems with estrogen building up in the body.

So what needs to be done to fix this?

First, diet. I explore the autoimmune paleo diet below. It's a protocol that works for leaky gut because it removes many of the offending foods that drive further destruction of the gut.

Gluten, dairy, soy, seeds, nuts, beans, other grains, nightshades (tomatoes, eggplants, peppers, and white potatoes), and many common medications (like antacids and NSAIDS) are all substances that are eliminated on this plan. Some people see this list as overly prohibitive and just want to give up—or they start negotiating how they can get around eliminating some of these things.

Well, think about it this way: What if I told you that you could make a single investment and double, triple, or even increase your money tenfold if you stuck with it? Wouldn't you want to make that investment? And if you did get such a good return on your investment, wouldn't you put more money into it?

That's what this diet is. It's a way of getting a great return on your investment.

Granted, it's not magic and there are other factors that can get in the way and make it less effective. Let's take a look at some of these.

FACTORS THAT UNDERMINE SUCCESS

Insulin resistance: We've already covered sugar issues. This is a key issue, because often people with Hashimoto's use sugar to attempt to overcome fatigue. They also use sugar or carbohydrates as comfort food to try and overcome emotional pain, anxiety, and depression.

I know, because I've done this myself and still struggle with it at times. But it can lead to adrenal stress, because the adrenals release cortisol to try and compensate for excess sugar, which ultimately undermines gut health.

Low stomach acid: We've already touched on this as well. Low stomach acid affects everything downstream. And one of the consequences is further destruction of the gut.

Adrenal stress: We'll explore this in depth in the chapters on the water element. High cortisol leads to further destruction of the immune barrier, can degenerate the intestinal walls, and can promote more inflammation in the gut. (Interesting side note: Steroid therapy used for inflammation can also do the same things.)

Imbalance of healthy bacteria: This is a huge issue in the way that it influences the thyroid and Hashimoto's. Toxins released by bacteria can reduce thyroid hormone levels, contribute to thyroid hormone receptor resistance, decrease TSH, increase the amount of inactive T3, and make Hashimoto's worse.

Problems with fat digestion: We'll take a more in-depth look at the gallbladder in the chapters on the wood element, but I want to mention it here. When fat isn't broken down and digested properly it can lead to further inflammation and breakdown in the gut, because undigested fats can become rancid.

In addition, good fat is important as a building block for steroid hormones like estrogen, progesterone, testosterone, and cortisol. It also transports important minerals and is essential for the absorption and storage of key vitamins including A, D, E, and K.

Slow transit through the gut: One factor that's very common for people with Hashimoto's is that everything slows down in the gut. This can result in constipation, more inflammation, and more problems with gut bacteria.

In the ecosystem of the gut everything is connected. And things slowing down can lead to fermentation, fats going rancid, and bacteria getting out of control and out of balance.

Too much estrogen: Another issue that you may think about being related to the gut and Hashimoto's is how it can contribute to excess estrogen in the body. A clogged liver due to excess sugar, gallbladder issues, and problems caused by poor digestion and bacterial overgrowth can lead to the buildup of excess estrogen to the point where it can actually become toxic.

This creates another vicious cycle, because excess estrogen can cause an increase in thyroid-binding globulin (TBG), which means less thyroid hormone can be freed to get into the cells. Then we wind up with another contributor to functional hypothyroidism.

WHAT HAPPENS WHEN THE INTESTINES BREAK DOWN?

As we have already discussed, leaky gut leads to bodywide inflammation and pain. The tissues that get inflamed vary with different people and seem to depend on genetics and environmental factors.

This cycle of suffering can lead to:

- Gluten sensitivity and celiac disease
- Food allergies

- Inflammatory bowel disease (IBD)

- Autoimmune diseases

- Neurological conditions

- Cognitive problems (depression, anxiety, schizophrenia, and others)

That last bullet is critical: Recent research has revealed the remarkably strong connection between the brain and the intestines. In fact, the brain and gut are highly integrated, and they communicate with each other mostly through the autonomic nervous system (ANS) and the hypothalamic-pituitary-adrenal (HPA) axis.

It is also interesting to note that the main area that controls the gut in the brain is the limbic system, which is very much connected to our emotions and feelings. The nervous system of the gut is so sophisticated it is sometimes referred to as a second brain.

And permeability and inflammation in the intestines has been shown to directly lead to permeability and inflammation in the brain.

"As above, so below" is certainly true of the brain and the intestines.

WHAT IS THE BEST TEST FOR LEAKY GUT?

Twenty years ago, many people tested for leaky gut by measuring leakage of a sugar molecule (lactalose) into the bloodstream. Since then, researchers and doctors in clinical practice have questioned this method, because very small molecules like sugar do not really challenge the immune system effectively.

Researchers decided that we needed a better way to look at the breakdown of the barrier system.

Cyrex Labs developed a test that does several things: It looks at what triggers the breakdown of the intestines, such as toxins produced by bacteria and antibodies produced against parts of the intestine's barrier system, such as occludin, zonulin, and actomyosin.

Here are the four things that we test for intestinal permeability and why they matter. I touched on this test in chapter 8. Cyrex Labs calls it **Array 2—the test for** leaky gut.

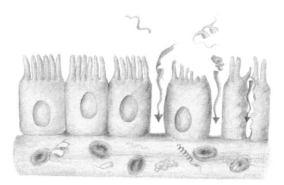

Various proteins provide valuable information on how the gut is breaking down.

1. **Lipopolysaccharides (LPS):** These are large molecules found in certain bacteria. They are toxins produced by gram-negative bacteria; if they are absorbed, they cause a strong immune response.

    If antibodies against LPS are found, this shows that large molecules have leaked through the intestinal barrier into the bloodstream.

2. **Occludin:** This is a protein that holds together the tight junctions of the intestines. It's like glue that binds cells together. If antibodies to occludin are found, it shows that these junctions are breaking down. This is a way to measure the breakdown of the intestinal barrier membrane.

3. **Zonulin:** This is a protein that regulates how easily things can pass through the walls of the intestines. It's like a zipper. If antibodies to zonulin are found, it shows that the normal process that regulates the passage of all kinds of stuff through the intestines is compromised.

    The zipper has opened up the cells. This can be a clue to what may be causing the damage to the barrier system.

    Zonulin has recently become popular in drug manufacturing, and a new generation of drugs will have this protein added to ensure that the medication is more easily absorbed. It's a bit frightening when you think about the implications.

4. **The Actomyosin Network:** This is a group of proteins that controls the intestines' barrier system by maintaining the flexibility of the tight junctions.

This is kind of like the anchor of the intestines. If antibodies to the actomyosin network are found, it shows there is a problem with the barrier system caused by infiltrating cells.

For example, 92 percent of celiac disease patients with flat intestinal mucosa have antibodies to actin. This test measures the mechanism involved in damaging the intestinal barrier.

Okay, that's a lot of information on leaky gut.

Let's shift gears and take a look at some solutions.

The Autoimmune Diet: An Excellent Foundation for Healing

Much has been written about the autoimmune paleo diet. It is a simplified approach that removes many of the most inflammatory foods from your diet.

In the beginning there is an elimination phase that cuts out gluten, dairy, soy, eggs, nuts, seeds, beans, all grains, and nightshades.

This is truly healing though subtraction, and it helps reduce systemic inflammation by eliminating (for a period of time) all the foods that may irritate and further exacerbate irritation and destruction of the intestinal lining.

Much of the difficulty that people have in healing Hashimoto's comes from its complexity. And simplifying and removing variables can be quite helpful in getting to the root of the problem.

This is difficult for many people to understand, because it is antithetical to a consumer culture where pills, supplements, and other quick solutions are being marketed and sold by the millions daily.

But despite the simplicity of the elimination diet and the challenge of cutting out many foods, it is remarkably effective in calming the immune system and providing the body with an opportunity to heal.

I advocate the elimination diet from the autoimmune paleo protocol as an excellent first step in calming immune function and beginning the process of healing the gut. This diet is recommended by my teacher, Dr. Datis Kharrazian, and by many others, including Dr. Sarah Ballantyne (a.k.a. The Paleo Mom).

Those of you who have worked with me know that I am also a big fan of Mickey Trescott, and we've been using her *Autoimmune Paleo Cookbook* as a starting point. It contains an excellent list of foods to include in your diet as well as foods to avoid.

The entire purpose of this approach is to get things back in balance. It is also an excellent time to use targeted nutrition to support the liver in detoxification, to heal the intestinal lining, and to restore the ecosystem of the gut. The elimination diet can be quite helpful as a foundation for reducing inflammation and neurodegeneration in the brain.

The Autoimmune Paleo Diet

- Eliminates a lot of foods that cause problems in the digestive tract

- Helps reset your body from the whole sugar burner/sugar addict mode to a fat-burning mode

- Gives you a chance to repair and rebuild your digestive tract as you do it

- Has the potential to dramatically improve the results of the supplements and medications you are taking because it also improves absorption and utilization of these nutrients.

It really is the foundation for success.

> People become so used to certain foods that they sometimes
> don't realize those foods are harming them.

Instead, they believe a foggy brain, skin rashes or rosacea, chronic respiratory issues, joint pain, water retention, a distended belly, chronic digestive issues, and lots of other symptoms are a normal part of life.

Foods that most commonly trigger these reactions are gluten, dairy, eggs, corn, soy, and yeast. Sometimes nuts are also a problem. And, technically, a person can develop an intolerance to any food, especially one that is eaten repeatedly when leaky gut is an issue.

So it is recommended to eliminate all of these foods and do a few more things, like some repairing and rebuilding. After that you can reintroduce foods slowly and systematically to identify which are triggers that lead to immune reactions. It is recommended to reintroduce one food at a time for three days and keep track of what happens.

IT'S IMPORTANT TO KEEP TRACK

This is why I asked you to keep a journal. You need to observe your reactions; these can be physical, psychological, and emotional. We've seen how emotions are so interconnected with our organ systems.

Another thing that's important to note is that adverse reactions aren't a bad thing. Everything is just a test, and whether something "works" and makes you feel better or "doesn't work" and makes you feel worse, that data is valuable because it is diagnostic.

This is the key component of the Reassess and Readjust part of the A.P.A.R.T. System. You have to evaluate what you're doing and keep track of what works and what doesn't.

For example, if you react to a food, then you know that food can't be part of your diet. It may be that you still need to do more work, or it might simply mean you just can't tolerate it.

You can revisit that food in a few more months, but you have to be prepared to say good-bye to some foods forever. Gluten, of course, is one of them.

Also, as we've established, digestive health is very much linked to blood sugar balance.

The other benefit of an elimination diet is that it is low in carbohydrates, which has the double benefit of repairing leaky gut and balancing blood sugar.

If you have any of the following key symptoms, you may need to get your carb intake under control: insomnia; routinely waking up at 3 or 4 A.M.; having an energy crash in the late afternoon; feeling spacey, irritable, or light-headed if you go too long without eating; constantly being hungry or craving sweets; and difficulty losing weight.

Sugar imbalance also leads to many hormonal problems, not just the thyroid. It impacts the adrenals, estrogen and progesterone levels, and more. If you have any of the symptoms mentioned above, you may have hypoglycemia, insulin resistance, or some combination of both.

And that's a lot to obsess about! (Remember, overthinking is a symptom of an out-of-balance earth element.)

OTHER INFECTIONS THAT CAN CAUSE PROBLEMS

Let's take a look at a couple of other factors related to digestive health that we haven't really covered yet.

Infections of the digestive tract can greatly complicate this whole process, and they're something that you need to look at and evaluate.

1. Parasites: These little critters are quite common. Some of the ones we have seen are amoeba, giardia, roundworms, and pinworms.

They can cause bowel irregularities such as diarrhea, constipation, or IBS-like symptoms; anemia; skin conditions, insomnia; emotional issues; and immune dysfunction, which can prevent healing processes from kicking in.

A stool test is the best laboratory test to determine whether you have parasites.

Herbs can sometimes be effective in treating parasitic infections. However, with a really tenacious parasite, you may need to use medication. It can sometimes be quicker, more effective, and easier on you in the long run.

CLINICAL PEARL:

As with any medical decision, you must always do a risk-benefit analysis. What's the risk of using a particular drug, herb, supplement, therapy, or surgery to address a problem? Then you need to ask what the benefit is.

The benefit should always outweigh the risk, and the best decisions are usually those in which the benefit outweighs the risk by a wide margin.

2. Candida (yeast overgrowth): Candida is a rather common diagnosis among many practitioners that has been linked to a number of health problems.

But, in my opinion, you have to be cautious when treating candida. Some of the antifungal treatments that are recommended are very hard on the liver and can wipe out some of the good flora in the gut.

This is an example of the benefit not always being as great as advertised, while the risk is that you can destroy some important good bacteria in the process.

My suggestion is to test for candida and act accordingly. Antibiotic overuse can lead to candida overgrowth and so can a high-carb, high-sugar diet.

Instead of the harsh candida attack, one of the best approaches to healing this condition is the elimination diet we've been discussing, with an added emphasis on eliminating sugars.

That's a simple approach where the benefit clearly outweighs the risk.

Don't you just love elegant solutions? As a practitioner, whenever I can find something that does multiple good things at once, I rejoice.

So let's take a moment to rejoice! Yay for elegant solutions!

3. H. pylori (bacterial overgrowth): A few different kinds of bacterial overgrowth are located in different places. Helicobacter pylori (H. pylori) bacteria is found in the stomach; it's linked to gastritis, heartburn, and nausea. More than 80 percent of people who have it are asymptomatic.

Some believe it actually has a purpose and can be beneficial if it doesn't get out of control. Herbs are effective in treating an overgrowth of H. pylori, particularly those containing berberine.

Small intestinal bacterial overgrowth (SIBO) is something we'll discuss further in the chapter on the fire element.

In an earlier chapter on the large intestine, we discussed the acronym FODMAP, which sounds a bit like a bad corporation. "Yes, I'm the senior VP over at FODMAP. We produce natural gas."

As you may recall, FODMAP foods are poorly digested in the small intestine, and bacteria love to ferment them so that they can have their own party!

Among other problems, this fermentation creates a lot of gas in the large intestine. I've included a whole article on it in the supplemental section on our website. A lot of the problem foods on that list can be addressed with an elimination diet.

But all of this begs the question: How do we figure out which intestinal condition we're suffering from? And what do we do about it?

The best way to start is to do a comprehensive stool test. A number of labs offer these; they test for all the critters that we mentioned above, and some test for gluten antibodies as well.

As the name implies, it's quite comprehensive and will give us a lot of helpful data about the state of the ecosystem that lives in your gut.

Then what do we do?

We do a four-step protocol I call "Farming Your Gut."

BEING A GOOD GUT FARMER

Here is a strategy for maintaining the gut's ecosystem, like a good farmer watches over his or her farm.

The four steps are:

1. **Weed:** Using herbs and supplements or medication, if necessary, remove the bad guys we mentioned above—parasites, fungi/yeast, and bad bacterial species.

2. **Compost:** Replace important stuff like enzymes, bile, and hydrochloric acid (HCL) in the ecosystem.

3. **Plant:** Repopulate the good guys, like more good bacteria.

4. **Heal the terrain:** Repair the ecosystem and the intestinal lining.

I strongly advocate healing *while* weeding, especially if you have identified that you have leaky gut.

—— **Important Takeways** ——

1. The earth element is the spleen/pancreas and stomach, and to some degree the entire digestive tract.

2. The negative emotion of the earth element is obsessive thinking or worry. The positive attributes are integrity and giving back in a healthy way.

3. Blood sugar balance is hugely important for healing Hashimoto's. Ignore this at your peril. I don't want to play with you if you won't fix this.

4. Leaky gut and other intestinal issues such as parasites, candida yeast, and bacterial overgrowth need to be evaluated and dealt with.

5. The elimination phase of the autoimmune paleo diet is an elegant solution in that it addresses so many of the issues we've talked about, and it is a great foundation for the other things we are doing. It's not the total answer, but it increases your chances of success dramatically.

6. There is no such thing as "sort of gluten-free." It's like being an alcoholic—you can't be "sort of sober."

Chapter 12

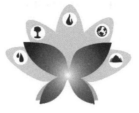

USING THE A.P.A.R.T. SYSTEM TO HEAL THE EARTH ELEMENT

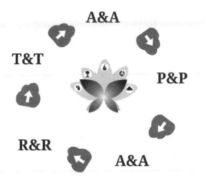

The A.P.A.R.T. System

APPLYING THE A.P.A.R.T. SYSTEM TO THE EARTH ELEMENT

All right, great stuff. Now let's apply the A.P.A.R.T. System to the earth element.

Take out your journal and look for symptoms of problems with the earth element. Note what they are, then create a plan for addressing them. After that, you must act on your plan; follow-through is crucial.

Next, take inventory of what you did. Look at what worked and what didn't. Both will provide valuable information.

Double down on what worked and change what didn't. Keep doing it.

Since the earth element is a kind of fulcrum, this should be an ongoing process that you do all year long.

1. A = Ask and Assess: Signs and Symptoms

Stomach: Both sets of symptoms could be caused by too little stomach acid.

TOO LITTLE STOMACH ACID:

Excessive belching, burping, or bloating; gas immediately following a meal; offensive breath; difficult bowel movements; sense of fullness during and after meals; difficulty digesting fruits and vegetables; undigested food found in stools.

TOO MUCH STOMACH ACID (THIS FEELING IS OFTEN CAUSED BY TOO LITTLE):

Stomach pain, burning, or aching one to four hours after eating; feeling hungry an hour or two after eating; heartburn when lying down or bending forward; temporary relief from antacids, food, milk, or carbonated beverages; digestive problems subside with rest and relaxation; heartburn from spicy foods, chocolate, citrus, peppers, alcohol, and caffeine.

These symptoms may, at their root, be caused by too little stomach acid. So boosting stomach acid is still an important part of the solution. But you may need to do some healing first. The autoimmune diet can be quite helpful.

BLOOD SUGAR ISSUES (HYPOGLYCEMIA):

Crave sweets during the day; irritable if meals are missed; depend on coffee to keep going/get started; get light-headed if meals are missed; eating relieves fatigue; feel shaky, jittery, or have tremors; being agitated, easily upset, or nervous; poor memory/forgetful; blurred vision.

INSULIN RESISTANCE:

Feeling fatigue after meals; craving sweets during the day; eating sweets does not relieve cravings for sugar; must have sweets after meals; waist girth is equal to or larger than hip girth; frequent urination; increased thirst and appetite; difficulty losing weight.

LEAKY GUT SYMPTOMS:

Leaky gut is often the foundation of much larger systemic problems and diseases. It can lead to:

- Digestive problems like gas, bloating, diarrhea, and IBS-like symptoms.

- Allergic reactions or hyperallergic responses.

- Autoimmune diseases. In fact, I would go so far as to say that leaky gut is ground zero for autoimmune disease. It is an essential ingredient for the formation and progression of these diseases.

- Chronic fatigue and fibromyalgia.

- Mood disorders and cognitive problems like anxiety, depression, ADD, and ADHD. Because there is such a strong connection between the brain and the gut, many neurological disorders are caused by leaky gut.

- Skin problems, rashes, dermatitis, acne, and more.

ORDER A COMPREHENSIVE STOOL TEST

Those are all the symptoms. As we discussed previously, a comprehensive stool test can also give you information on parasites, yeast/fungi, problem bacterial species, leaky gut, malabsorption, and more.

2. P = Prioritize and Plan

Not everything has the same level of importance. This is what 80/20 teaches us. Some things are having more of an impact than others. Figure out which they are (the positive feedback loops) and make a plan to fix them.

You must determine which of the earth systems have been compromised: the stomach, the spleen/pancreas, or the gut?

Here's the thing; it could be all of them. If it is, you can heal all of them.

3. A = Act and Adapt

Act and put your plan into motion, then observe the results. Double down on what works; change what doesn't. Results should be apparent relatively quickly. If they aren't, you need to make changes.

BLOOD SUGAR REGULATION

HOW TO KEEP BLOOD SUGAR IN A HEALTHY RANGE

When balancing blood sugar, there are two things to think about. The first is fasting blood glucose, which you can measure first thing in the morning before eating or drinking anything.

In functional medicine we define a normal range for fasting blood glucose as somewhere between 75 and 95 milligrams per deciliter (mg/dL). Although 100 is often considered the top of the range for normal, studies have shown that fasting blood sugar levels at the high end of normal may set you up for diabetes in the future.[52] This is another one of those instances where numbers are numbers, and there are various factors that can impact what the numbers mean.

And although 80 mg/dL is often defined as the low end of the range, there are healthy people with a fasting blood sugar in the mid-to-high 70s (especially if they follow a low-carb diet—all you paleo fans, time to do the wave).

The second and more important thing to do is measure your blood sugar one to two hours after a meal. This is called postprandial blood glucose.

Studies have shown that postprandial blood glucose may be a more accurate predictor of future diabetes (as well as cardiovascular disease) and may also be a

---

52   "Normal fasting plasma glucose levels and type 2 diabetes in young men," by A. Tirosh et al, 2005, *New England Journal of Medicine*, 353(14), pp. 1454–1462.

better initial marker before blood tests like fasting blood glucose and hemoglobin A1c (HbA1c) to indicate blood sugar imbalances.[53]

Normal blood sugar one to two hours after a meal is 120 mg/dL, but most healthy people are under 100 mg/dL two hours after a meal.

HOW THIS APPLIES TO YOU

How does this apply to you? If you're hypoglycemic, your challenge is to keep your blood sugar above 75 throughout the day.

The best way to do this is to eat a low-to-moderate-carbohydrate diet. The autoimmune paleo diet is ideal for preventing the blood sugar spikes and crashes I discussed earlier, as is eating frequent, small meals every two to three hours (to ensure a continuous supply of energy to the body).

If you're insulin resistant, your challenge is to keep your blood sugar below 120 two hours after a meal.

The only way you're going to be able to do this is to restrict carbohydrates.

BUY A BLOOD GLUCOSE METER

Everyone should buy a blood glucose meter. The technology has gotten to the point where they are very precise and quite inexpensive.

HOW LOW-CARB DO YOU NEED TO GO?

It's different for everyone. But for most people with Hashimoto's, a significant reduction in carbs is recommended.

That being said, as with most things there are exceptions to the rule, and some people may find that they need a certain amount of carbohydrates to function properly.

If this is the case, it is recommended to incorporate resistant starches, which are starches that release sugar more slowly and don't give you a dramatic spike in blood sugar.

---

53   "Postchallenge glucose concentration and coronary heart disease in men of Japanese ancestry. Honolulu Heart Program," by R. P. Donahue et al, 1987, *Diabetes*, *36*(6), pp. 689–692.

First, figure out your carbohydrate tolerance by buying a blood glucose meter and testing your blood sugar after various meals.

If you've eaten too many carbs, your blood sugar will remain above 120 mg/dL two hours after your meal.

Again, if you have Hashimoto's, it's important that you take steps to make sure your thyroid is properly balanced as well.

As you have seen, this thing works in both directions.

Sugar problems can mess with thyroid function, and thyroid disorders like Hashimoto's can cause sugar problems, putting you at greater risk for hypoglycemia, insulin resistance, and—if nothing is corrected—diabetes.

So take blood sugar balance seriously. I mean it.

SOME FOODS THAT BENEFIT THE EARTH ELEMENT

STOMACH FOOD SUGGESTIONS

Acid reflux ("stomach fire"): Often simply avoiding gluten and dairy can improve symptoms. Other foods to avoid if you have reflux or an ulcer are alcohol, coffee, anything fried, poor-quality vegetable oils, excessive salt, red meat, hot spices (such as cinnamon, chili peppers, black peppers, and mustard), citrus fruit, and plums.

Inflamed stomach lining: To heal an inflamed stomach lining, use foods that are mucilaginous and soothing, like soups made from gluten-free oats or rice, avocado, banana, tofu, water kefir, cucumber, cabbage (raw cabbage juice is more effective than cooked), microalgae and chlorophyll-rich products.

Also, herbs like slippery elm, licorice root, red raspberry leaf, marshmallow root, and chamomile can be helpful made as tea or taken in powder or capsule form.

Hypochlorhydria (too little stomach acid): Vinegar, as I mentioned above, can exacerbate acid reflux symptoms; however, because the real problem is often too little stomach acid (not too much), having a little apple cider vinegar before your meal (one to three teaspoons) can actually help this issue.

Supplementing with betaine HCL can also be helpful, but use with caution if you have acid reflux. In some cases, you may need to soothe the stomach between meals and boost stomach acid prior or during meals to heal. (Consult a qualified practitioner if you are unsure how to do this.)

SPLEEN/PANCREAS FOOD SUGGESTIONS

Deficient spleen-pancreas *qi*: congee (soup made from rice); oats; sweet rice; pounded sweet rice; carb-rich vegetables such as winter squash, carrot, rutabaga, parsnip, turnip, sweet potato, yam, and pumpkin; legumes such as garbanzo beans, black beans, and peas; pungent vegetables and spices such as onion, leek, black pepper, ginger, cinnamon, fennel, garlic, and nutmeg; and small amounts of certain sweeteners and cooked fruits such as rice syrup, molasses, cherry, and date.

For severe deficiency: small amounts of animal protein such as mackerel, tuna, halibut, anchovy, beef, beef liver or kidney, chicken, turkey, or lamb prepared in soup or congee.

Foods that dry dampness (overproduction of mucus): aduki beans, celery, lettuce, pumpkin, scallion, alfalfa, turnip, kohlrabi, white pepper, raw honey.

CLINICAL PEARL:

Soup and broth, like bone broth, are some of the most healing foods for the earth element. If you want to heal your gut, eat more soup.

BLOOD SUGAR REGULATION

FOODS COMMONLY USED IN THE TREATMENT OF DIABETES

- Grains and legumes (not recommended during the elimination phase of the autoimmune diet): millet, rice, sweet rice, oats, fresh corn, mung bean, garbanzo bean

- Chlorophyll foods: spirulina, chlorella, liquid chlorphyll

- Vegetables and fruits: string bean, carrot, radish, Jerusalem artichoke, turnip, asparagus, yam, spinach, avocado, pear, plum, lemon, grapefruit, lime, blueberry, huckleberry

- Herbs: dandelion root and leaf, cedar berries, yarrow flowers, blueberry/
  huckleberry leaf

- Sweeteners: licorice tea or powder

- Animal products: Clams; abalone; lamb pancreas; pork, beef, or fowl;
  lamb kidney; chicken or goose

QI GONG FOR THE EARTH ELEMENT: BETWEEN HEAVEN AND EARTH

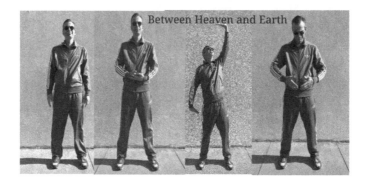

This exercise balances, harmonizes, and heals the entire digestive system. The movement of the hands in opposite directions pulls and lifts the stomach, spleen, liver, and gallbladder. It is an effective exercise for constipation, because it stimulates peristalsis and helps to bring blood flow to the intestines.

Begin in a natural standing position, feet shoulder-width apart, hands relaxed at your sides. Bring your hands up to your belly, just below your navel, gathering a ball of energy.

Inhale and continue to bring your hands up to your solar plexus (just below your heart). As you exhale, separate your palms.

Rotate your right palm up toward the sky and your left palm down toward the ground. Rise up on your tiptoes if your balance allows. Your eyes and your head should follow your right hand upward.

Move the palms in opposite directions until the right arm is fully extended above the head. Point your fingers toward the left and bend your palm at a 90-degree angle, as though you were holding a small stone in your hand.

The left hand should also be at a 90-degree angle and should be extended down toward the earth, pointing forward. Try to get your hands to 90 degrees; if you aren't flexible enough, just go as far as you can comfortably.

In your mind visualize your opposite hands connecting energetically to heaven and earth. In Chinese medicine, man (or woman) is considered to exist in the space between heaven and earth.

Inhale as you return your arms toward your body, facing both palms down toward the ground.

Exhale and gently push both hands down, visualizing negative energy flowing out of you and down into the earth.

Finish by returning your hands to the starting position, just below your navel, one palm on top of the other.

Repeat the entire exercise on the opposite side.

Do this exercise three times on each side one to three times per day.

4. R = Reassess and Readjust

Retest, reassess, and ask all over again. Figure out what worked and what didn't. Double down on what worked and either eliminate or re-create a plan for what didn't.

With the earth element, journaling is an absolute necessity. Once you remove foods for a period of time, you'll want to keep track of the process of reintroducing them.

It is best to reintroduce one food at a time, so that is your only variable, and to test it for three consecutive days. Note anything and everything in your journal. You will know if it is a food that you can't reintroduce, because you will feel absolutely terrible after eating it.

5. T = Try and Try Again

Keep doing it, keep refining, keep building on the positive results, and keep looking for the remaining positive feedback loops that are causing vicious cycles.

Build on all of your victories. Celebrate them and use them to create more positive momentum.

Chapter 13

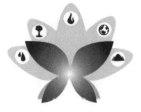

The Water Element:
THE ROOT OF HEALING

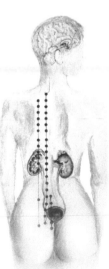

In this chapter, you will learn about the water element—another system that is incredibly important for healing. The water element includes the kidneys, adrenals, and urinary bladder.

The kidneys and adrenals play a huge role in solving the Hashimoto's puzzle.

With the water element, an entirely different set of vicious cycles are at work; a systematical approach will help to unwind them.

By now you should be starting to get a real sense of what we're up against.

Hashimoto's is a formidable foe. You aren't going to fix it with some cookie-cutter approach. No one supplement or medication is going to fix it; the disease is too involved, too complicated, and not always linear.

The vicious cycles that we have discussed so far all feed on one another, so there are times when you have exponential decline, and if you start repairing and unwinding them and you stay vigilant and committed, you start to see exponential progress as well.

But it doesn't end when you put down this book. First of all, what I have shared with you has taken years and years of research, study, and clinical experience.

You need to review this material and keep learning. Visit our supplemental section and go deeper.

We have only begun to start unwinding these various systems and their vicious cycles. This takes committed work and—dare I say it—devotion.

DON'T BE DISCOURAGED; IF I CAN DO IT, SO CAN YOU!

If you're feeling discouraged or overwhelmed, I totally get that, because I have been there. I have experienced many of these symptoms and challenges and I have been forced to walk the talk. So I understand the challenge.

A few years ago I hit a major wall and I crashed. I was in pain all the time. I had no energy, I was depressed, and I had such bad brain fog and memory issues that I really thought I was losing it.

I had to go through this process myself, do the evaluations, and change my diet. To this day, I follow the diet I introduced to you in this book. I journal, take some supplements, and constantly have to be vigilant and committed. So I get it.

But I can also tell you this: The rewards are amazing. I feel so much better today. As long as I stay on track, I generally feel the best I have in 20 years or more.

And I want this for you, too! But I also want you to know it takes work. There are going to be challenges and setbacks.

You're going to need support and encouragement, so don't try and do it all alone. Reach out and ask for help when you need it.

Now, let's get into this chapter.

HERE'S WHAT YOU'LL LEARN:

- How thyroid health is intertwined with adrenal health. We'll explore the understanding of the endocrine system in Chinese medicine and how this impacts you emotionally and spiritually.
- We'll look at how the thyroid impacts kidney function.
- And you'll learn how blood sugar balance is critical for adrenal health and how the adrenals and the pancreas are also interconnected.

Like I said in the last chapter, you can't escape the blood sugar reality. It is always going to be there, and it has to be dealt with on a daily basis.

THE KIDNEYS

THE WATER ELEMENT

In Chinese medicine, the water element includes the kidneys and the urinary bladder. Both organs primarily function using liquids and water. So it's not a big leap to see how that connection was made.

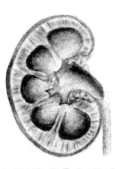

Let's start with the kidneys. What do they do? A lot.

Once again, when you really have a look, it's astonishing how our bodies work. The kidneys are considered perhaps the most important organs for homeostasis (natural balance) in the body.

They are two of the body's elimination channels, as well as two of its regulatory organs. If the kidneys cannot remove waste, toxins stay in the body and the body is forced to try and eliminate them through other channels.

One example of those channels is the skin. The skin is also an organ of elimination, excreting uric acid and waste products in sweat and oil.

If the kidneys are not functioning at full strength, toxins will be eliminated through the skin. This may result in rashes, as irritating toxins are excreted through the skin. This may also result in strong urine that smells like body odor.

KIDNEYS REGULATE CHEMICAL BALANCE

The kidneys also regulate chemical balance and water content in the body. If the kidneys are not performing that job, numerous health problems and symptoms can arise.

Some examples of these types of conditions are: gout (formation of uric acid crystals in the joints and kidneys), acidosis (a systemic problem of too much acid throughout the body), kidney and urinary bladder infections, and kidney stones.

The kidneys also provide an important function in maintaining fluid and electrolyte balance. Electrolytes are substances, such as salts, that dissolve or break down into ions when mixed with water. Optimal health depends on maintaining proper water and electrolyte balance.

Our bodies are 75 percent water. Water is used by every cell in the body and is essential for proper metabolism because it provides the medium in which virtually all chemical reactions take place.

If there's too much water in the body, the kidneys excrete it. If there's too little, the kidneys conserve it by retaining it. It really is the organ of the water element.

It is interesting to note that dehydration can cause you to experience pain in your kidneys. Some people incorrectly think that they have a lower-back problem because of muscle stiffness or spinal problems when in reality they just need to drink more water.

WATER BENEFITS THE WATER ELEMENT: GO FIGURE!

So next time your back hurts, try drinking water instead of reaching for ibuprofen or acetaminophen (both of which can damage the kidneys, liver, and intestines).

The kidneys maintain the sensitive balance of electrolytes in our body fluids. They regulate the levels of many chemical substances in the blood such as chloride, sodium, potassium, and bicarbonate.

The kidneys also regulate the balance between water and salt in the body by selectively keeping or excreting both substances as the body demands.

The kidneys maintain the blood's acid-alkaline balance, as do the lungs. Normal blood pH is between 7.35 and 7.45, which is slightly alkaline. If the blood becomes too acidic or too alkaline, serious health consequences and even death may result.

The kidneys maintain this balance by controlling the absorption and replacement of certain ions (e.g., bicarbonate). Our diet and lifestyle choices can influence our body's acidity.

THE KIDNEYS REGULATE BLOOD PRESSURE

The kidneys also function in blood pressure regulation. When blood pressure is low, cells in the kidneys release a hormone that initiates a process resulting in the constriction of blood vessels. This is part of the renin-angiotensin system (RAS).

RAS is a hormone system that regulates blood pressure and fluid balance. When blood volume is low, the kidneys secrete renin. Renin stimulates the production of angiotensin.

Angiotensin causes blood vessels to constrict, resulting in increased blood pressure. Erythropoietin is produced in the kidneys; when it passes through the bone marrow, erythropoietin binds to certain cells, stimulating them to create red blood cells.

THE KIDNEYS ACTIVATE VITAMIN D

Vitamin D is a group of fat-soluble hormones.

Its major role is to increase the flow of calcium into the bloodstream by promoting absorption of calcium and phosphorus from food in the intestines, and reabsorption of calcium in the kidneys, enabling normal mineralization of bone and preventing conditions caused by too little calcium. It is also necessary for bone growth and bone remodeling.

So why is vitamin D important for Hashimoto's?

Because research studies have linked vitamin D deficiency to numerous autoimmune diseases such as rheumatoid arthritis, lupus, diabetes, multiple sclerosis, and others.

Vitamin D plays an important role in balancing the Th1 (cell-mediated) and Th2 (humoral) arms of the immune system. It does this by influencing T-regulatory (Th3) cells, which govern the expression and differentiation of Th1 and Th2 cells.

Remember, Th3 is like the general of the immune system, calling back and calming down the troops. We need it to strengthen the command-and-control structure of the immune system.

Vitamin D deficiency is also specifically associated with autoimmune thyroid disease (AITD), and has been shown to benefit autoimmune-mediated thyroid problems.

Vitamin D also has another, lesser-known, role: It regulates insulin secretion and sensitivity, and it balances blood sugar. As previously explained, insulin resistance and blood sugar problems mess with the thyroid in a number of ways.

THINGS THAT REDUCE VITAMIN D

Research over the past 20 years has identified a number of things that reduce the absorption, production, and activity of vitamin D in the body, including latitude, air pollution, sunscreen, skin color, age, weight, skin temperature, and the health of the kidneys, liver, and gut.

Since vitamin D is absorbed in the small intestine, guess what impacts its absorption? Yes, it's true, leaky gut can slow absorption of vitamin D.

High cortisol levels (caused by stress or medications like steroids) are also linked to lower vitamin D levels. The synthesis of active vitamin D from sunlight depends on cholesterol.

Stress hormones are also made from cholesterol. When the body is in an active stress response, most of the cholesterol is used to make cortisol, and not enough cholesterol is left over for vitamin D production.

Obesity reduces the activity of vitamin D. Obese people have lower serum levels of vitamin D because it gets taken up by fat cells.

Not eating enough fat or not digesting fat properly reduces absorption of vitamin D. Vitamin D is fat-soluble, which means it requires fat to be absorbed.

People on low-fat diets and people with conditions that impair fat absorption (like IBS, IBD, gallbladder, or liver disease) are more likely to have low levels of vitamin D.

A variety of medications reduce absorption or biologic activity of vitamin D. Unfortunately, these include drugs that are among the most popular and frequently prescribed, including antacids, replacement hormones, corticosteroids, anticoagulants, and blood thinners.

Aging reduces the conversion of sunlight to vitamin D because as the skin ages it can't synthesize vitamin D as efficiently.[54] In addition, once in the bloodstream, vita-

---

54   "Vitamin D deficiency, muscle function, and falls in elderly people," by H. C. J. P. Janssen et al, 2002, *The American Journal of Clinical Nutrition*, 75(4), pp. 611–615.

min D must be converted in the liver (called hydroxylation) and it is further metabolized in the kidneys. These processes can be compromised with age.

Inflammation of any type reduces the utilization of vitamin D in the body. And as we have learned, inflammation is at the root of our problems.

BUT WAIT, THERE'S MORE

To further complicate matters, we now know that certain people with normal levels of vitamin D still suffer from deficiency symptoms.

How is this possible?

For circulating vitamin D to perform its functions, it must first activate the vitamin D receptor (VDR). The problem is that many people with autoimmune disease have a genetic defect that affects the expression and activation of the VDR and reduces the biologic activity of vitamin D.

Studies have shown that a significant number of patients with autoimmune Hashimoto's disease have VDR defects.[55] And we've seen this clinically many times as well.

Here's what this means: If you have low thyroid function, you might be experiencing vitamin D deficiency, even if your blood levels of vitamin D are normal.

It also means that if you have a VDR polymorphism, it's likely you'll need to maintain higher than normal blood levels of vitamin D to avoid the effects of vitamin D deficiency.

But it's important to be cautious here, because too much vitamin D can also be problematic. So this needs to be monitored. You need to assess and reassess.

As with many things in the body, there is a "Goldilocks" or "just right" zone we're aiming for. Determining where your ideal zone is may take some trial and error, but a good general benchmark for 25 OH vitamin D is between 55 to 70 NG/ml (the common standard of measurement for Vitamin D blood tests).

Yup, so much more than a thyroid problem, people.

---

55   "Association of vitamin D receptor gene 3'-variants with Hashimoto's thyroiditis in the Croatian population," by M. Stefanić et al, 2008, *International Journal of Immunogenetics*, *35*(2), pp. 125–131.

Quick Recap

The kidneys do a whole lot:

1. They maintain fluid, electrolyte, and acid-alkaline balance.

2. They eliminate metabolic waste.

3. They help regulate blood pressure.

4. They produce erythropoietin (EPO), a hormone that stimulates red blood cell production.

5. They activate vitamin D.

URINARY BLADDER

What about the urinary bladder? Its job is pretty straightforward.

The bladder is a hollow, muscular organ shaped like a balloon. It sits in your pelvis and is held in place by ligaments attached to other organs and the pelvic bones.

The bladder stores urine until you are ready to go to the bathroom. It swells into a round shape when it is full and gets smaller when empty. If the urinary system is healthy, the bladder can hold up to 16 ounces (two cups) of urine comfortably for two to five hours.

THE HASHIMOTO'S CONNECTION

What do the kidney and urinary bladder have to do with Hashimoto's?

You guessed it, Hashimoto's and hypothyroidism can have a big impact on both kidney and urinary bladder function.

Hypothyroidism & Hashimoto's can cause:

- Less blood flow to the kidneys, which can cause creatinine to build up and not be excreted. Creatinine is a chemical waste molecule that is generated from muscle metabolism.

- Increased amounts of uric acid. Some 20–30 percent of gout patients have hypothyroidism. This is often linked to higher levels of creatinine.

- High blood pressure. According to one study, up to 40 percent of hypothyroid patients had high blood pressure.[56]

If the kidneys fail to filter waste products from your body properly when your pressure is low, then angiotensin is produced, which raises your blood pressure.

Also, a rise in cortisol from your adrenals can raise your blood pressure. Hypothyroidism can also cause edema. You can see this swelling under the eyes, or as mild swelling of the hands and feet. This is a very common symptom for people with Hashimoto's.

Swelling is caused by several things: decreased kidney function, capillaries becoming more permeable, poor lymphatic drainage, and salt and water retention by the kidneys.

RECAP: HYPOTHYROIDISM AND THE KIDNEYS

Hypothyroidism can lead to alterations in salt, water, calcium, phosphate, vitamin D, and uric acid levels; high blood pressure; and edema.

It's all connected. Kidneys are the water organ.

The endocrine gland of the water element is the adrenals. Now let's take a look at the adrenal glands.

---

56   "Cardiovascular involvement in general medical conditions: Thyroid disease and the heart," by I. Klein and S. Danzi, 2007, *Circulation, 116*(15), pp. 1725–1735.

Chapter 14

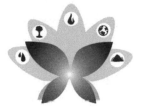

THE ADRENALS

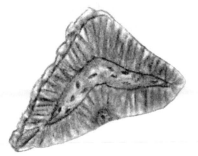

The adrenals are two little glands about the size of an almond that sit on top of the kidneys. The one on the right kidney has a triangular shape; the one on the left kidney has a sort of half-moon shape. (Perhaps this difference in shape of the two kidneys is what led ancient doctors to give one kidney yin attributes and the other yang attributes.)

Each of the adrenals has two different zones. The inner zone (the medulla) secretes adrenaline, norepinephrine, and just the right amount of dopamine. These are the stress hormones.

The outer zone . . .

(Imagine Rod Serling of *The Twilight Zone* doing the voice-over for this next passage.)

You're traveling through another dimension, a dimension not only of sight and sound but of mind; a journey into a wondrous land whose boundaries are that of the imagination. There's a signpost up ahead—your next stop . . .

. . . the outer zone—the adrenal cortex.

This is where three different types of hormones are secreted: glucocorticoids, mineralocorticoids, and androgens. These hormones are all made from cholesterol and are critical to everyday function.

Of the glucocorticoids, cortisol is the star. It is stimulated by ACTH from the pituitary. This is very much like the relationship between TSH (also secreted by the pituitary) and T4. ACTH and cortisol are the analogous hormones of the adrenals.

What does cortisol do? It regulates blood sugar levels, increases body fat, defends the body against infections, and helps the body adapt to stress. It also helps to convert food into energy and is anti-inflammatory.

What *doesn't* it do might be a better question. It's the body's fixer.

Aldosterone is the main mineralocorticoid. It helps regulate blood volume, blood pressure, and the body's sodium and potassium levels.

ANDROGEN HORMONES

The androgen hormones are testosterone and DHEA (which stands for the impossible-to-pronounce dehydroepiandrosterone).

These are present in both men and women. DHEA is popular for being the "youth hormone." It does have antiaging effects. It also helps the body fight infections and helps protect the body from the effects of cortisol and stress.

Cholesterol gets converted into pregnenolone, the precursor for all of those hormones. Pregnenolone is also a precursor for cortisol.

With chronic stress—the kind that causes a host of health problems, including hypothyroidism—something called a "pregnenolone steal" happens.

This is when the body says, "Sorry, DHEA and testosterone, we need to borrow pregnenolone for a little while and use it to make more cortisol."

This is the body's way of conserving resources to help us survive stressful situations, like living with Hashimoto's. The problem with chronic stress (a perpetual state of "pregnenolone steal") is that it ends up draining the adrenals.

Remember that, because we're going to come back to it in a moment. I want to digress quickly into the brain. In chapters 2 and 3, we talked a bit about the hypothalamus, where the ancient Taoists tapped into the energy of the Big Dipper.

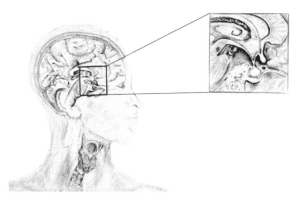

Hypothalamus: The boss of the boss.

The hypothalamus is really like the boss of the boss. You know, like when the boss is really arrogant and always doing bossy things and then, all of a sudden, the boss's boss shows up and puts him in his place?

Well, the relationship between the pituitary and the hypothalamus is nothing like that. (I just wanted to make sure you were paying attention.) Their relationship is more like, "Hey, we have this amazingly complex, super complicated body to run. Do you want to help each other? Cool!"

The hypothalamus is the pituitary's boss.

It says, "Hey, pituitary, tell the liver to get his act together, and while you're at it, tell the thyroid and the adrenals and the mammary glands and the ovaries, too. Tell them all the boss is back in town."

With the adrenals, this benevolent enlightened dictatorship is called the hypothalamic-pituitary-adrenal (HPA) axis. These three run the whole show.

The HPA axis plays a major role in regulating immune function, digestion, energy use, mood, and—thrill of thrills—sexuality. The HPA axis is controlled by hormones (in a nonlinear fashion) and is totally manipulated by stress.

THE FEMME FATALE OF THE HPA AXIS

Stress is like the femme fatale of the HPA axis. It's the mean wife of the boss' boss—the Leona Helmsley (the "Queen of Mean") of the body. (She left $12 million to her dog, named Trouble, when she died—$12 million to a dog!)

Anyway, where am I going with all of this? A dysfunctional HPA axis, like a troubled empire ruled by the Queen of Mean, can cause all kinds of problems.

With Hashimoto's, one of the biggest reasons why people continue to feel exhausted even though they are taking thyroid hormones is because of a messed-up HPA axis.

Here you may feel better initially and then you start feeling worse and worse, until you are right back to where you started, feeling like crap. And guess what?

The blood work looks normal or you have a low TSH and a low or low-normal T4.

Okay, so let's take a look at a few different ways that stress causes hypothyroid symptoms.

Most people are aware of the obvious forms of stress that affect the adrenal glands: very full schedules, financial problems, divorce, losing a job, moving, being stuck in traffic, and the many other challenges of modern life.

But other things you may not think of can also compromise the adrenal glands, such as blood sugar spikes and falls, problems in the gut, food intolerances (especially gluten), environmental toxins, chronic infections (like Epstein-Barr), autoimmune problems, and inflammation.

All of these conditions cause stress and signal the adrenals to pump out more "fight or flight" hormones.

Adrenal stress is one of the most common problems we encounter clinically, because nearly everyone is dealing with at least one of the stressors I just discussed.

The irony is that many conventional doctors don't recognize adrenal issues as a real medical condition. Often this is because adrenal issues aren't limited to the adrenals. They impact many other systems and can be centered in the brain and the HPA axis.

Symptoms of adrenal stress are many and nonspecific because the adrenals, like the thyroid, can affect every system in the body.

COMMON SYMPTOMS OF ADRENAL STRESS

Some of the more common symptoms are:

- Fatigue (also a thyroid symptom)

- Eating to relieve fatigue (another blood sugar problem)

- Irritability or light-headedness between meals (a blood sugar and adrenal problem)

- Mood swings

- Decreased immunity

- Dizziness when moving from sitting or lying to standing, which affects blood pressure

- Headaches (especially splitting headaches)

- Sleep issues, such as difficulty falling asleep and/or staying asleep, and waking up feeling exhausted even after you've had enough sleep

- Sugar and caffeine cravings (have a hankering for an iced Frappuccino?— it could be your adrenals)

- Gastric ulcers (ulcers in the stomach can be caused by the adrenals)

Weak adrenals can cause hypothyroid symptoms even if there isn't a problem in the thyroid gland itself. In such cases, working on the adrenals is key to improving thyroid function.

The most significant indirect effect the adrenals have on thyroid function is via their influence on blood sugar.

High or low cortisol, caused by any of the chronic stressors listed above, can cause hypoglycemia, hyperglycemia, or both. And, as you learned in a previous chapter, blood sugar imbalances cause hypothyroid symptoms in a variety of ways.

But adrenal stress also has more direct impacts on thyroid function.

CASE STUDY:
ADRENALS AS THE ROOT OF THE PROBLEM

One of our clients, a woman named "Ashley," suffered from fatigue, brain fog, concentration problems, muscle aches, and hip and shoulder pain. She also suffered mild depression and thinning hair and nails.

She had elevated Graves' and Hashimoto's antibodies, and a high TSH level (above 16 at one point). Her symptoms fluctuated from hyper to hypo (Ashley reported that these were "crazy cycles" for about 15 months).

She also could not tolerate thyroid replacement hormone at all. She had a very bad reaction to both Synthroid and Armour.

Further investigation revealed signs and symptoms of leaky gut, hypoglycemia, adrenal issues, and high homocysteine levels.

We put her on an autoimmune diet, treated her hypoglycemia by making sure she started the day by eating a good combination of protein and fat, and didn't let her sugar crash throughout the day by having her eat at regular intervals.

We also treated her leaky gut and worked on the adrenals by helping her adapt to stressors. We worked aggressively to reduce the systemic inflammation that was at the root of her problems.

After working with us for three months, Ashley experienced considerable improvement.

She returned to her primary physician, reported what she had done, and requested a follow-up blood test. The doctor initially refused because he said that it wasn't possible that there could be any improvement with the type of treatment she reported.

He said diet and the adrenals didn't matter, and so on. She insisted, and finally he relented and ordered the tests.

Everything came back within the normal range (all the antibodies, the TSH, and everything else).

Ashley was, of course, elated.

Here is an e-mail Ashley sent us:

"Hello Marc!
I know you didn't ask me for an update, but everyone deserves praise every now and then.
:)
Well . . . if you remember, you helped me about 18 months ago. I had horrible antibodies, leaky gut, adrenal problems, etc. All of this came after a pregnancy.
Anyway, my thyroid antibodies have not come back, my gut feels amazing (unless I accidentally ingest gluten) and I assume my adrenals are working just fine! In fact, I'm pregnant again with my second, and my thyroid is looking good and I'm feeling amazing!!!
I owe this all to you!
So once again, thank you so much, you literally changed my life, and keep the Facebook posts coming. I love learning all I can about the latest updates!
Wishing you wisdom and happiness!"
Ashley G., Breckinridge, Mo.

I'm not going to pretend this happens with everyone, nor do I deserve all the credit. She deserves the credit for persevering, following the plan, and believing that something else was possible.

There are also some really important takeaways here.

First, the answer wasn't just thyroid replacement hormone. This is the answer for some people, but not for everyone—especially postpartum, when things are really in flux and the body is adapting to a new normal.

There are also fillers in thyroid medication that may be problematic for some people.

Ashley's case also shows that sometimes the thyroid isn't the direct cause of the problems. Here it was the inflammatory process, the adrenals, and an immune system that was out of balance.

It took some digging and detective work to look elsewhere for solutions, but there were pretty clear indications about where they were. What's also really encouraging about this case is that the changes were sustained over more than a year.

That's a very good sign.

So if you're struggling and the solution that has been offered to you isn't working, don't be afraid to dig deeper and look for solutions in other systems of the body.

Chapter 15

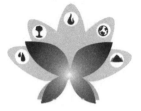

THE THYROID
AND THE ADRENALS

How the Adrenals and the Thyroid Interact

THYROXINE TREATMENT CAN CAUSE ADRENAL PROBLEMS

One of the things that doctors rarely discuss is that treatment with T4, like Synthroid or levothyroxine, can have a major impact on the adrenals.

If someone has adrenal insufficiency, they are at risk for thyroxine making the problem worse!

Even if the adrenal insufficiency is mild to moderate, it may have an effect on thyroid conversion, tissue uptake, and thyroid response—and not in a good way.

If the T4 to T3 conversion doesn't happen as it should, the body can become overloaded with unused T4.

If it is converted but the T3 cannot enter the cell walls due to adrenal insufficiency or iron deficiency, then the T3 cannot be used and may pool or build up in the blood.

When this happens, you may suddenly feel all the hyper symptoms, like heart palpitations, insomnia, and nervousness. This is one of the reasons why some Hashimoto's people may experience hyper to hypo cycles.

In many cases, T4 and TSH blood tests will appear normal, but the patient will feel really lousy.

If a doctor raises the thyroxine dose in this situation, things may become worse. How bad depends on the degree of adrenal insufficiency.

Symptoms may include all the symptoms mentioned above.

Here's what is written on the warning label for Synthroid (but is true of all synthetic T4 drugs):

"Patients with concomitant adrenal insufficiency should be treated with replacement glucocorticoids prior to initiation of treatment with levothyroxine sodium.

Failure to do so may precipitate an acute adrenal crisis when thyroid hormone therapy is initiated, due to increased metabolic clearance of glucocorticoids by thyroid hormone."[57]

What this means, in plain English, is that in cases of hypothyroidism, the adrenals need to be evaluated before patients are put on thyroid replacement hormone.

How many people with Hashimoto's and hypothyroidism do you think have adrenal insufficiency?

I put this question to my Facebook support group and 100 percent of the 85 respondents with Hashimoto's said they had most of the symptoms of adrenal insufficiency mentioned in the list I shared above.

Granted, that's not a scientific study, but it certainly is emblematic of the problem.

Have you ever heard of a doctor checking for this prior to beginning treatment?

It's not very common, believe me. Many doctors dismiss adrenal insufficiency as one of those make-believe disorders.

THE FLIP SIDE

The other side of this is the many ways that adrenal stress can cause hypothyroidism.

As we discussed earlier, it affects the HPA axis and this, in turn, disrupts the hypothalamus-pituitary-thyroid (HPT) axis. Communication gets garbled all around.

---

57   "Synthroid," Drugs.com, Retrieved from www.drugs.com/pro/synthroid.html

And we all know how important good communication is, especially when you have a super-complicated body to run.

ADRENAL STRESS CAN LEAD TO AUTOIMMUNITY

The inside of the body has three main barriers, the blood-brain barrier, the digestive tract, and the lungs.

These barriers prevent the bad guys from getting into the bloodstream and the brain. As we discussed in the chapter on leaky gut, when they break down, a whole cascade of trouble can follow.

Cortisol can be one of the factors leading to the breakdown of these barriers, which can impact immune function in a couple of different ways.

Since cortisol calms the immune system, too little cortisol can lead to too much immune stimulation and an overaggressive immune reaction.

Too much cortisol can weaken the immune system and make it harder for you to defend yourself against infections. This immune system suppression can lead to further breakdown of the intestinal lining, because the immune system is not strong enough to defend itself.

When the barrier systems break down, proteins, bacteria, viruses, fungi, and other large particles can leak into the bloodstream or the brain, where they don't belong. Over time, this positive feedback loop repeats over and over again, and the immune system is put on high alert.

This is the process that leads to allergies, sensitivities, intolerances, and eventually autoimmune diseases like Hashimoto's.

ADRENAL STRESS LEADS TO THYROID HORMONE RESISTANCE

Thyroid hormone doesn't work in the body if it can't turn on receptors inside of our cells.

One factor that makes receptors less sensitive is the systemic inflammation that is at the root of Hashimoto's. The immune proteins that we looked at in the chapters on the metal element are responsible for this. This inflammation blocks thyroid hormone from getting into the cells and it clogs the receptors.

It's like thyroid hormone is a little dog barking outside the door of the cell, and the inflammation is making so much noise that the cell can't hear it, so it just gets ignored.

This is another cause of functional hypothyroidism. In this situation, the person may be taking thyroid hormone medication but still have all the hypothyroid symptoms. And raising the dose doesn't help (or only helps temporarily) because the problem isn't too little thyroid hormone, it's unresponsive thyroid hormone receptors.

Blood test results for these patients may look perfect; TSH, T3, and T4 can all be normal.

ADRENAL STRESS REDUCES CONVERSION OF T4 TO T3

As we learned in the chapters on the thyroid, 93 percent of the hormone produced in the thyroid gland is T4. But T4 must be converted into T3 before it can be used by the cells in the body.

The immune proteins that cause receptor problems can also affect conversion of T4 to T3. This transformation is made possible by an enzyme called 5 alpha deiodinase. This happens in the liver, gut, and peripheral tissues of the body.

Some of the Th1 and Th2 proteins (e.g., IL-6, TNF-alpha and IL-1) that we discussed earlier have been shown to suppress thyroid hormone conversion. In fact, studies have shown that IL-6 (which is often found in abdominal fat) can reduce T3. There's a direct link: So as IL-6 levels go up, T3 levels go down.

The immune cells mentioned earlier can make T3 levels go down and reverse T3 levels go up. Reverse T3 is a form of T3 that is inactive, because it doesn't work on the cells of the body.

So as you can see, this one process can lead to thyroid receptors not working properly and thyroid hormone not getting converted; the result is that it doesn't work the way it should.

ADRENAL STRESS CAN ALSO CAUSE HORMONAL IMBALANCES

And as if that weren't enough, cortisol also has a powerful effect on the liver. High cortisol caused by chronic stress impairs liver function by slowing down certain pathways.

This can prevent the liver from being able to clear out hormones like estrogen, which causes more thyroid-binding globulin (TBG) to be produced in the body. TBG is a protein that attaches to thyroid hormone. It's kind of like a subway train that shuttles thyroid hormone through the blood.

When thyroid hormone is catching a ride with thyroid-binding globulin, it is inactive, which means it doesn't work. It has to get off the train and be freed before it can activate receptors on the cells. These are the free-fraction thyroid hormones such as free T3 and free T4 that you see on lab tests.

When TBG levels are high, there are fewer free thyroid hormones. This will show up on a lab test as low T3 uptake and low free T3 or free T4.

WHAT TO DO?

Here's the thing: With Hashimoto's, we are constantly under a great deal of physiological stress. You can't just take something for the adrenals and hope for the best. You can't just treat this one child in the family.

Adrenal stress has many causes, including anemias; blood sugar imbalances; gut inflammation; food intolerances (like gluten); vitamin, nutrient, and essential fatty acid deficiencies; environmental toxins; and chronic emotional and psychological stress.

Sound familiar?

These are also all the things that make Hashimoto's worse.

You can't ignore them or pretend like they aren't there (like so many doctors do). They all have to be dealt with.

All of them. Half measures don't lead to half results; they often lead to no results.

When these conditions exist, they must be addressed, or any attempt to support the adrenals directly will either fail or be only partially successful.

This is so much more than a thyroid problem. It's a multisystem problem.

We'll cover what to do for your adrenals in a moment.

All right, wow, we covered a ton there.

QUICK RECAP

The adrenals are extremely important. They must be properly assessed and treated.
Five things that can lead to hypothyroidism that are caused by stress and the adrenals are:

1. Disruption of the HPA axis. The "Queen of Mean" ruins everybody's evening.

2. Compromised conversion of T4 to T3.

3. Autoimmunity.

4. Thyroid hormone resistance.

5. Hormone imbalances.

It's all connected, it's not linear, and it's not a one-size-fits-all solution. You can do it, but only if you tackle all of these contributing factors. And it might just take more than reading this book to do it.

That's a lot to take in! Let's just sit in silence for the next few minutes and meditate. All together now, "Ommmmmm . . . ommmmmm."

HASHIMOMENT: KNOW YOUR LIMITATIONS

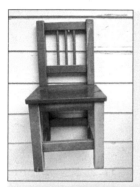

When we have Hashimoto's, we have to understand our limitations.

Sometimes you just need to take a seat and rest. When making plans, be sure to give yourself an opportunity to do less if you need to.

Sometimes it's okay to say no. It will all get done in due time.

Saying no requires the skill of detachment, and there's no better way to develop that skill than to do some sort of breathing or meditation exercise that helps you let go.

Here's a nice, simple meditation that I learned from the Taoist Master Hua-Ching Ni.

Sit quietly and repeat this sentence to yourself:

"I am complete."

Inhale as you say "I" silently to yourself.

Hold your breath for a second or two as you say "am."

And exhale as you say "complete."

It's okay to say no, because you already have everything you need.

Repeat this meditation over and over again until you start to believe it.

And give yourself permission to just let go for a few minutes each day.

Chapter 16

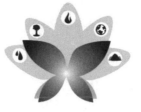

THE CHINESE MEDICINE VIEW
OF THE WATER ELEMENT

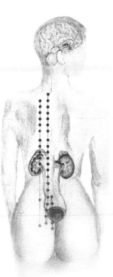

THE WATER ELEMENT

The Chinese medical view of the kidney includes two completely different sets of characteristics.

The yin organ of the water element is the kidney, but the kidneys themselves have two aspects. There is kidney yin and kidney yang.

Each of the kidneys has a slightly different shape and location in our body; they aren't exactly symmetrical.

That may be one possible explanation why the ancient Chinese had different ways of looking at them. Kidney yin is the organ itself; kidney yang, in my opinion, sounds like the endocrine system.

And the various adrenal hormones can also be viewed as yin and yang. Cortisol and DHEA are more yin; norepinephrine and epinephrine are more yang.

The water element's yang organ is the urinary bladder, which doesn't do a lot in Western physiology, but in Chinese medical physiology, the urinary bladder channel is hugely important.

It can be used to treat all the major organs of the body and a host of psychological and emotional conditions. It taps into every major nerve coming out of the spinal cord. (You can see the urinary bladder channel depicted as dots in the graphic at the beginning of the chapter.)

The tissue related to the kidneys is the bones, which makes sense given what we know about the kidneys' role in activating vitamin D for bone growth and bone remodeling.

The sense organ is the ear. In fact, in a developing fetus, the ears and kidneys develop in the fifth to eighth week of pregnancy.

The water element's negative emotion is fear. This is interesting, because the body's stress response is all about fear. Fear is what drives fight or flight.

The kidneys are thought to be responsible for will or aspiration. They store refined substances known as *jing*, which is linked to reproduction and inherited traits. The ancient Chinese identified the concept of DNA and genes, which is what *jing* embodies.

Fear in the kidneys is associated with cold, producing chills and shivering. This has a physiological basis in that cold stimulates the adrenal glands and, in turn, produces the stress reactions of fear, fright, shock, and alarm.

The hormones that correlate to the kidney yang are adrenaline, epinephrine, a little bit of dopamine, and some endogenous opiates.

These hormones, as we have discussed, come from the medulla and respond to stimuli from the nervous system.

What do these yang hormones do? Give you yang energy! They increase metabolism, heart rate, blood pressure, blood flow to the legs, lung function, and metabolic functions in the liver.

The kidney yin aspect of the adrenals is the adrenal cortex and the corticosteroids that influence blood sugar and mineral metabolism. Sex hormones are also released under the influence of ACTH.

Aldosterone has a role in sodium, potassium, and water balance. Cortisol is anti-inflammatory; the Chinese identified cortisol imbalances as "false heat," or an improper inflammatory condition.

This is found in kidney yin deficiency. Interestingly, cortisol is also responsible for the anti-inflammatory effects of acupuncture. From a spiritual and emotional level, the water element has profound influence.

WATER IS THE HIGHEST FORM OF GOODNESS

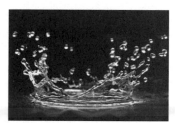

The Taoists hold water in very high esteem.

In chapter 8 of the *Tao Teh Ching,* water is spoken of in this way: "The highest form of goodness is like water. Water knows how to benefit all things without striving with them. It stays in places loathed by all men. Therefore it comes near the Tao."[58]

So the irony of the water element is that, at its heart, it teaches us that true power comes from wisdom, which results in the cultivation of our resources.

Resources are our energy, our time, our emotions, all of that. Right? If you get overextended, then you deplete those resources.

But a chronic reaction to fear, the chronic stress response, drives the kidneys and bladder officials to either over- or underutilize willpower to control the use of our resources.

If we are reckless with the resources that we have, ambition may push us to exhaustion as we try to make our way in the world. With every new project we complete, the feelings of success and accomplishment are fleeting, and fear shows up again as we're off to the next project.

Have you ever experienced that? Jeez, I sure have. And where does it get us? Burned out.

Remember when I cited that statistic about 80 percent of people with autoimmune disease having experienced some very stressful event prior to its onset?

---

58   *Tao teh ching,* by L. Tzu (J. C. H. Wu, Trans.), 1990, p. 10. Boston, MA: Shambhala Publications.

On the other hand, if we are very conservative with our resources, we may get frozen by this fear and do very little. Every project is potentially rewarding, but when fear kicks in, we may react by pulling back and stopping midstream.

So the wisdom inherent in the water element teaches us how to balance these two extremes so we don't get burned out, and so we don't let fear paralyze us into inactivity. There has to be a happy medium.

The bladder is involved in the storage and usage of things we acquire during our lives, such as the experiences, the wisdom, and whatever else we collect along the way.

So another way of understanding the resources that the kidneys help us use and save is the idea of our inherited constitution. This is called *jing*, which relates to DNA but also to our inherited emotional and spiritual essence.

JING IS A METAPHOR FOR OUR OWN WELL

Jing is the water in our well. *Jing* is distributed to all the other yin organs by the kidneys. *Jing* also stores all of our life's potential—our destiny, in a sense. This potential must be conserved and used wisely over the course of our lives as our destiny unfolds.

The general idea is to draw only as much as you need for the task at hand and save the rest. You want to live off the interest of what you collect along the way and do your best to save your inheritance.

The life issues of those of us with problems involving this yang energy revolve around the general theme of utilizing our resources appropriately.

Hashimoto's involves a deficiency of yang. We see this in various endocrine glands: the adrenals, pancreas, thyroid, and pituitary.

So when our kidney energy is not functioning harmoniously, we overspend, overwork, overplay, just overdo it in general.

In his book *Nourishing Destiny,* Lonny Jarrett tells a great story that sums up this concept beautifully.[59] I've paraphrased and embellished it a bit here.

There's a beggar who lives on the street in a marketplace in ancient China. A genie sees the beggar and decides to help him.

---

59   "Water-the great," 1998, in *Nourishing destiny: The inner tradition of Chinese medicine,* by L. Jarrett, pp. 185–186. Stockbridge, MA: Spirit Path Press.

He approaches the beggar and asks, "How much money would be enough to help a poor man?" The beggar says, "500 yuan" (that's the currency). Of course, after a few days the money is spent and the beggar is back on the street sleeping in the marketplace.

Once again the genie sees him and asks, "How much money would be enough to help you?" The beggar thinks about it, revises his calculation, and says, "10,000 yuan."

This time he is able to buy a small house and hire servants. But he doesn't save his money. He spends it here, there, and everywhere and loses it all and winds up back in the marketplace, sleeping on the street.

The genie approaches him a third time and asks the same question. The beggar reflects on his previous two experiences and says, "100,000 yuan will last me for a lifetime, I know it."

So now, he's a little more savvy. He buys nice clothes, gets married, has a family. This was a lot of money in those days, so he has prestige, people take notice, and he gets appointed to a high-ranking position in the court.

But he is who he is. He hasn't learned the fundamental lesson from the water element. So he lives large and spends big, and because of his excessive lifestyle and some bad investments, he descends into misery, winding up in the marketplace once again, sleeping on the street.

When the genie sees the beggar, he takes pity on him and decides to help one last time. When the beggar sees the genie walking toward him, he gets up and runs for the hills.

So that's the lesson of the water element: We must learn how to care for and save what we are given. That is really key and may be the most important lesson of this entire book.

If we want to heal our Hashimoto's, not depleting what we have is hugely important. But what does that mean in real life?

Just like we need to take the sugar balance problem seriously, we really need to take the impact of stress on our bodies, minds, and souls seriously. Living that type A, hard-running lifestyle will, over time, result in you squandering your reserves. There is no question about it.

Okay, now that we've covered the water element, let's rest. Take a little break to think about this in our own lives. When we come back, we'll look at how the bladder energy and spirit figures in.

SAVINGS IN THE BANK

We looked at the kidney's role in preserving our inheritance. Now let's take a look at the bladder's role in saving and using what we collect along the way.

According to the *Yellow Emperor's Classic* the bladder is responsible for regions of the body, and it stores body fluids.

As we have seen with other yang partners to the yin organ, the function of the yang organ is to assist the yin partner and kind of be a conduit to the outside world.

The spirit of the kidneys is the will. When the kidney and bladder are working together harmoniously, wisdom is manifest in everything you do.

The bladder orchestrates your inheritance—your natural talents, abilities, and genetic predisposition—and, like a good accountant, it helps you manage what your life brings you.

Money, experiences, relationships, etc., are like a reservoir. A reservoir needs to be able to hold water without losing it and be able to expand when there's lots of rain, so it can provide water when you need it.

The healthy function of the bladder is to empower us to adequately assess both the quantity and quality of our reserves. Like the will, the bladder must guide us to spend our resources the right way, not to just blow our savings impulsively.

So, when the water element is out of balance, fear rules. Chronic stress takes over. Even though no immediate threat is there, we live in a constant state that we won't have enough or that we are going to lose what we do have.

This causes a separation of the heart and mind, which prevents the bladder from accessing innate wisdom. Without that wisdom, you lose perspective.

This is why anxiety is a very common symptom of adrenal problems. Fear takes over and it's out of context, present even when there is no real threat.

When this happens, the kidneys can't communicate with the outside world, so they become secretive and paranoid. Fear is the result.

Another analogy regarding how the bladder functions is that it's like when a person driving a car sees their gas light turn on, but then they see a sign that says, "Next gas 10 miles." Has this ever happened to you?

You start asking yourself, "Is the gas tank really almost empty?" Then you rationalize that the warning light must be designed to come on long before that happens. And yet you berate yourself for not filling up when you had the chance.

And to the person driving along next to you, your car looks fine. They can't see all of your internal chatter and anxiety. They don't know that your reserves are severely depleted.

Right? They don't realize that you're driving fast because you're freaking out.

This happens when you have an urgent need to pee, too. You get nervous and anxious, you can't focus on other stuff—you've got to go. That overstimulated feeling is common with the bladder in general.

> **The feeling of being overstimulated is also very common with Hashimoto's.**
> **We are under so much physiological stress all the time that it's really easy to get overstimulated.**

Remember when I spoke about the bladder channel running down the back and accessing virtually the entire nervous system via the spinal cord?

That's a bladder problem: overstimulation of the nervous system.

Quick Recap

Okay, let's recap.

The water element and the kidneys are about our natural wisdom and our will.

The yin organ is the kidney; the yang organ is the bladder. The adrenals are the endocrine glands that also have their own yin and yang character.

Fear is the dominant emotion of the water element. And when fear drives your life, you suffer the consequences and eventually burn out.

We have seen how many ways the adrenals and stress can lead to problems with Hashimoto's and our health; this organ system cannot be ignored.

We need to heal the water element. We need to get a handle on our fears and conserve our resources so that we have enough in the tank when we need it.

We also need to calm our nervous systems and support the adrenals.

There are three basic stages of adrenal fatigue and exhaustion.

In this final part of the chapter, we will discuss those and look at some testing that's available for the adrenals.

But before we get there, let's look at a few things that you can do to support and heal your adrenals.

HOW TO SUPPORT AND HEAL YOUR ADRENALS

Numero uno: Avoid stimulants, especially supercaffeinated, sugar-based coffee and energy drinks. These are the physiological equivalent of running up credit card debt and putting nothing in your bank account.

Talk about emptying your reserve! You will definitely need a bailout after consuming these drinks; they do nothing for you nutritionally. They destroy your adrenals and quickly rob you of any energy savings you may have.

Have a little green tea if you need a pick-me-up. Other things to avoid include ephedra, caffeine, guarana, kola nut, and prescription stimulants like Adderall, Ritalin, Concerta, and that new superexpensive diet drug Qsymia (phentermine).

BALANCE YOUR BLOOD SUGAR

To minimize stress on the adrenal system and ensure maximum energy, consider a low-glycemic (low-sugar) diet consisting of sufficient protein and fat along with low-glycemic carbohydrates eaten in smaller, more frequent meals throughout the day.

This is precisely why I advocate the autoimmune paleo diet that we've spoken about in previous chapters.

Practice stress management and relaxation techniques such as meditation, yoga, and qi gong.

Also, make sure you have at least one day a week when you do nothing. I mean *nothing.* Schedule downtime. Many people have lives that are so busy that even their time off is overloaded. I was one of those people. Trust me, you can't sustain it.

Have fun, laugh, and make pleasure a regular part of your life. Have fun, people! We need to laugh.

Avoid dietary causes of inflammation. These drain your adrenals; they include refined flours, high-fructose corn syrup, and industrial seed oils in particular. You can control what you put in your mouth.

Ensure adequate intake of DHA and EPA. These are omega-3 fatty acids, and they're very beneficial for the adrenal glands. Natural sources include fish oil, flaxseed oil, krill oil, and hemp seed oil.

Toxicity issues can also undermine adrenal health. If you are having an immune reaction to environmental toxins such as heavy metals, mold, or chemicals and you don't work on addressing it, you won't get anywhere with your adrenals.

Something else that can be beneficial for the adrenals and kidneys are a group of herbs called adaptogens. In the 1940s, a Soviet scientist named Dr. Nikolai Lazarev coined the term *adaptogen*.[60]

The original definition is as follows:

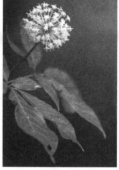

- The adaptogenic effect is nonspecific in that the adaptogen increases resistance to a very broad spectrum of harmful factors ("stressors") of different physical, chemical, and biological natures.

- An adaptogen is to have a normalizing effect, that is, it counteracts or prevents disturbances brought about by stressors.

- An adaptogen must be innocuous to have a broad range of therapeutical effects without causing any disturbance (other than very marginally) to the normal functioning of the organism.[61]

Adaptogenic herbs have been used in Chinese medicine for hundreds of years. From a Chinese medical perspective, the beauty of these herbs is that they can be combined into powerful adaptogenic formulas for healing the adrenals and helping the body adapt to stress.

Adaptogens are thought to work on normalizing the hypothalamic-pituitary-adrenal (HPA) axis. I have provided a more complete list in the following chapter.

Let's take a look at one adaptogenic herb and examine its pharmacology, so you can see an example of how this works.

60 "Plant adaptogens. III. Earlier and more recent aspects and concepts on their mode of action," by A. Panossian et al, 1999, *Phytomedicine*, 6(4), pp. 287–300.
61 "Plant adaptogens. III," by A. Panossian et al.

In Chinese, this herb is called Ci Wu Jia. Its botanical name is *Eleutherococcus senticosus*. It is traditionally a spleen and kidney tonic used for low-back and knee pain, physical weakness, insomnia, and anorexia.

Pharmacologically it does a lot:

It is a mild sedative for the central nervous system, so it's calming.

It increases endurance and lessens fatigue, so it can give you energy in a nutritious way, unlike an energy drink.

It protects the body from radiation.

It enhances immune function in a number of different ways.

It is anticancer.

It is anti-inflammatory.

It increases coronary blood flow.

It is anti-bacterial.[62]

And in cases of low resistance or extra demand on physical strength and mental work, such as high-altitude flying, long-distance sailing, working in high or low temperature or in deep water (all very stressful environments), this herb was found to increase physical strength, improve mental power, and increase vision, color vision, and hearing.

Wow! Do you think that might be beneficial for adrenal fatigue or stress? Yes, indeed.

---

62   *Chinese medical herbology and pharmacology,* by J. K. Chen and T. T. Chen, pp. 864–866.

Recap: Healing the Water Element

In the water element, the kidney is yin; the urinary bladder is yang. The adrenals have both yin and yang aspects.

The negative emotion of the water element is fear. We must learn not to let fear control us, dictate our decisions, and manipulate our will.

This can block us from our innate wisdom, separate our hearts from our minds, and force us to lose our way.

Some keys to healing the adrenals are:

1. Avoiding stimulants.

2. Balancing blood sugar.

3. Practicing stress management (not just thinking about it, but actually doing things like meditation, yoga, qi gong, taking days off, having down time, etc.).

4. Having fun. We need to play.

5. Avoiding dietary causes of inflammation. Gut infections and inflammation are chronic adrenal stressors all by themselves.

6. Making sure we're getting enough omega-3s in our diet.

7. Adding adaptogenic herbs to our mix of supplements.

Chapter 17

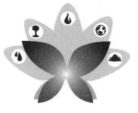

USING THE A.P.A.R.T. SYSTEM TO HEAL THE WATER ELEMENT

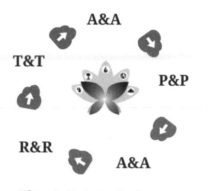

The A.P.A.R.T. System

1. A = ASK AND ASSESS

Open your journal and look for symptoms of problems with the water element. Note what they are, then create a plan for addressing them. After that, you must act on your plan; follow-through is crucial.

Next, take inventory of what you did. Look at what worked and what didn't. Both will provide valuable information.

Double down on what worked and change what didn't. Keep at it.

Winter is an excellent time to heal water element issues. But don't wait to deal with stress and heal the adrenals; they are just too important.

Signs and Symptoms of Adrenal Fatigue

ADRENALS – SYMPTOMS ASSOCIATED WITH LOW CORTISOL

- Cannot stay asleep
- Crave salt
- Slow starter in the morning
- Afternoon fatigue
- Dizziness when standing up quickly
- Afternoon headaches
- Headaches with exertion or stress
- Weak nails

ADRENALS – SYMPTOMS ASSOCIATED WITH HIGH CORTISOL

- Cannot fall asleep
- Perspire easily
- Under high amount of stress
- Weight gain when under stress
- Wake up tired even after six or more hours of sleep
- Excessive perspiration or perspiration with little or no activity

KIDNEY SYMPTOMS CAUSED BY HYPOTHYROIDISM

The kidneys are a perfect place to see how the different systems of the body are impacted by hypothyroidism and Hashimoto's.

HYPOTHYROIDISM CAN CAUSE:

- **Less blood flow to the kidneys.** This can cause creatinine to build up and not be excreted. Creatinine is a chemical-waste molecule that is generated from muscle metabolism.

- **Increased amounts of uric acid. As many as** 20–30 percent of gout patients have hypothyroidism. This is often linked with higher levels of creatinine.

- **High blood pressure.** According to one study, up to 40 percent of hypothyroid patients had high blood pressure.[63]

Hypothyroidism can cause blood pressure to be low. Over time, the kidneys may fail to filter waste products sufficiently from your body properly when your pressure is low and, as a result, angiotensin is produced, which raises your blood pressure.

Also, a rise in cortisol from your adrenals can raise your blood pressure.

HYPOTHYROIDISM CAN ALSO CAUSE EDEMA.

You can see this swelling under the eyes or as mild swelling of the hands and feet.

This is caused by several things: decreased kidney function, capillaries becoming more permeable, poor lymphatic drainage, and salt and water retention by the kidneys.

In turn, these changes can lead to some serious problems with the heart and kidneys.

GENERAL SYMPTOMS OF KIDNEY IMBALANCE FROM A TCM POINT OF VIEW

- All bone problems, especially those of the knees, lower back, and teeth
- Back pain, especially in the area of the kidneys, which are located midway down the back just below the lower rib cage
- Hearing loss and ear infections and diseases
- Head-hair problems such as hair loss, split ends, and premature graying

---

63 "Effects of thyroid function on blood pressure. Recognition of hypothyroid hypertension," by D. H. Streeten et al, 1988, *Hypertension, 11*(1), pp. 78–83.

- Any urinary, reproductive, and/or sexual issues

- Poor growth and development

- Excessive fear and insecurity

TESTING THE ADRENALS

In this last section, I'd like to take a look at some testing we can do for the adrenals and also talk about the three stages of adrenal burnout.

Like virtually everything in our body, things don't usually happen overnight; they develop over time and progress from "okay" to "sort of bad" to "really bad" if you don't do anything to stop the progression.

We see this with the progression of type 2 diabetes, which goes from dysglycemia to insulin resistance to metabolic syndrome to full-blown diabetes.

The same is true with autoimmune disease. It goes from silent autoimmunity to reactive autoimmunity to full-blown autoimmune disease.

The adrenals are no exception. Adrenal problems also go through a progression. It looks like this:

THREE STAGES OF ADRENAL DYSFUNCTION

1. **Alarm reaction:** This happens in normal life. The adrenal glands become hyperactive to increase cortisol levels in order to adapt to the demands of stress.

2. **Resistance stage:** This is the "pregnenolone steal" that occurs in response to prolonged stress, when the body steals pregnenolone from cholesterol to make cortisol.

   When this happens, hormonal imbalances arise because there isn't enough cholesterol to use them. It can cause PMS, infertility, male menopause, and polycystic ovary syndrome (PCOS).

3. **Exhaustion stage:** This is the point when the adrenals are saying "uncle" and they can no longer adapt to stress.

The cofactors needed to make cortisol become depleted and cortisol levels drop too low. Because the adrenals no longer produce sufficient cortisol, the pregnenolone steal cycle also stops.

There are a few tests that you can do at home, and I've included these in the supplemental materials.

HOW TO TEST YOUR ADRENALS AT HOME

Basically, let me give you a quick rundown of what they are.

The first is to test your blood pressure.

You'll want to take and compare two blood pressure readings—one while lying down or sitting and another while standing. (Rest for five minutes in a relaxed position before taking the first reading.)

Once the first reading is complete, stand up and immediately check your blood pressure again. If your pressure is lower after standing, you may have reduced adrenal gland function and, more specifically, an aldosterone issue. (Aldosterone is an adrenal hormone; hypothyroidism can lead to low levels of aldosterone in the blood.)

Normal adrenal function will elevate your blood pressure upon standing in order to push blood to the brain.

It's also a good idea to do this test both in the morning and in the evening, because you can appear normal one time and not another.

A SECOND ADRENAL TEST

The second test you can do is called the pupil test; it also tests aldosterone levels.

You need to be in a dark room with a mirror. From the side (not the front), shine a bright light like a flashlight or penlight toward your pupils and hold it there for about a minute. Carefully observe what happens to your pupil.

With healthy adrenals (and specifically, healthy levels of aldosterone), your pupils will constrict and stay small the entire time you shine the light from the side.

The light causes them to constrict, which is a natural response.

In someone who has adrenal fatigue, the pupil will get small but within 30 seconds it will begin to get larger again—or it will obviously start to flutter as it tries to stay small.

Why does this happen?

Because when you have adrenal insufficiency, you can also have low aldosterone, which can cause an imbalance whereby you have too little sodium and too much potassium in your system.

This imbalance is what causes the sphincter muscles of your eye to be weak and dilate in response to light.

So the fluttering struggle to keep the pupil small may mean you have adrenal challenges.

ADRENAL LAB TEST

In terms of laboratory tests, by far the best one is the adrenal salivary index (ASI). This provides the most accurate, useful, and comprehensive test for the adrenals.

One important thing to understand (and this is true of a number of different tests) is that the most important test is the second or third.

One test is useless, because we are establishing a baseline and then we are going to take action. And we need to know if what we are doing is helping.

The second and third tests give us that information. We must always reassess and readjust.

The adrenals generally respond pretty well to treatment. If they don't, you need to look for something deeper, such as a parasite, heavy-metal toxicity, a chronic viral infection, or some food intolerance.

Sometimes you have to be a detective and rule out infections or intolerances.

The ASI tells us how a person's adrenals are working throughout the day. It's a 24-hour test. Cortisol is secreted in a specific pattern over a 24-hour period and by measuring saliva at different intervals throughout the day, we can chart cortisol levels accurately.

Being in a chronic state of alarm or prolonged stress will mess with this rhythm. One example of this is people who are night owls, have trouble falling or staying asleep, or wake up really tired after getting enough sleep. Their rhythm has been disrupted.

The ASI shows abnormalities in the circadian rhythm since it charts key hormone levels and pinpoints where problems arise along the way. It can be a really valuable test.

You can learn more about herbs and nutritional support for each stage of adrenal dysfunction in the next section.

Okay, let's wrap it up; we covered an awful lot in this section.

ADRENAL TESTING RECAP

Some of the tests you can do for the adrenals are:

1. The blood pressure test. Take two measurements, one seated or lying down and one standing. Compare them. If there is a big difference, this may point to adrenal problems.

2. The pupil test. Point a light at your pupils. Watch them constrict, then watch as they return to normal. If they get small and then quickly go back to normal or flutter, then this is positive for adrenal issues.

3. The best laboratory test available is the adrenal salivary index (ASI), which involves taking multiple saliva tests throughout the day to track your circadian rhythm. It can be very helpful not only for identifying the problem but also for tracking your progress in fixing it.

Awesome!

We've covered a lot in these chapters on the water element. The kidneys, bladder, and adrenals all contribute to fear and loathing in your body.

We have to deal with stress. It can be very destructive, and it does real damage. It is something we really have to take seriously.

If we want to heal our Hashimoto's, we absolutely *have* to heal our adrenals. The reality is that the whole process of healing these multiple systems is, without question, going to take longer than it takes you to read this book.

I am teaching you about what is going on. Correcting it takes time, patience, vigilance, and devotion.

But it is so worth it, people.

All right! (I love this stuff. It's so fascinating to me.)

2. P = Prioritize and Plan

Not everything has the same level of importance. This is what 80/20 teaches us. Some things are having more of an impact than others. Figure out which they are (the positive feedback loops) and make a plan to fix them.

What does that mean when it comes to the water element? Check kidney and adrenal function. Adrenal health is very important if you are taking thyroid replacement hormone.

Remember the warning label for Synthroid that we discussed earlier in the chapter. Clearly, evaluating and treating the adrenals, if necessary, is a major priority.

3. A = Act and Adapt

WATER: KIDNEYS, URINARY BLADDER, AND ADRENALS

FOODS:

Foods that nurture kidney yin: string beans, black beans, mung beans and their sprouts, kidney beans, most other beans, kuzu root, watermelons and other melons, blackberries, muleberries, blueberries, huckleberries, water chestnuts, seaweed, spirulina, chlorella, black sesame seeds, sardines, crab, clams, eggs, and pork

For kidney yang deficiency: cloves, black peppercorns, ginger, cinnamon bark, walnuts, black beans, onion family, quinoa, chicken, lamb, trout, and salmon

For treating damp heat in the bladder (bladder infections): aduki beans, lima beans, celery, carrots, winter squash, asparagus, mushrooms and other vegetables that are not warming, diluted lemon juice, diluted cranberry juice or cranberry tablets, huckleberries

For building *jing*: micro-algae, fish, liver, kidney, brain, bone and bone marrow, human placenta, cereal grass, chicken, mussels

HERBS/SUPPLEMENTS:

Herbs that nurture kidney yin: marshmallow root, prepared rehmannia root, mandarin, asparagus root, aloe vera gel, silver colloid

For deficient kidney *qi*: rose hips, oyster shell, clam shell, schisandra fruit, raspberries, blackberry leaves, gravel root

For treating damp heat in the bladder (bladder infections): uva ursi herbal tea, dandelion leaf, plantain leaf, pipsissewa, flaxseed, watermelon seed

For building *jing*: nettle, royal jelly, bee pollen, dodder seed, deer antler, mandarin, tortoise shell

ADAPTOGENIC HERBS:

There are quite a few herbs that have adaptogenic properties, meaning that they help your body adapt to stress.

But as with everything, there is a risk/benefit analysis that must be done with them, especially when autoimmunity is involved. You must be cautious about stimulating the immune system when taking adaptogenic herbs.

Here's a list of herbs that can be helpful, but it may be best to introduce them one at a time rather than in a mixed formula. That way, if you have a reaction you'll know which herb was responsible.

- Acanthopanax
- American ginseng
- Ashwagandha (this plant is a nightshade and may cause a reaction)
- Cordyceps
- Codonopsis
- Eleuthrococcus
- He shou wu (also excellent for helping promote hair growth)
- Holy basil
- Jiaogulan (also excellent for reducing cholesterol)
- Licorice
- Maca
- Panax ginseng
- Rhodiola
- Schisandra

Herbs that influence ACTH: ACTH is to the adrenals what TSH is to the thyroid. It regulates cortisol production. High ACTH may mean the adrenals aren't producing enough cortisol. Low ACTH may mean the pituitary isn't producing enough adrenal hormones.

ACTH INCREASING:

- Ginko

- Panax ginseng

- Tripterygium

ACTH REDUCING:

- Acanthopanax

- Hypercium

- Licorice

SUGGESTIONS FOR DIFFERENT STAGES OF ADRENAL FATIGUE/EXHAUSTION

1. Alarm Stage:

Balance blood sugar and support healthy response to insulin resistance: alpha-lipoic acid, biotin, chromium, gymnema sylvestre, inositol, magnesium, zinc

Adaptogens **(see above)**

Essential fatty acids: fish oil, evening primrose oil

2. Resistance Stage:

Balance blood sugar and support healthy response to insulin resistance: alpha-lipoic acid, biotin, chromium, gymnema sylvestre, inositol, magnesium, zinc

Adaptogens **(see above)**

Essential fatty acids: fish oil, evening primrose oil

Add licorice and B vitamins **(see food sources below)**

3. Adrenal Exhaustion:

Chromium, adrenal, pancreas glands, choline bitartrate, coenzyme Q10, inositol, rubidium chelate, vanadium.

Adaptogens **(see above)**

Essential fatty acids: fish oil, evening primrose oil

Add licorice and B vitamins **(see food sources below)**

In cases of extreme exhaustion, consider consulting a physician or practitioner. You may benefit by adding pregnenolone and DHEA.

COMMON ISSUES

Bladder infection: Broth ingredients can be chosen from aduki beans, lima beans, celery, carrots, winter squash, asparagus, mushrooms, and other vegetables that are not warming. Recommended fruit: lemon (diluted juice), cranberry (diluted juice or tablets), huckleberries.

Chronic bladder infection: watermelon; pears; carrots; celery; corn silk; squash; oranges; cantaloupe; grapes; strawberries; lotus root; loquats; plenty of water; and, in general, cooling, diuretic foods (see edema below)

Edema (swelling and water retention): ginger skin, winter melon, winter melon skin, squash, apples, mulberries, peaches, tangerines, coconuts, seaweeds, fish, celery, green onions, garlic, bamboo shoots, spinach, water chestnuts, carrots, watermelon, beef

HERE ARE SOME FOOD SOURCES OF B VITAMINS.

Vitamin B1: rice bran, pinto beans, peas, millet, lentils, almonds, turnip greens, collard greens, kale, asparagus

Vitamin B2: salmon, trout, cod, mackerel, perch, oysters, mushrooms, almonds, hijiki

Vitamin B3: rice bran, red pepper, wild rice, kelp, sesame seeds, peaches, brown rice, mushrooms, barley, almonds, apricots

Vitamin B5 (pantothenic acid): beef, chicken, salmon, mackerel, sardines, barley, rice, avocados, plums, raisins, almonds, dates

Vitamin B6: bananas, barley, brewer's yeast, molasses, brown rice, liver, beef, cabbage, carrots, potato, yams

Vitamin B12: beef liver, beef kidney, ham, sole, scallops, eggs, oats, pickles, amasake, algae, spirulina and chlorella, brewer's yeast

Folic acid: liver, asparagus, lima beans, spinach, Swiss chard, kale, cabbage, sweet corn

AN EXCELLENT KIDNEY CLEANSE

Here is a simple formula that is effective for cleansing the kidneys and dissolving kidney stones.

1 quart pure apple juice (must be organic)

2 ounces hydrangea root (chopped)

Soak the hydrangea root in the apple juice for 12 hours. Bring the mixture to a boil. Slowly simmer for 30 minutes. Let the mixture cool, strain out the hydrangea root, and bottle. Keep the juice in the refrigerator. Drink a cupful 3 to 4 times per day for 3 to 7 days.

Note: Hydrangea root can be purchased whole at most health food stores. It has been used by both Western and Chinese herbalists. It promotes detoxification, clears dampness and damp heat, dissolves deposits, promotes urination, and reduces infections.

It is a gentle, yet effective remedy. However, it should not be taken for a prolonged period of time, and if you have kidney or liver problems, you should consult a licensed herbalist before using.

Also, it is a mild diuretic, so if you are taking diuretics or blood pressure medication you should consult your doctor before using. It is not recommended for women who are pregnant or nursing.

Hydrangea root can be obtained as a tincture, which is the herb in liquid extract form. If you want to use this form, modify the recipe by filling a cup with apple juice and adding 20 to 30 drops of hydrangea tincture. Drink warm or cold.

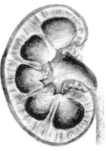

QI GONG EXERCISE FOR THE WATER ELEMENT

Bending for Health

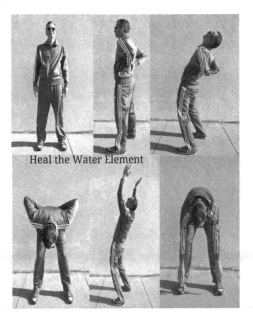

Heal the Water Element

Purpose and effect: In your mind, when you are doing this exercise, imagine that you are gathering the purest energy from heaven and earth. As you do so, visualize it flowing into you and nurturing your own energy reserves.

The point of these movements is to stimulate the kidneys, adrenaline glands, and circulation in your abdomen, especially the lower third. Focus on the waist and lower abdomen as you do this.

As we learned in the chapters about the water element, the kidneys' sphere of influence includes the teeth, ears, urinary bladder, and adrenals. Bringing energy to the adrenals can have an effect on both the urinary and respiratory systems.

The area of the lower back and abdomen also includes important nerve centers like the lumbar nerve plexus and the solar plexus. These are also positively impacted by this exercise.

As you lean backward, guide the energy up from the bottom of your feet, through your body, and out the top of your head. The forward and backward bending brings blood flow to your brain.

The brain, of course, is also connected to the nervous system, so this exercise can help balance your body's metabolism and improve communication among all of your nerves and internal organs.

This exercise also tones your abdominal muscles and improves libido, mental clarity, and concentration. It can also help with reproductive problems in women and prostate issues in men.

CAUTION: If you have heart disease or high blood pressure, please be cautious when doing this exercise and don't overdo the forward or backward bends. Listen to your body and don't push too hard. If you start to feel light-headed or dizzy, you may be overdoing it.

How to begin: Start with your feet a little wider than shoulder-width apart.

As you inhale, bring your hands to the front of the abdomen across from where your kidneys are (a little above the navel). Imagine you are holding a ball of energy there.

As you exhale, bring your palms to your kidneys (mid-back, just below your rib cage); point your thumbs to the front and your fingers to the back, as you would if you were to put your hands on your hips.

Keep your knees relaxed and your legs slightly bent. (Note: If you have wrist or hand issues, you may place your hands a little lower on your back to reduce pressure on the wrist and finger joints.)

Next, inhale again and lengthen your spine, leaning backward as far as you can without causing discomfort. Try to gently stretch and bend your entire spine. (The goal of this exercise is to make your spine stronger and straighter.)

Then, as you exhale, bend forward and let your head hang down in front of your body. Make sure you keep both your back muscles and your waist as relaxed and loose as possible.

Next, inhale again, returning to an upright position with your palms on your kidneys. This time, make your spine long and look up and back, leaning backward as far as you can without causing discomfort.

Finally, exhale, come back to standing, and sweep your arms slightly over and in front of your head. Now bend forward again as far as you can without causing discomfort, allowing your hands to sweep downward without moving your arm muscles.

If you are loose enough, reach down and hold your toes. If this is too difficult, no worries—just relax into the forward bend and hold your lower legs or knees.

Modifications for people who are especially weak and/or fatigued: If this exercise is difficult, you can change the breathing so that each step is done with an inhale and an exhale.

Also, instead of reaching all the way to your toes, place your palms (thumbs on the inside, fingers on the outside) on your thighs and massage down the outside of your legs toward your toes (this is where the kidney and liver channels run, so by doing this you will be massaging these channels).

Repeat the exercise three times one to two times per day.

From *The Healing Art of Qi Gong* by Master Hong Liu

4. R = Reassess and Readjust

Retest, reassess, and ask all over again. Figure out what worked and what didn't. Double down on what worked and either eliminate or re-create a plan for what didn't.

This an area that is rarely looked at by doctors, but as we've discussed, Hashimoto's can have far-reaching effects on both kidney and heart functions.

It is very important to check kidney function. Order a simple renal panel and test uric acid levels and electrolytes.

Try some things and reassess.

5. T = Try and Try Again

Keep doing it, keep refining, keep building on the positive results, and keep looking for the remaining positive feedback loops that are causing vicious cycles.

The water element is the root of our health. We must continually revisit it.

Chapter 18

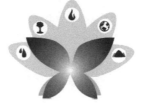

HASHIMOTO'S AND THE BRAIN

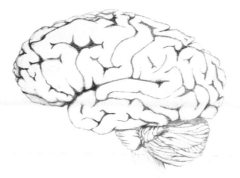

Hashimoto's and hypothyroidism have a profound impact on our brains. This is an area that I'm really passionate about.

It's also an area that almost no one talks about or does anything about, which I'm totally baffled by. This is arguably the most important part of our body to talk about and treat.

Several of the most common symptoms of Hashimoto's are brain-related. Some are obvious, such as brain fog and memory loss; others are less so, like depression and neurological disorders, which can resemble or develop into Alzheimer's and Parkinson's disease.

Regardless of how obvious they are, all of these brain-related symptoms are a sign of degeneration of the brain. This is not a good thing.

But before we dive into your brain, let's recap what we've learned in the previous chapters, because what we have learned also applies to the brain.

In chapter 2, we covered the thyroid and looked at how many people are functionally hypothyroid.

In other words, they have enough thyroid hormone but it's not getting converted properly and/or isn't getting absorbed into the cells of the body.

There are many reasons for this, and we've covered some of them. But the important thing to realize when it comes to the brain is that if thyroid hormone isn't getting properly converted and absorbed, then this might make brain-related symptoms worse. (More on that below.)

Then we looked at the metal element and the immune system. Hashimoto's is an autoimmune disease, which is an area that conventional medicine often ignores or takes the "let's wait and see" approach.

Which really means, let's wait until 70–90 percent of that part of your body is destroyed before we do anything.

Common sense tells us that waiting for that much tissue destruction is a bad idea.

It turns out that one thing that people with Hashimoto's are at risk for is brain autoimmunity. And this can be really destructive to brain cells.

Finally, we looked at the water element—the kidneys, urinary bladder, and adrenals.

And we saw how destructive stress can be for people with Hashimoto's. Because our bodies are under so much physiological stress, we just can't afford additional emotional stress and abnormally stressful events.

They are too costly.

Well, it turns out that stress is really costly for brain cells, too. So, let's dive in and have a look at what's going on upstairs.

Thyroid health and brain health are linked from our earliest development in the womb.

BRAIN AND THYROID HEALTH START IN THE WOMB

One of the truths that unfortunately gets little attention is the impact of a healthy thyroid on the development of a healthy baby, especially on a developing baby's brain.

If you have Hashimoto's and you want to get pregnant, it is very important for you to test your thyroid early and often.

There is a very real risk of retardation or poor brain development, and studies have shown that women who are hypothyroid during pregnancy are four times more likely to have a child with autism.[64]

It is important to realize that if you are taking thyroid replacement hormone, you may need to adjust your dosage in order to ensure that your baby's brain develops properly.

It is also vitally important to be as thyroid healthy as possible *prior* to trying to conceive.

Because this condition is not only a risk to the baby's brain. One of the leading causes of miscarriage is hypothyroidism. A thyroid workup should be a routine part of any woman's prenatal care. Unfortunately, this is rarely done.

HYPOTHYROIDISM CAN CAUSE PROBLEMS IN A CHILD'S BRAIN, TOO

These risks are not only present in the developing brain of a fetus. Once a child is born, if they have too little thyroid hormone, they can experience issues with learning language and have memory problems.

This may be caused by a number of factors. Some environmental toxins have been shown to negatively impact thyroid hormone production.

In fact, studies have shown that polychlorinated biphenyls (PCBs) alter the expression of thyroid hormone-responsive genes in children's brains.

HYPOTHYROIDISM IN ADULTS CAN LEAD TO ALL KINDS OF COGNITIVE DISORDERS

In adults, thyroid hormone has been shown to have major influences over virtually every brain activity.

T3 and T4 are involved in the formation of neurons, neuronal migration, axonal and dendritic growth (these are different kinds of nerve fibers), myelination, and more.

Hashimoto's and hypothyroidism can lead to various disorders, including lethargy, hyporeflexia, and poor motor coordination.

---

64   "The role of thyroid hormone in fetal neurodevelopment," by E. G. de Morreale, 2001, *Journal of Pediatric Endocrinology Metabolism, 14* (Suppl 6), pp. 1453–1462.

They are also linked to bipolar disorders, depression, and loss of cognitive functions, especially in the elderly.

And in the most extreme cases, Hashimoto's can lead to a condition called Hashimoto's encephalopathy, which can cause severe changes in the brain that look very much like the destruction caused by Alzheimer's.

The brain actually loses massive amounts of brain tissue with Hashimoto's encephalopathy.

Clearly, thyroid hormone has a powerful effect on the brain. And hypothyroidism and brain inflammation can cause serious and lasting damage to the brain.

BRAIN FOG IS BRAIN INFLAMMATION

One of the most common symptoms of Hashimoto's is brain fog: that feeling like you are thinking through a haze, like you can't quite focus or concentrate no matter how hard you try.

Brain fog is an indication of inflammation in your brain. Immune cells in the brain, called microglia, are responsible for this.

The immune system in the brain is different from the immune system in the rest of the body. In the body it is much more complex; there are many different parts and they balance and regulate each other.

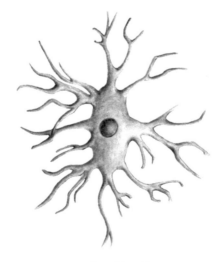

Microglia cell

In your brain, the immune system is simpler. It's like one of those people who has only two speeds: sleeping or balls to the wall.

Microglial cells have an extremely sensitive hair trigger.

And they are capable of inflicting major damage. (Think Chihuahua with an automatic rifle.) Frighten them or make them mad and there's carnage everywhere.

These cells are responsible for causing Alzheimer's, Parkinson's, cardiovascular disease, and more.

These cells also respond quickly to pathogens and injury, accumulate in regions of degeneration, and produce a wide variety of pro-inflammatory molecules.

That's right, they cause inflammation.

Thyroid hormone has a major influence on them. It can help keep them calm and modulate them.

This is why some people with Hashimoto's notice that their brain fog really improves once they are given thyroid hormone.

For many others, this doesn't help at all. If that's the case, there is something else driving the inflammation and the immune attack. (More on this in a moment.)

FATIGUE IS OFTEN BRAIN-BASED

Another common symptom for people with Hashimoto's is fatigue, and in many cases this is being caused by the same brain inflammation.

When these people perform activities that require mental activity, such as reading or driving for long periods of time, they get tired.

Even after they start taking thyroid hormones, they may continue to have these symptoms.

Their brain has less endurance, so they get tired when they use their brains for extended periods of time.

If you have fatigue when you read, drive, or have long conversations, this is brain-based fatigue.

You cannot get brain endurance back unless you support your brain. At this point it is not simply a thyroid hormone problem anymore.

OTHER FACTORS LEAD TO BRAIN DEGENERATION

The thing to realize is that inflammation and subsequent fatigue may be caused by an autoimmune response. In addition, things that trigger your immune system may also trigger your brain inflammation and neurodegeneration.

Let's take a look at a couple of the usual suspects. One is gluten, the other is leaky gut. Together they equal leaky brain and brain inflammation.

LEAKY GUT CAN ALSO MEAN LEAKY BRAIN

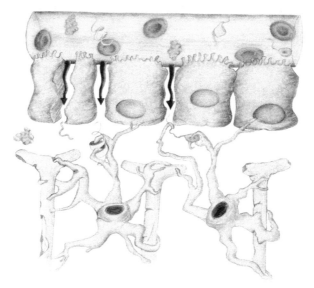

Microglia cells attack neurons after being stimulated by foreign particles.

Zonulin, a protein found in connection with gluten consumption (the "zipper" we discussed earlier) is linked to leaky gut (intestinal permeability)—the very thing that commonly leads to antibody reactions to foods, which leads to sensitivities, allergies, and eventually to conditions like Hashimoto's.

There is a direct link between inflammation in the gut (commonly generated by irritants such as gluten), microglial activation (as a result of these foreign compounds getting into the bloodstream), and brain degeneration.

Gluten has also been linked to the destruction of cerebellar tissue and is a known cause of ataxia, the loss of control of bodily movements. In fact, some researchers have found that a gluten-free diet is helpful in treating this condition.[65]

If you have leaky gut, you may also have leaky brain. These same proteins are found in the blood-brain barrier. So gluten and other proteins and foreign matter can get into the bloodstream and may wind up in your brain.

This is why some people's brain fog doesn't improve with thyroid hormone. It's not just a thyroid hormone problem, because other factors are leading to inflammation in the brain.

In order to improve brain fog, you must reduce brain inflammation and heal the barrier systems, because when things enter the brain that shouldn't, the microglia respond. If that response is severe the tissue around it can be collateral damage.

A LEAKY BRAIN MEANS MORE BRAIN CELLS GET CHEWED UP

The microglial cells also make up the blood-brain barrier, which is a thin barrier that lines the brain and allows only tiny, necessary substances to pass through.

The blood-brain barrier is important for keeping the bad guys (foreign invaders such as viruses or bacteria) and environmental toxins out of the brain.

Unfortunately, according to Dr. Datis Kharrazian, the blood-brain barrier can develop leaks for a variety of reasons.[66]

These include poor blood sugar stability (particularly insulin resistance), chronic stress, chronic inflammation, poor gut health, poor diet with unhealthy fats, and unchecked autoimmune activity such as Hashimoto's disease. (Alcohol use and high homocysteine are also recognized factors.)

BRAIN DEGENERATION CAN ALSO BE AUTOIMMUNE

Autoimmune attacks on parts of the brain have also been noted with Hashimoto's patients.

---

65 "Gluten ataxia in perspective: Epidemiology, genetic susceptibility and clinical characteristics," M. Hadjivassiliou et al, 2003, *Brain*, 126, pp. 685–691.

66 *Why isn't my brain working?* by D. Kharrazian, 2013. Carlsbad, CA: Elephant Press.

One part of the brain that has been observed to be vulnerable in patients with Hashimoto's is the cerebellum. And as we have already discussed, research has also shown that gluten can lead to destruction of the cerebellum (the Purkinje cells, in particular) through molecular mimicry (these cells resemble gluten proteins in structure).

Coincidence?

Regarding the immune system in the brain, it's important to understand that it has no "off" switch.

If there is an immune response in the brain, there is nothing to call off the attack, and the microglial cells create brain inflammation and chew up brain tissue in the process.

WHAT DOES A HEALTHY BRAIN NEED?

A healthy brain needs three things:

1. Oxygen

2. Glucose

3. Stimulation

1. Oxygen: In order to get sufficient amounts of oxygen to the brain, you need to make sure you are getting sufficient blood flow to the brain. So things that inhibit blood flow can impact brain health.

Anemias, especially iron-deficiency anemia, can lead to too little oxygen. If you are iron deficient, this must be corrected.

Low blood pressure can also reduce blood flow to the brain. If your blood pressure is too low, you may want to increase your salt consumption.

Smoking can reduce blood flow to your brain.

Your blood carries everything your brain needs: oxygen, glucose, nutrients, hormones, and neurotransmitters.

Exercise is really important for improving brain health and circulation. High intensity for short duration may be most beneficial. About five minutes of high intensity per day is a good place to start.

2. Glucose: Up to half of the body's glucose supply fuels your brain.

If you are hypoglycemic and you go too long without eating, then you experience the effects of low glucose on the brain: feeling spacey, light-headed, dull, or slow-witted.

On the other hand, if you are a sugar addict and you have developed insulin resistance (the most common symptom of this is fatigue after meals), then glucose can't get into your cells and do its job.

Either way, your brain suffers, and brain cells get killed as a result.

So, if you are hypoglycemic you must start the day with a good protein and fat combination, and you must eat frequently throughout the day.

Your goal must be to never experience that spacey, light-headed feeling again. By the time you experience that, it's too late. The damage has already been done.

For sugar addicts and those with hypoglycemia, a low-carb diet like the autoimmune paleo approach is absolutely imperative.

3. Stimulation: For stimulation, you need to do things that stimulate your brain in a variety of ways. Exercise is one way.

Games are another: Crossword puzzles, chess, memory games, and other activities that require you to be engaged mentally are helpful. Web-based brain games like Lumosity.com can provide various kinds of brain stimulation.

HASHIMOTO'S AND BRAIN DEGENERATION ARE BOTH MULTISYSTEM PROBLEMS

One of the things that I frequently discuss in my writing and consultations is that Hashimoto's is a multisystem disorder.

It's not just a thyroid problem or just an immune system problem.

It extends into all the major systems of the body, including the liver, adrenals, pancreas, stomach, digestive tract, and, yes, the brain.

Often this is why people don't get better. Their doctors ignore all the other systems that are breaking down and keep increasing the dosage of their thyroid hormone.

Well, a lot of times that just doesn't work. You need to have a multisystem strategy.

We really need a strategy for first determining where the problems are and then a program designed to fix them.

The A.P.A.R.T. System is designed to help you do this.

WHAT CAN YOU DO ABOUT BRAIN DEGENERATION?

You have to start by addressing the areas that caused a leaky blood-brain barrier if you want to restore brain integrity.

That's why we recommend the elimination phase of an autoimmune paleo diet to determine whether other foods besides gluten, such as dairy or eggs, are provoking the immune system.

Then we work on the other systems that are involved—balancing blood sugar, addressing gut health and gut infections, and supporting adrenal health so your adrenal hormones are neither too high nor too low.

All of these will help put out the fires of inflammation, the killer of brain cells.

In addition, we use supplements created specifically for blood-brain barrier integrity that heal the leaky brain, reduce brain inflammation, and increase blood flow to the brain. The brain needs oxygen.

And we may also work on other strategies, like enhancing the liver's methylation pathway and supplementing with alpha-lipoic acid.

And below you'll find some important questions to ask in order to properly evaluate your brain and brain nutrition.

The good news is that many of the things we've discussed that are really beneficial for healing Hashimoto's are also really beneficial for the brain.

Before we dig deeper, let's do a quick recap.

Hashimoto's and the Brain Recap

1. A lot of common symptoms of Hashimoto's—fatigue, brain fog, memory issues, and poor concentration—as well as emotional issues like depression, anxiety, and moodiness, in general are all brain-related. We're going to look more deeply at that next.

2. Some brain-related issues have to do with hypothyroidism or functional hypothyroidism (not getting enough active thyroid hormone to brain cells).

3. Other issues are related to autoimmunity in the brain. Gluten is a major player in this, as is dairy, by the way. Dairy is very similar in protein structure to myelin, which is what surrounds nerves and neurons in the brain. If your immune system attacks dairy, it can attack your brain.

4. The brain needs three things to be healthy: oxygen, sugar, and stimulation. Make sure you are not anemic or have too-low blood pressure. Also, be sure you balance your blood sugar and get plenty of stimulation through games and other mentally challenging activities.

5. Lastly, all the things that make Hashimoto's worse also make brain degeneration and inflammation of the brain worse. So we have to work on this.

Now we're going to take a look at some of the ways that Hashimoto's can impact the brain and how that can affect us emotionally and psychologically.

This is really important, because a lot of people with this disease struggle with feeling like they're crazy, or they blame themselves for the way they feel. A lot of times the reasons they feel this way are rooted in what's happening to their brain.

Chapter 19

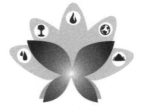

NEUROTRANSMITTERS: MOLECULES OF EMOTION

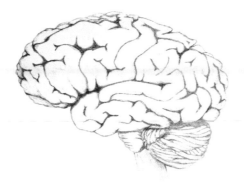

In this section, we're going to examine how all of this affects your emotions and outlook.

In the other chapters, I also explore the Chinese medical perspective, but there isn't a whole lot related to the brain or the nervous system in Chinese medicine.

Traditionally, the brain is known as the sea of marrow or the sea of neural tissue.

In the Taoist tradition, the glands in the brain have important spiritual meaning and power. The pituitary and hypothalamus, which we learned were so important for the adrenals and thyroid, are thought to be what is activated in meditation.

This area of the brain is thought to give and receive light and to awaken our inner knowledge. It's here that we can get in touch with our deepest potentials.

So there was a sense from the Taoists of the mystical power of the brain. And I think we're really starting to see that with modern neuroscience.

I recently read a fascinating book called *The Emotional Life of Your Brain* by Richard Davidson. (I highly recommend it.)

Davidson has done a lot of really interesting research on neuroscience and the brain over the past 30 years. His research looks at the role of emotions in the brain.

The first thing he writes in the book is that no two brains are alike and therefore, no two *people* are alike.

I know this from clinical experience, and if you've observed any of the Hashimoto's or thyroid support groups, you'll see this playing out every day.

Nothing works for everyone. No medication, no supplements, no diet is foolproof. And it all happens in degrees, right?

Sometimes they work perfectly, sometimes they work a little, sometimes they work great and then stop working, and sometimes they don't work at all.

You see it over and over and over again. And one of the key reasons is because of the different ways that people's brains are wired.

One of the things Davidson's book makes clear is how complex this is. Like everything else, there are all of these different factors that affect the way you deal with things.

One of the most important aspects in dealing with Hashimoto's and the process of healing it is how you deal with the challenges and the adversity of the disease.

As it progresses, you will have plenty of opportunities for failure and disappointment.

I've worked with a lot of different people at different stages of Hashimoto's, and what's interesting is that some get results and some don't.

Or maybe a better way to say it is that some people with the same set of symptoms just get *better* results.

And as someone who has this disease and who has been through a good deal of adversity, I really want to help others avoid the same fate.

The thing this book really helped me to see is that the reason different people have different results is really dependent on the wiring of their brains.

EMOTIONAL STYLE: WHAT'S YOURS?

There's a concept Davidson calls "emotional style," and it's comprised of six characteristics: how fast you recover from adversity (how resilient you are), what your outlook tends to be (are you generally positive or negative), how adept you are at picking up social cues from those around you, how self-aware you are; how emotionally sensitive you are; and how well you focus.

When you see it all laid out, it makes sense. This is a big part of why some people get better faster. It's not one thing.

Just like working on the physical part of Hashimoto's, there are all these different factors.

So first you have to figure out where you are in this spectrum, and that will give you a much better sense of where you need to go.

I just want you to think about that and realize that there are a number of different reasons why your brain wiring may be preventing you from getting the results you want.

And, as you begin to figure out your emotional style—what's really unique to you—there are a few general truths that can be quite helpful.

The first one has to do with learning.

Because one of the most important things that Hashimoto's has taught me is that I have to learn how to do things differently.

And real learning involves changing my behavior.

I can get some great advice about changes that I need to make in my life, but if I don't change my behavior, I haven't learned anything. A perfect example of this is an alcoholic.

An alcoholic most likely knows that at some point he or she has to stop drinking. It becomes pretty obvious.

They have to have enough self-awareness to admit it, and eventually, if they do, they know they have to change. And one of the best tools for changing the lives of alcoholics is Alcoholics Anonymous.

Because AA is a program that is entirely devoted to changing behavior, it's a system for real learning.

The people who stay sober are those who learn how to live differently.

The same is true with Hashimoto's. You have to learn—and be willing—to change your behavior.

This is true of several different things.

Food: Being 100 percent gluten-free and balancing your blood sugar are two important behavioral changes.

Language: The way you talk is a behavior that often needs changing, too. How you speak to others and to yourself about your Hashimoto's can make a big difference.

Thinking: The default thoughts you have and the negative self-talk you engage in can undermine your faith and progress. I have found that changing this behavior, in particular, can be the difference between success and failure in healing Hashimoto's.

HOW YOU IDENTIFY YOURSELF MATTERS

How do you identify yourself? Do you say things like "I'm a Hashi's"? Well, stop for a second.

Are you really? If that's the case, then you are really strongly identifying yourself with the disease.

What can you say instead? I don't like using the word *Hashi's*. To me, it's too cute. I don't want to get that close to it. It's always going to be Hashimoto's. I'd rather distance myself.

"I have Hashimoto's." Or even better, "I'm working on getting Hashimoto's in remission."

I often talk about that because it's my goal and my focus. "In remission" is somewhere over there, outside of me. That's where I want it.

I've observed people who use all-or-nothing language: "I will never lose a pound, even if I live on celery!"

Or "I'm always tired, and nothing helps."

"I've tried everything. I've spent thousands of dollars. Nothing works!"

Talking like this wires your brain and reinforces these beliefs. It creates neural pathways that when reinforced often enough can create a positive feedback loop. And the negative messages can become self-fulfilling.

What you keep saying out loud becomes your default thought. And if it becomes your default thought, then it becomes your reality.

Even if you're frustrated and you're not happy with where you are, you have to find a different way of expressing it.

"I'm not where I'd like to be yet." Something like that has a grain of hope.

Because it won't get better if you can't change your relationship to it. And I guarantee you, there is something that is better.

Something.

That's why a gratitude list can be a valuable habit to cultivate. Think about what you have to be grateful for and focus on it. That can dramatically change your relationship to this process.

The last thing I want to talk about in this section is stress.

STRESS AND THE BRAIN

We touched on this when we looked at the water element. When we release too much cortisol as a result of being stressed, it can actually damage the brain and the body.

Hashimoto's is, at its root, a disease of inflammation. And inflammatory markers like plasma fibrinogen rise during stressful events.

Stress is a major trigger of autoimmunity. And in terms of the brain, emotion plays a big role in impacting the immune system. Some neurons in the brain, called sympathetic fibers, connect all the way to the thymus and lymph nodes.

So activating these neurons in the brain with positive emotions like joy, happiness, enthusiasm, silliness, fun (is that an emotion?) has been shown to modulate the endocrine and immune systems.

That's our wheelhouse. Hashimoto's is an autoimmune disease of the endocrine gland.

How your brain is wired can have a big impact on healing. And what's really interesting is that with the mind-body connection, it's not just a one-way thing.

What happens in your brain affects your body, and what happens in your body affects your brain. So everything you're learning is not just woo woo or theoretical—it's grounded in science.

I also want to look at how hypothyroidism and Hashimoto's can lead to deficiencies in important neurotransmitters.

MOLECULES OF EMOTION

These are the "molecules of emotion," as researcher and scientist Candace Pert, who discovered the opiate receptor in the brain, called them in her book of the same name, *Molecules of Emotion*.

Why should you care about all of this?

Because as we learn about your emotional style, we can discover whether you're resilient, hopeful, or focused. Deficiencies in any of these neurotransmitters can affect emotions and behaviors.

If you have these deficiencies, then your odds of improving your thinking or your behavior are greatly reduced.

If you want to succeed, you have to work to make the odds in your favor. Right?

I don't know about you, but I'd rather go to the track knowing which horse has the advantage.

I like to win, because it's more fun.

So if you want to be more resilient and have a better outlook or be more focused, you should make sure you have enough of the neurotransmitters that make these things happen.

There are many, but the ones that we're going to look at are serotonin, dopamine, acetylcholine, and GABA.

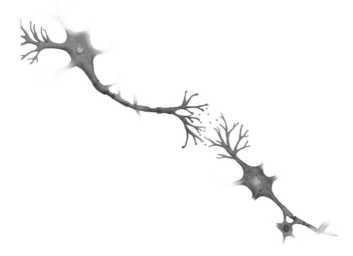

WHAT IS A NEUROTRANSMITTER?

A neurotransmitter is a compound released from a nerve terminal.

When an electrical impulse travels to the end of a nerve cell, it stimulates the terminal of the cell to secrete a chemical-signaling molecule at a special place between nerve cells called a synapse.

These signaling chemicals make it possible for us to have feelings, emotions, passions, and instincts. And with hypothyroidism, we can easily become deficient in them.

This is what makes your emotions go all over the map. As we have discussed, depression and anxiety are very common with Hashimoto's patients.

The reason these people are feeling this way is because of this connection between thyroid hormone and these neurotransmitters.

SEROTONIN

Too little serotonin can lead to feelings of sadness, rage, and joylessness, or you may just feel like giving up. It makes you less resilient.

Serotonin is also used as a messenger to release TSH, and it modulates the production of T3 inside cells using an enzyme called 5 alpha-deodinase. It actually may influence the rate of T3 conversion.

And it works the other way, too. Thyroid hormone has a direct effect on the amount of serotonin in your body, and if you have too little thyroid hormone, this slows the synthesis of serotonin.

This is one reason that some people with hypothyroidism and functional hypothyroidism get depressed.

There's always a physiological reason, people. It's not because you're just depressed.

This depression can be caused by too little serotonin.

And a lot of antidepressants work by blocking the reuptake of serotonin. It floods your body with more of it.

DOPAMINE

Too little dopamine can lead to self-destructive thoughts and feelings of isolation, anger, and irritability. It's the reward and pleasure molecule.

Being a dopamine fiend is the same as having a drug addiction.

Too little dopamine makes you feel like *Why bother?* There's no reward. With serotonin deficiency, you can't find joy. With dopamine deficiency, you can find joy, but you just feel like *What's the point?*

Thyroid hormones play an important role in the release of dopamine. And studies have shown that reduced dopamine can actually raise TSH. This is yet another reason why testing TSH is sometimes not reliable for determining how well your thyroid is functioning.

Your thyroid doesn't exist in a vacuum. It's interacting with all of these other things—neurotransmitters; other endocrine glands like the adrenals, pituitary, and pancreas; and the brain.

ACETYLCHOLINE

This is a really important neurotransmitter for brain activity. It's responsible for nerve firing.

Too little acetylcholine can cause memory issues, slow recall, difficulty calculating, and problems with focus. Having trouble paying attention right now?

Could be you are deficient in acetylcholine.

When you are hypothyroid, your brain uses acetylcholine to make up for insufficient amounts of thyroid hormone. It's like borrowing from Peter to pay Paul.

T3 has been found to directly stimulate acetylcholine.

This is one of those neurotransmitters that I take supplements for on a regular basis. It's great for ADD or ADHD.

GABA

GABA stands for gamma-aminobutyric acid.

Too little GABA can make you feel anxious, panicked, and restless. It's a calming agent. Therefore, too little of it makes you uptight and not in a good way.

It also affects TSH release in the pituitary. It affects how much TSH is released. It also affects thyroid hormones that are stimulated by TSH.

Like T4.

And thyroid hormones keep GABA in your system after it is released and make more of it get released.

Again, this all goes both ways.

YOU'RE NOT CRAZY!

You're not losing your mind; it's the impact of hypothyroidism on your brain and these neurotransmitters.

If you have too little serotonin, that will impact your ability to bounce back and determine whether or not you get enjoyment and pleasure from things.

Too little dopamine is going to impact your outlook and motivation.

Too little acetylcholine means you can't focus or concentrate and finish tasks. Making changes requires focus.

Too little GABA will make you unable to handle stressors. You may freak out on a regular basis over trivial things. This can lead to anxiety or worry.

We have to look for these things. We can't pretend this isn't happening. It's happening all the time.

All of these neurotransmitters can be nourished. You can take the raw materials for them to help your body produce more of them when you're deficient.

(I've put a list of some of the food sources of the building blocks of these neurotransmitters in the final chapter of this section.)

This is way more than a thyroid problem. It's an all-over-your-body problem, and that's where the answers are.

You see? It is all connected: all the physical issues, all the emotional issues, the way you feel.

It's all happening for a reason, and that reason is the impact it's having on your mind, your body, and your spirit.

So take a moment and forgive yourself. It's not your fault.

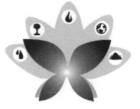

Chapter 20

USING THE A.P.A.R.T. SYSTEM TO SAVE YOUR BRAIN

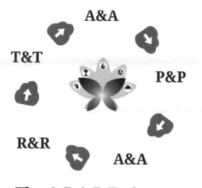

The A.P.A.R.T. System

1. A = Ask and Assess

Grab your journal and look for symptoms of problems with the brain. Note what they are, then create a plan for addressing them. After that, you must act on your plan; follow-through is crucial.

Next, take inventory of what you did. Look at what worked and what didn't. Both will provide valuable information.

Double down on what worked and change what didn't. Don't ever stop this process. Your brain is too important.

BRAIN-RELATED SYMPTOMS

Low circulation: low blood pressure, low brain endurance for focus and concentration, cold hands and feet, poor nail health, fungal growth on toenails, tip of the nose is cold.

Essential fatty acid deficiency: dry and unhealthy skin, dandruff or a flaky scalp, difficulty consuming fried foods, difficulty consuming raw nuts or seeds, difficulty consuming fish (not fried). Also a diet high in processed foods may not have sufficient essential fatty acids.

If you have gallbladder issues, you may have difficulty consuming olive oil, avocados, flaxseed oil, or natural fats, which can lead to deficiencies in these natural fats.

Hypoglycemia: irritable, nervous, shaky, or light-headed between meals; feel energized after meals; difficulty eating large meals in the morning; energy level drops in the afternoon; crave sugar and sweets in the afternoon; wake up in the middle of the night; difficulty concentrating before eating; depend on coffee and sugar for energy.

Insulin resistance: fatigue after meals, cravings for sugar and sweets after meals, need for stimulant (such as coffee) after meals, difficulty losing weight, increased frequency of urination, difficulty losing weight, difficulty falling asleep, increased appetite.

NEUROTRANSMITTER SYMPTOMS

The best way to assess neurotransmitters is to look at the symptoms associated with them. There is saliva testing available for neurotransmitters, but the science on it is questionable.

Instead, get out your journal and write down the symptoms that you have. Determine which neurotransmitters might be deficient, and try some of the recommendations below.

Key symptoms of serotonin deficiency: loss of pleasure in hobbies and interests; feeling overwhelmed with ideas to manage; feelings of inner rage or unprovoked anger, paranoia, or sadness for no reason; loss of enjoyment in favorite activities, favorite foods, friendships, and relationships; feelings of susceptibility to pain.

Key symptoms of dopamine deficiency: feeling like *What's the point?—there's nothing in it for me*, feelings of worthlessness and hopelessness, self-destructive thoughts, inability to handle stress (or getting angry and aggressive when stressed), desire to isolate from others, unexplained lack of concern for family and friends, inability to finish tasks, feelings of anger for minor reasons.

Key symptoms of acetylcholine deficiency: memory issues (especially short term), decrease in visual memory (shapes and images) and verbal memory, occurrence of memory lapses, difficulty calculating numbers, difficulty recognizing objects and faces, slow mental recall.

Key symptoms of catecholamine deficiency: needing coffee or caffeine sources to improve mental function, decrease in mental alertness and speed, increase in distractedness, decrease in concentration quality, slow cognitive processing.

Key symptoms of GABA deficiency: feelings of nervousness or panic for no reason, feelings of dread or a "knot" in the stomach, feelings of being overwhelmed for no reason, inability to turn off the mind when relaxing, disorganized attention, worry over things you never thought about before, feelings of inner tension and inner excitability.

2. P = Prioritize and Plan

Not everything has the same level of importance. This is what 80/20 teaches us. Some things are having more of an impact than others. Figure out which ones they are, then make a plan to fix them.

There is an awful lot to unpack when it comes to the brain. There's inflammation, autoimmunity, neurotransmitters, and possible permeability to the blood-brain barrier.

All of these things need to be evaluated and treated. Without question, this is a top priority.

3. A = Act and Adapt

Act and put your plan into motion, then observe the results. First step? The autoimmune paleo diet.

Why is the autoimmune paleo protocol a good diet for the brain?

So glad you asked. It helps address the major needs of a healthy brain. The brain needs three things:

1. Oxygen

2. Sugar

3. Blood flow

1. Oxygen: In order to get oxygen to the brain, you must have healthy blood pressure and good blood flow.

If you haven't done so, check your blood pressure. Normal range is 120/80. If you are 10 points or lower than that, you may need to do something to raise your blood pressure.

A little sea salt or Himalayan salt can be helpful.

Check below for other important recommendations.

2. Sugar: Sugar is a huge issue for the brain, and it can be a problem both if you have too much or too little.

If you are hypoglycemic, you cannot skip meals or go long periods without eating. When you do this, you deprive your brain of important fuel.

That spacey, irritable feeling is your brain saying, "What are you doing to me?" That can cause brain inflammation, which by now I hope you realize is not good.

The flip side is too much sugar or insulin resistance. While your brain definitely needs sugar, too much of it is brain poison.

It is also inflammatory; if you routinely take in too much sugar, you may develop insulin resistance. This means insulin can't get into your cells, and sugar can't get in and do its job either.

Researchers now believe that excess sugar is a major causative factor in Alzheimer's. In fact, they are actually calling it "brain diabetes" or "type 3 diabetes."

In a review of the literature published in the *Journal of Diabetes Science and Technology*, researchers concluded: "Altogether, the results from these studies provide strong evidence in support of the hypothesis that AD [Alzheimer's disease] represents a form of diabetes mellitus that selectively afflicts the brain."[67]

It's no joke. You have to take sugar seriously. We've seen how it can make Hashimoto's so much worse. Well, if that's not incentive enough, knowing that it can also destroy your brain should be.

The autoimmune paleo diet can really help. It takes all refined sugar out of your diet and helps to convert you from a sugar burner to a fat burner.

67　"Alzheimer's disease is type 3 diabetes—Evidence reviewed," by S. M. de la Monte and J. R. Wands, 2008, *Journal of Diabetes Science and Technology, 2*(6): pp. 1101–1113.

3. Blood flow: The last point is also hugely important for the brain. The brain needs blood flow. If you are anemic or deficient in iron, B12, or B6, your brain is compromised.

You don't get essential nutrients or enough red blood cells (which carry oxygen) to your brain.

> YOU CANNOT BE ANEMIC AT ALL!

Not even a little. Seriously, this is super important.

FOODS FOR THE BRAIN AND NEUROTRANSMITTERS

DIETARY SOURCES OF DHA AND EPA: FISH, FISH OILS, MARINE SOURCES

DHA: FISH, FISH OILS, SPECIALTY EGG/DAIRY PRODUCTS

Fish: Anchovy, carp, catfish, cod, eel, flatfish, haddock, halibut, herring, mackerel, mullet, perch, pike, pollock, salmon, sardine, sea bass, shark, snapper, swordfish, trout, tuna, whiting

Crustaceans: Crab, shrimp, spiny lobster

Mollusks: Clam, conch, mussel, octopus, oyster, scallop

Be cautious with fish; make sure to have variety in your diet and to eat more small fish, which are lower on the food chain and are less likely to have accumulated heavy metals and other environmental toxins.

Serotonin

Foods that are high in the amino acid tryptophan (a precursor for serotonin): avocado, wild game, chicken, duck, pork, turkey

VITAMINS AND SUPPLEMENTS

Calcium, fish oils, 5-HTP, magnesium, melatonin, passionflower, pyridoxine, SAM-e, St. John's wort, tryptophan, zinc

Avoid: PCBs and pesticides. Rinse all produce thoroughly; opt for grass-fed, organic meat.

Dopamine

Foods: chicken, duck, turkey

Avoid (during the elimination phase of the diet): dark chocolate, walnuts, eggs

VITAMINS AND SUPPLEMENTS

Phenylalanine, tyrosine, methionine, rhodiola, pyridoxine, B complex, phosphatidylserine, ginkgo biloba

Rhodiola is an adaptogen. It can enhance concentration and endurance, uplift one's mental state, and support optimal immune, adrenal, and cardiovascular function (even under conditions of severe stress).

Avoid: cigarette smoke and quit smoking, as cadmium in cigarettes reduces dopamine

Acetylcholine

Foods: avocados, artichokes, beef, broccoli, brussels sprouts, cabbage, cucumbers, eggs, fish, liver, lettuce, zucchini

VITAMINS AND SUPPLEMENTS

These are best taken early in the morning through the afternoon.

Choline, phosphatidylcholine, phosphatidylserine, acetyl-L-carnitine, DHA, thiamine, pantothenic acid, vitamin B12, taurine, huperzine A, ginkgo biloba, Korean ginseng

Avoid: aluminum; fluorescent lighting (change to full-spectrum lights); electromagnetic fields from computers, cell phones, power lines, microwaves, and other devices

GABA

Foods that are high in glutamic acid/glutamate: banana, beef liver, broccoli, spinach, oranges, halibut

Avoid: simple carbohydrates, such as simple sugars, white flour, and wheat products

VITAMINS AND SUPPLEMENTS

Inositol, GABA, glutamic acid, thiamine, niacinamide, pyridoxine, valerian root, passionflower

Avoid: lead and toxic chemicals

EXERCISES FOR THE BRAIN

SIMPLE QI GONG EXERCISE FOR THE BRAIN:

Beating the Heavenly Drum: Place your palms over your ears with your fingers spread over the back of your head. Overlap and snap the index and middle fingers over each other and gently hit the back of your skull with your index finger. Repeat nine times.

This exercise stimulates the brain, prevents stroke, and improves memory.

OTHER IDEAS FOR BOOSTING NEUROTRANSMITTERS

Serotonin: aerobic exercise, prayer, meditation, yoga, chanting

Dopamine: weight lifting, meditation and relaxation, alternate nostril breathing

Acetylcholine: aerobic exercise, soft lighting, gentle music, pleasant scents

GABA: aerobic exercise, play and recreation, allow others to take care of you

4. R = Reassess and Readjust

Retest, reassess, and ask all over again. Figure out what worked and what didn't. Double down on what worked and either eliminate or re-create a plan for what didn't.

Since there are no reliable laboratory tests for neurotransmitters, the best way to asses them is by looking at the symptoms associated with them.

Use your journal to get an initial assessment. Then try some of the things suggested and ask about those symptoms again.

5. T = Try and Try Again

Keep doing it, keep refining, keep building on the positive results, and keep looking for the remaining positive feedback loops that are causing vicious cycles.

Chapter 21

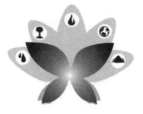

The Wood Element:
LIVER AND GALLBLADDER

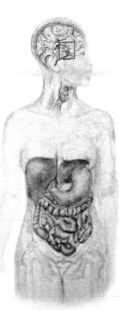

In this chapter, we'll be looking at the wood element, which is the liver and gall-bladder in Chinese medicine.

You'll discover how the thyroid and liver are so dependent on one another.
You'll learn which hormone medication can torpedo thyroid health, and how important healthy liver function is for clearing out these hormones.

You'll discover how to detoxify your liver and gallbladder in a gentle way so that they can effectively clear hormones, environmental toxins, and pathogens that can make your symptoms worse.

THE YIN AND YANG OF THE WOOD ELEMENT

The wood element's yin organ is the liver, and the yang organ is the gallbladder. It's not hard to see how these two are related. They live together just underneath your ribcage on the right side of your torso.

Let's start with the liver. What an amazing organ this is!

OUR AMAZING LIVER

In Chinese medicine, the liver was traditionally regarded as "the general" of the body because of its role in orchestrating so many important activities.

In fact, the liver is probably the most diverse and active organ in the body.

It performs many important functions and is the location where most of the major biochemical pathways used for both anabolic (building) and catabolic (breaking down) activity takes place.

The liver also functions as a filter to remove toxins and waste products from the body, and it stores nutrients such as vitamins, minerals, and iron.

In addition, it plays a role in managing levels of certain chemicals in the body, such as cholesterol, hormones, and sugars. A healthy liver filters about 1.5 quarts of blood per minute.

The liver is centrally involved with carbohydrate, fat, and protein metabolism. The liver's role in carbohydrate metabolism is to help the body maintain adequate levels of sugar.

The liver's role in fat metabolism involves a number of important reactions. First, the liver is very active in oxidizing triglycerides (sugars stored as fat) to produce energy.

The liver is also responsible for the bulk of lipoprotein production and lipogenesis (the process by which simple sugars such as glucose are converted to fatty acids) The liver also synthesizes large quantities of cholesterol and phospholipids.

It is interesting to note that low-fat diets and products that have been heavily marketed for years do not actually address the real problem—sugar.

FAT IN THE LIVER IS CAUSED BY TOO MUCH SUGAR

The reason why we have so many problems regarding fat accumulation in the liver (fatty liver) is because of the excessive amounts of sugar in the typical American diet.

Even many "low-fat" foods have lots of sugar added to them, most of which is often in the form of high-fructose corn syrup that is almost entirely converted into fat in the liver.

Hopefully you've already gotten a sense of how destructive sugar imbalances can be for people with Hashimoto's. But if you need extra incentive to get off of sugar, you should know that it's also the major cause of fatty liver disease and elevated fats like triglycerides, cholesterol, and LDL.

CASE STUDY:
HOW IMPROVING LIVER FUNCTION
CAN HELP LOWER CHOLESTEROL

Anita, a 57-year-old woman with Hashimoto's, also had high cholesterol, high LDL, and triglycerides.

Her main concerns were weight gain, difficulty sleeping, shortness of breath, and upper-back pain.

Anita was also experiencing constipation and exhaustion in the morning (in fact, she sometimes felt like she didn't get any sleep even when she had). She would get winded and tired very easily. Sometimes walking uphill would wipe her out.

She was prescribed Armour Thyroid and all of her thyroid numbers were in the normal range. In the past, Anita had tried Synthroid and did not react well to it.

After a workup of all the systems of her body, we elected to focus on healing the gut, nourishing detoxification pathways in the liver, reducing systemic inflammation, and healing the adrenals.

The goal was to improve function in these areas first and then to revisit the cholesterol issues.

About 60 days after we got started, Anita got another blood test and her cholesterol had dropped more than 100 points (it went from 320 to 218).

What did we do?

Got her on a strict autoimmune paleo diet, which effectively eliminated all the refined sugars that were driving her high cholesterol.

We improved liver function and reduced systemic inflammation, thereby helping her thyroid medication work better.

And we worked on healing her adrenals so she had some energy.

This is yet another example of how when you find the mechanism that is causing something to happen, you can work to reverse the negative effect of that positive feedback loop. Boom! Sometimes you get some amazing results.

Of course we can't promise this with every person with high cholesterol, but I can tell you that this is fairly common when the person is really compliant and they cut out the sugars and carbohydrates that lead to elevated cholesterol in the first place.

Anita R., Alaska

LIVER AND PROTEIN METABOLISM

The liver is involved in some important aspects of protein metabolism. First, it is active in the breakdown of amino acids, and it is because of this that liver transaminase enzymes such as ALT are measured to assess liver disease.

Liver cells are also responsible for the synthesis of plasma proteins such as albumin. Albumin and clotting factor are only made in the liver, so tests measuring serum albumin and prothombin time are also excellent for assessing liver function and health.

In addition, the liver plays an important role in the removal of waste products of protein such as ammonia. When the liver fails to function properly, the body fills with excess amounts of ammonia, which can lead to advanced liver damage and impaired brain function.

The liver is also very important in dealing with environmental toxins. In medical literature the process is called biotransformation, but most other folks know it as detoxification or detox.[68] We'll get deeper into this in a moment.

---

68   "The Transformer database: Biotransformation of xenobiotics," by M. F. Hoffman et al, 2014, *Nucleic Acids Research*, 42 (Database issue), pp. D1113–D1117.

LIVER AND HASHIMOTO'S

As always we must ask, How does this relate to Hashimoto's?

The body is not a machine. Rather, like our earth, it is a group of interacting ecosystems that all talk to and influence one another in both good and bad ways.

The liver and the thyroid are a perfect example of this. Here is a brief breakdown of how they interact:

- The liver is where 60 percent of thyroid hormone is converted from T4 to T3. Both T3 and T4 are glucuronidated and sulfated there. (More on that in a minute.)

- Thyroid hormone influences the way cholesterol and other lipids are synthesized and broken down. (And where does this happen? Yes, the liver.)

- With Hashimoto's and hypothyroidism, this process is often slowed down, which results in high cholesterol and other lipids like LDL and triglycerides.

- Thyroid hormone affects detoxification pathways in the liver and affects insulin growth factor and cytochrome P450 enzymes, which metabolize drugs and environmental toxins. When this slows, toxins can build up.

- On the autoimmune side, researchers have noted that there is a link between autoimmune thyroid and autoimmune liver diseases, and that the liver and thyroid are mutually responsible for proper function in one another.[69]

- Very high levels of thyroid hormone (T3) can raise bilirubin levels, which can actually be toxic to the liver because bilirubin damages mitochondria.

HOW IS THYROID HORMONE CONVERTED IN THE LIVER?

The liver is where 60 percent of thyroid hormones are converted into their usable form. So you can see how low thyroid function can create a vicious cycle.

---

69   "Clinical associations between thyroid and liver diseases," M. J. Huang and Y. F. Liaw, 1995, *Journal of Gastroenterology and Hepatology, 10*(3), pp. 344–350.

Hypothyroidism impairs liver function so that fewer thyroid hormones become active. So it goes until you have all the common symptoms of too little thyroid hormone: fatigue, brain fog, joint pain, hair loss, weight gain, depression, etc.

Thyroid hormone is converted primarily through two processes: glucuronidation and sulfation. So let's break these down.

GLUCURONIDATION

Glucuronidation is an important process for converting thyroid hormone. This pathway is supported by B vitamins, magnesium, and glassine.

SULFATION

Sulfation involves binding things that are partially broken down in the liver with sulfur-containing compounds. It is one of the major detoxification pathways for neurotransmitters, toxins, and hormones (like thyroid hormones).

Vitamin B6 and magnesium are important for sulfur amino acid metabolism, as are foods containing sulfur such as eggs, meat, poultry, nuts, and legumes.

It's important to choose animals products wisely and buy organic whenever possible, because organic foods have far fewer toxins like antibiotics, hormones, and pesticides (all of which can cause liver problems).

Another important point about sulfating is that it requires sulfate, which is often poorly absorbed by the digestive system, especially by people with Hashimoto's, who often suffer from leaky gut syndrome.

Sulfate is the oxidized, inorganic form of sulfur produced by an oxidation step called—you guessed it—sulfoxidation.

This step is made possible by an enzyme called sulfite oxidase, which uses the essential mineral molybdenum. Problems with sulfoxidation can be seen in people who are sensitive to foods that naturally contain sulfites (such as garlic) or to medications and foods to which sulfites have been added as a preservative (such as dried fruits, herbs, and some salad bar vegetables).

(These people may also have an abnormally strong odor in their urine after eating asparagus. If you experience this, molybdenum supplementation or organic sulfates like sodium sulfate or magnesium sulfate may be something to try.)

The liver is such a valuable organ that takes such a beating in today's world. So many things give it a hard time.

Chemicals, heavy metals, drugs, food additives—jeez, poor thing. I love you, liver! (I'm just going to come out and say it. I don't care who knows.)

RECAP: WHAT THE LIVER DOES

1. The liver is like the general of the body. It is involved in orchestrating protein, carbohydrate, and fat storage and production.

2. It is heavily involved in biotransformation (commonly referred to as detoxification), and lord knows we need to understand how to detox our poor livers.

3. The liver does all kinds of stuff related to the thyroid: It is where most of the conversion of T4 to T3 happens (60 percent).

4. Thyroid hormone has a big impact on activities in the liver: It affects cholesterol production and metabolism and it affects detoxification. Too much T3 can actually be toxic to the liver.

5. Thyroid hormone is converted via two main pathways: glucuronidation and sulfation.

Love your liver. Be a liver lover. Love you, liver!

Chapter 22

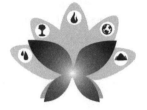

THE GALLBLADDER
AND LIVER DETOXIFICATION

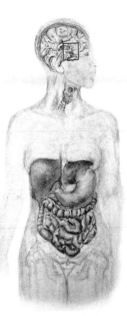

Let's take a look at the gallbladder's role in all of this: The gallbladder is a small, pear-shape sac located just below the liver that stores and concentrates bile. It is connected to the liver (which produces the bile) by the hepatic duct.

When food that contains fat reaches the small intestine, a hormone is produced by cells in the intestinal wall and carried to the gallbladder via the bloodstream.

The hormone (cholecystokinin, for you curious readers) causes the gallbladder to contract, forcing bile into the common bile duct.

A valve, which opens only when food is present in the intestine, allows bile to flow from the common bile duct to the duodenum (located in the upper small intestine) where it functions in the process of fat digestion.

Sometimes substances contained in bile crystallize in the gallbladder, forming gallstones. These small, hard objects are more common in persons over 40, especially women and patients who are obese.

These stones can cause inflammation in the gallbladder, a disorder that produces symptoms similar to indigestion that are often worse after a fatty meal.

HOW DOES THE GALLBLADDER FIT IN?

The liver has several pathways through which it metabolizes hormones, filters toxins, and cleans the blood. By-products from these processes are dumped into the gallbladder to help get them out of the body.

Low thyroid function slows down the whole process, making the liver and gallbladder sluggish and congested and helping to make gallstones.

X-rays of hypothyroid patients often show a bloated gallbladder that contracts sluggishly.

This can slow down the flow of bile, which can lead to slower breakdown of fats, cholesterol, and other toxins that are broken down in the liver.

This whole process can encourage the formation of gallstones. Many people with Hashimoto's have gallbladder issues.

Another important area for Hashimoto's folks is liver detoxification. If liver detoxification is not addressed, treatment will often not work or success will be severely limited.

For example, as many of us know, much of conventional health-care treatment looks at lab test results to determine which hormones a person is deficient in.

With Hashimoto's, as we've learned, it's usually TSH and sometimes T4, if you're lucky.

Most care is aimed at giving the same hormone therapies to everyone. As we have also seen, it's usually synthetic T4. The truth is, however, that many hormonal imbalances are caused by compromised detoxification function.

This is especially true when a patient's blood work does not match their symptoms or if they have a previous history of toxic overload in the form of chemical or drug exposure.

In addition, if people have detoxification issues that are causing their problems, using hormones or drugs may make their problems worse.

Unfortunately, a very common approach used by many physicians is to ignore detoxification issues and just continue to increase the dosage of thyroid hormone.

If your liver is not functioning properly, this can result in adverse reactions like increased hair loss, loss of bone density, palpitations, irregular heartbeat, insomnia, anxiety, and much more.

And this is not limited to hormonal issues but may be true for a number of different health problems.

For example, many studies have shown that poor detoxification can lead to neurological disorders, chemical sensitivities, adverse drug reactions, fatigue, and autoimmune disorders.

If proper liver detoxification is not restored, the chances of returning a person back to optimal health are really low. This is not to say that the process is simple, because there are many factors involved.

LIVER DETOXIFICATION

Liver detoxification involves two basic steps: phase I and phase II. A third step (phase III) involves the gallbladder.

PHASE I DETOXIFICATION

The ultimate goal of detoxification in the liver is to take fat-soluble compounds and change them into water-soluble compounds so that they can be excreted by the kidneys in the urine, in sweat, and through the bowels as feces.

These compounds, called lipophilic (meaning fat-loving) chemicals, come from sources inside the body, such as hormones, neurotransmitters, micronutrients (calcium, sodium, potassium), and also from bacteria, toxins produced by intestinal bacteria, and broken down immune complexes (like antibodies and antigens).

The liver also transforms chemicals from outside the body—drugs, pesticides, environmental toxins—into these same water-soluble compounds so that they can be eliminated from the body.

Phase I detoxification involves cytochrome P450 enzymes. In a normal phase I reaction, these enzymes use oxygen and NADH to neutralize toxic compounds—to make them ready to react and bind to a phase II enzyme.

Phase II enzymes will then complete the process and make the toxin more easily excreted from the body. Phase I enzymes directly neutralize some chemicals, but most others are changed into these intermediate forms that are then converted by phase II enzymes.

The process is called conjugation. It is interesting to note that once a compound has been converted by a phase I enzyme into its in-between form, it becomes much more active and toxic.

Okay? Stay with me.

So, some people have very active phase I detoxification systems and slow or inactive phase II enzymes.

These are the people who may have severe reactions to toxins and often suffer some chronic pain or illness. One side effect of phase I deactivation of toxic compounds is free radical production.

For every molecule of toxin metabolized by phase I, one molecule of free radical is generated. This is why antioxidants are so important. They neutralize free radicals.

One of the most important antioxidants is . . . *wait for it* . . . glutathione, of which we have already sung the praises.

It is extremely important in neutralizing phase I side effects and serving as a platform for phase II conjugation. The stuff is incredible.

PHASE II DETOXIFICATION

Phase II liver detoxification usually involves the conjugation of phase I half-detoxed metabolites, but some toxins are also directly acted upon by phase II enzymes.

This conjugation reaction either neutralizes the toxin or makes it more easily eliminated through the urine, bile, or sweat.

There are six main phase II pathways: glutathione conjugation, glycine conjugation, methylation, sulfation, acetylation, and glucuronidation.

We've already looked at two of them—glucuronidation and sulfation; they are the pathways that convert thyroid hormone.

You see how all of this is connected?

PHASE III DETOXIFICATION

This involves the gallbladder. Once the liver has detoxified chemicals, they are delivered to the bile for elimination via the feces.

If there are problems with bile synthesis or secretion, toxins, nasty chemicals, and hormones will not be eliminated.

Improving bile function should be considered with anyone who complains of gallstone-type symptoms, such as problems digesting fried foods, flatulence several hours after meals, excessive burping after meals, etc.

This should also be considered in people who have had their gallbladders removed. When this organ is removed, the cystic duct acts as a reservoir for bile.

Therefore, it is very important to have proper elimination of bile.

People often ask me, "Hey, if I had my gallbladder removed do I still need to worry about this?"

Here's the thing: Just because a surgeon decided to remove an organ from your body does *not* mean that millions of years of evolution are magically made to disappear.

Your body still continues to function and need the services performed by that now-missing body part.

Some other part of your body must compensate. In the case of your gallbladder, a portion of the duct is usually left, and the liver adapts and takes up the functions previously done by the gallbladder.

Another interesting thing to note is that the body reabsorbs approximately 96 percent of the bile we produce. If this bile is still full of toxins, you can continually recycle toxic bile.

Bile is made primarily of lecithin. So to build bile, eat more lecithin if you can tolerate it.

BILE SYNTHESIS HELPS CLEAR HORMONES FROM THE BODY

Bile synthesis and elimination can be very helpful when balancing hormones because bile can help clear hormones out of the body.

And that brings me to one heck of a segue.

I want to talk about some medications that can really adversely affect thyroid function. The first being birth control, which can stay in the body for a prolonged period and just keep circulating. When this happens you can accumulate an excess amount of estrogen that can cause problems with thyroid hormone absorption.

A year or so ago, I interviewed Dr. Izabella Wentz about her book, *Hashimoto's Thyroditis: Lifestyle Interventions for Finding and Treating the Root Cause.*[70] And one thing that came up was birth control.

BIRTH CONTROL AND HASHIMOTO'S

Here's some information that I learned from her, which comes from her book. Birth control pills can have a big impact on thyroid and immune health and can be a major trigger for Hashimoto's.

They deplete the body of important nutrients that are essential for thyroid function, like zinc, selenium, and the amino acid tyrosine. In addition, they deplete the body of folic acid and vitamins B12 and B6.

Depletions of these vitamins can lead to anemias or depression. Because these vitamins are necessary for conversion of T4 to T3, they and can impact how thyroid hormone is metabolized in the liver.

Many oral contraceptives also contain lactose as an inactive filler. This may be a problem for women with Hashimoto's, because many have dairy intolerances that can cause a flare-up of symptoms.

In addition, birth control pills can impact intestinal bacteria, allowing yeast and disruptive species to take over.

As we have discussed, healthy intestinal bacteria is essential for proper thyroid hormone conversion, so disruptions in the ecosystems of your gut can lead to additional immune dysfunction.

---

70   *Hashimoto's thyroiditis: Lifestyle interventions for finding and treating the toot cause*, by I. Wentz, 2013.

And finally, oral contraceptives actually simulate a shift from Th1 to Th2, because they create a state that is similar to pregnancy in the body. This can encourage more instability and confusion in the immune system.

And that's just one drug and that's only part of the impact it has on the body. These are the unintended consequences of medication.

CLINICAL PEARL:

The best laboratory test for determining the impact of synthetic hormones and other synthetic drugs that can affect the thyroid is resin T3 uptake.

This test measures the number of receptor sites available for unbound T3 to bind on. This is critical for thyroid hormone to do its job. If there aren't enough of these sites available, thyroid hormone may not work properly.

This may be high or low: High T3 uptake may be caused by heparin, anabolic steroids (testosterone), phenytoin, and large doses of salicylates (aspirin). High T3 uptake is found in hyperthyroidism.

Low T3 uptake may be caused by normal pregnancy, heparin, estrogen, methadone, and antiovulatory drugs. Low T3 uptake is found in hypothyroidism.

There are other drugs that may reduce TSH secretion, decrease thyroid hormone secretions, and decrease T4 absorption, such as antacids.

When you take antacids that contain calcium carbonate with the thyroid medication levothyroxine, it may form a new compound that can't be properly broken down.

This means it can't be absorbed. We already discussed how common issues with acid reflux are for people with Hashimoto's. It is common for people to take antacids.

The same is true with ferrous sulfate, an iron supplement, which may also hamper thyroid hormone absorption.

Other drugs, like phenobarbital, actually increase the liver's degradation of levothyroxine. This means you may need a higher dosage to get the same result.

Metformin, a popular drug used for diabetes, has been found to cross the blood-brain barrier and impact the pituitary gland. It may suppress pituitary TSH to subnormal levels in hypothyroid patients.

And this is by no means a complete list.

In conclusion, we have two important things to think about in regard to medication and the liver.

First, a clogged liver may have difficulty metabolizing and detoxifying hormones and medication, which means you may have more of it circulating in your body or you may have more toxic metabolites that can intensify inflammation.

Second, you must always consider the effect of other medications that you have been prescribed on thyroid hormone. An excellent website for researching drug interactions is RxList.com.

Wow, we've covered a lot of information. Okay, let's recap.

RECAP

1. Gallbladder function can be compromised with Hashimoto's. If you've had your gallbladder removed, the remaining duct and the liver must do the work of the old gallbladder.

In either case, supplements that help with bile flow (I've listed them in the supplemental materials) can really help.

2. Liver detox: It's huge.

Phase I: Changes fat-soluble substances into potent "in-between" supertoxins that wait to be further transformed into water-soluble substances so that your body can say, "Buh bye."

These "in-between" metabolites can cause real damage. Antioxidants help. Our buddy glutathione is the champ among champs in this regard.

Phase II: Six different pathways to neutralize those scary in-between toxins or to just plain get them outta here!

Phase III: Bile gets in on the action. If you have a compromised gallbladder or a surgeon has decided to remove yours, then eliminating toxins may not happen as well as it should. And you could be recycling these toxins.

Taking herbs and other things that help with bile flow may be a really good idea for these folks.

Last, many problems with medications and hormones are caused by poor detoxification. If they can't be metabolized or eliminated properly, they can stay in circulation and continue to be biologically and chemically active.

So let's work on it, people! Give those livers and gallbladders some love.

HASHIMOMENT: DON'T STOP LOVING

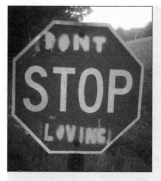

With Hashimoto's, we sometimes get frustrated and angry—both at ourselves and others. It's a natural response to being out of control.

Hashimoto's has a profound impact on our brains and neurotransmitters, the molecules of emotion in our bodies.

This can make us moody, short-tempered, and inclined to lash out. Or the fatigue, brain fog, and pain we're experiencing can make us not want to hang out and socialize because it's just too much effort.

But when you hurt others or yourself, you create another type of vicious cycle, one that can be hard to break.

It feeds on itself.

One simple way to break it is to be kind and loving in spite of it all.

Don't forget to be compassionate to everyone, including yourself.

Chapter 23

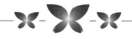

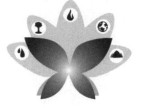

THE CHINESE MEDICINE VIEW
OF THE WOOD ELEMENT

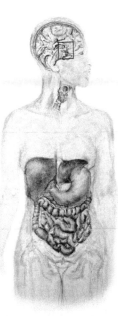

Now let's take a look at the wood element in the context of Chinese medicine. The liver is the yin organ and the gallbladder is the yang organ.

SPHERE OF INFLUENCE OF THE LIVER

The nervous system, tendons, ligaments, and eyes are thought to be part of the sphere of influence of the liver.

And so many people with Hashimoto's also have issues in all of these areas: eye problems, tendon issues, and cognitive issues affecting the brain.

Most people associate eye issues with Graves' disease, but they are also a big problem for people with Hashimoto's. Severe eye pain was what first led me to my diagnosis.

Carpal tunnel syndrome is the most common tendon-related issue connected to Hashimoto's. Oftentimes getting off of gluten, dairy, and soy can dramatically improve symptoms.

And, of course, brain issues are a huge problem for people with Hashimoto's. As we have discussed, the familiar brain fog is often a sign of inflammation of the brain, but some people develop serious complications and brain degeneration from a condition called Hashimoto's encephalitis.

As you know, Chinese medicine views interactions in the body in the context of body, mind, and spirit.

This can be really helpful in seeing how physical problems can affect you emotionally and psychologically.

In Chinese medicine, the liver is sometimes described as something like a military commander in the body. It formulates tactics and strategies, moving blood and energy (*qi*) throughout the body.

As we have learned, the thyroid is part of the endocrine system (which is viewed as *qi*) and is derived from the yang energy of the kidneys.

The ancient Chinese recognized this relationship and how important one is for the other.

The liver needs that *qi* to have the energy to do its job, and if it is clogged or blocked, it can't facilitate the movement of energy throughout the body. When the liver gets stuck or clogged, the most common emotion that people experience is anger.

Anger can be directed outward at people you know (usually those closest to you: family, friends, co-workers), or it can be directed inward and result in depression, self-hatred, and low self-worth.

Or sometimes you can experience a combination of the two.

In fact, depression is one of the most common symptoms associated with Hashimoto's, and antidepressants are some of the most commonly prescribed drugs for people with hypothyroid issues.

THE GALLBLADDER

The gallbladder is the yang organ of the wood element. It stores and secretes bile, which stimulates flow through the stomach and intestines and is very important in helping us to absorb and eliminate different foods, as well as different ideas and concepts.

Proper bile flow and production also help us with good judgment, clear thinking, and decision making.

If there are liver/gallbladder issues, we can end up taking actions without thinking them through, making decisions and not following through on them, or simply getting stuck, unable to decide what to do.

According to Deke Kendall in his book *Dao of Chinese Medicine*, the endocrine gland associated with the wood element is the pineal gland.[71]

He makes the connection via the spirit of the liver (*hun* in Chinese).

Functional activities in the liver—like the breakdown of carbs, fats, and protein—are influenced by natural cycles in the body.

Many metabolic activities in the liver are inhibited at night and reactivated the next morning by daylight.

These events are now known to be controlled by melatonin, the hormone produced by the pineal gland that is made from central serotonin.

Central serotonin levels have a direct influence on our moods. If you have too much melatonin or a diet low in tryptophan, which is a precursor to serotonin, you may develop symptoms like depression, an inability to concentrate, mental fatigue, PMS, carb cravings, obesity, reduced libido, and chronic pain.

Many of the symptoms mentioned above are worse for people who live in higher northern or southern latitudes where there is less sunlight.

The pineal gland sets the body's internal clock based on available light. The liver's sense organ is the eyes; perhaps that is the connection.

---

71 *Dao of Chinese medicine*, by D. E. Kendall.

CLINICAL PEARL:

It's also interesting to note that melatonin rhythm has its own internal clock with a monthly or lunar cycle, which may influence hormones released by the hypothalamus.

Taking melatonin as a supplement can disrupt natural cortisol rhythms and sleep patterns.

Another interesting thing to note about melatonin is that it is a Th1 stimulant. Some people with Th1 dominance have flare-ups of their symptoms at night, especially between the hours of 1 and 5 a.m. (when melatonin peaks).

THE LIVER'S IMPACT ON THE BODY'S INTERNAL ENVIRONMENT

The environmental condition associated with the wood element is wind. In nature, wind moves in an unpredictable fashion.

When external events are rapidly changing, the facility of the liver and gallbladder are to make decisions and implement plans so that we can adapt to our circumstances.

If the wood element is out of balance and we habitually react in anger, we might develop internal wind.

Symptoms of internal wind are usually neurological, such as convulsions, muscle twitches and spasms, headaches, or pains that change location rapidly.

Emotionally, wind can become anger that blows up like a storm whenever we are faced with a surprise change or unexpected circumstance.

This can result in indecisiveness that makes it difficult for us to put together a coherent plan of action.

Like wind, anger can confuse your vision and make it difficult to overcome life's challenges.

On the other hand, if you suppress your anger, this may cause stagnation as resentment builds up inside of you.

KINDNESS IS KEY TO HEALING THE WOOD ELEMENT

One of my favorite expressions about resentment is that it is like taking poison and waiting for the other person (the person you resent) to die.

What this ultimately does is stop you from growing. If every obstacle or unexpected event makes you angry, this distracts you from adapting and moving forward.

In some ways, the opposite of that anger is benevolence and kindness. When we can see events from that point of view, we are able to see the big picture of how external circumstances complement our own internal plans.

The sage is the enlightened being; he or she moves through life in a calm, unattached manner, not controlled by their emotions.

This detachment allows us not to blame ourselves or anyone else. This is when life starts to fire on all cylinders. Now the gallbladder can manifest the inner plan and read external events appropriately so that everything lines up.

It's a beautiful thing.

THE LIFE OF A SAGE: THEY FORGET THE LIVER

This is how Chinese philosopher Chuang Tzu described the life of the sage . . .

"They forget the liver and gall, cast aside eyes and ears, turning and revolving, ending and beginning again, unaware of where they start or finish.

Idly, they roam beyond dust and dirt; they wander free and easy in the service of inaction . . ."[72]

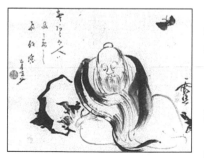

There is a concept in Taoism called *wu wei* (pronounced woo way), which can be translated to "doing without doing." It all becomes that effortless.

Man, that's what I want! *Wu wei* for days!

To summarize, it really comes down to this: Do you want to be right, or do you want to be happy?

The habitual reaction of anger drives the liver and gallbladder to either under- or overuse their natural

---

72   *The complete works of Chuang Tzu*, by C. Tzu (B. Watson, Trans.), 1968, p. 87. New York, NY: Columbia University Press.

creativity in directing the process of growth. You never feel fulfilled, because everything becomes an obstacle that feeds your anger.

Or you feel so defeated by every challenge that you just give up and don't make any progress.

Only when you can feel love and kindness for yourself and others can that natural wood energy flow.

Wu wei, all the way!

Let it go. Love yourself, then you can love others, and then it just flows. It takes practice. It really does.

And that's where we're going to leave it. Just *wu wei*. Effortless doing without doing.

Try to imagine living your life like that.

Or better yet, start living your life like that and see what happens.

Chapter 24

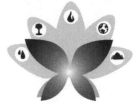

USING THE A.P.A.R.T. SYSTEM TO HEAL THE WOOD ELEMENT

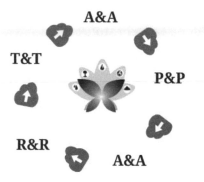

The A.P.A.R.T. System

1. A = Ask and Asses

Your journal should be filling up by now. This time, look for symptoms of problems with the wood element. Note what they are, then create a plan for addressing them. After that, you must act on your plan; follow-through is crucial.

Next, take inventory of what you did. Look at what worked and what didn't. Both will provide valuable information.

Double down on what worked and change what didn't. Once a year, during the spring, revisit healing the wood element.

GALLBLADDER AND LIVER: WOOD SYMPTOMS

GALLBLADDER:

- Greasy or high-fat foods cause distress
- Lower-bowel gas and/or bloating several hours after eating
- Bitter metallic taste in mouth, especially in the morning
- Unexplained itchy skin
- Yellowish cast to eyes
- Stool color alternates from clay to normal brown
- Reddened skin, especially palms
- Dry or flaky skin and/or hair
- History of gallbladder attacks or stones
- History of gallbladder removal

LIVER DETOXIFICATION:

- Acne and unhealthy skin
- Excessive hair loss
- Overall sense of bloating
- Bodily swelling for no reason
- Hormone imbalances
- Weight gain
- Poor bowel function
- Excessively foul-smelling sweat

SYMPTOMS OF LIVER IMBALANCE IN CHINESE MEDICINE

Emotions of the Wood Element: One of the most common signs of disharmony of the liver is showing symptoms related to anger. Feeling rage, being short-tempered, mean, cruel, sadistic, easily frustrated, rude, impatient, arrogant, or flying off the handle at the slightest provocation—these can all be signs of a dysfunctional liver.

It's no accident that drinking alcohol can often accompany these emotions, because alcohol is toxic to the liver and must be metabolized and detoxified. Oftentimes this kind of behavior is followed by guilt, self-loathing, depression, and excessive self-criticism. That's another manifestation of this energy turned inward.

COMMON SYNDROMES OF THE LIVER

Liver Stagnation: Excesses of one kind or another are common with the liver. Eating too much—especially greasy, fried foods—and consuming too much alcohol and/or sugar can all clog the liver and cause significant health problems.

Since the liver is the conductor of blood and energy flow in the body, one of the consequences of these excesses can be cysts and lumps throughout the body. They can be found anywhere but are sometimes found in the thyroid.

We've seen the important connections between the liver and the thyroid. When the liver is stagnant, a lump may be felt in the throat, even though one cannot physically be found.

A goiter—an enlarged thyroid, visible as swelling in the neck—may also be a sign of a congested liver.

The chest or abdomen may become distended or breasts enlarged. Swelling or lumps can occur in the neck, groin, sides of the body, and lateral portion of the thighs.

THE LIVER ALSO RULES THE TENDONS AND EYES

When there is too little energy and blood flow in the body then the tendons are not nourished and can easily become compromised.

Many tendon issues are caused not by swelling, but rather by tears and fraying. This is often the cause of tendon pain in conditions like carpal tunnel syndrome or lateral epicondylitis (better known as tennis elbow).

In fact, it's interesting to note that a recent review in the *Muscles, Ligaments and Tendons Journal* found that there are thyroid receptors in tendons and that thyroid hormone plays an important role in keeping tendons healthy and strong.[73]

This is yet another interesting connection between Hashimoto's and carpal tunnel syndrome, and other common tendon-related issues.

It is not clear why this is true. One theory is that myxedema could impact the median nerve sheath and lead to compression and impairment of the nerve. Because of its impact on peripheral vascular flow, hypothyroidism can lead to poor nourishment of tendons and may also cause this type of problem.

In my opinion, every patient who is diagnosed with carpal tunnel should have a thyroid workup to rule out thyroid disease.

Eye conditions are also commonly related to the liver. The eyes become inflamed, swollen, or pulled out of focus by the muscles that control them.

Much like tendons, the eyes rely on small capillaries and blood flow for their health and nourishment.

Thyroid eye disease is very common, and while Graves' is more often associated with eye issues, Hashimoto's patients also suffer from serious eye problems. It was my own eye issues that led to my initial diagnosis.

Many eye conditions such as glaucoma, macular degeneration, cataracts, redness, dryness, and near- and farsightedness are thought to be related to the condition of the liver.

Corneal disease has been linked to Wilson's disease, cirrhosis, hepatitis, and more. Glaucoma has been identified in liver diseases such as Maroteaux-Lamy syndrome and Scheie syndrome.

Vitamin A deficiency and problems with the rods of the retina have been noted in biliary cirrhosis. Other issues involving the optic and cranial nerves have also been linked to liver diseases.

One treatment strategy for eye issues is to heal and detoxify the liver. In fact, many writers and therapists who teach vision correction suggest a dietary method that uses this approach.

---

73   "Thyroid hormones and tendon: Current views and future perspectives," by F. Oliva et al, *Muscles, Ligaments and Tendons Journal*, 3(3): pp. 201–203.

The strategy includes a vegetarian diet with an emphasis on fresh, raw vegetables and sprouts. Meals are small, and eating the last meal in the early evening is recommended.

Eating moderate amounts of food and avoiding late meals can allow the liver and gallbladder time to prepare for regeneration when the energy of the body circulates through them. According to Chinese medicine this happens from 11 P.M. to 3 A.M.

In addition, the B vitamin known as folic acid is considered an important nutrient in the treatment and correction of myopia (nearsightedness). Folic acid is found in green leafy vegetables and sprouts.

LIVER BLOOD ISSUES

As we've discussed, the liver is an important filter in the body. In Chinese medicine the liver is also thought to store and purify the blood. When the liver is clogged and full of fatty tissue (as it is in metabolic syndrome, which is caused by eating too much sugar) then toxins can build up.

The buildup of toxins in the blood is thought to be the cause of acne, eczema, carbuncles, boils, and even some allergies. And, as we discussed earlier, problems with phase II liver detoxification can lead to the buildup of highly toxic substances in the body.

These toxins can contribute to degenerative disease and diseases of inflammation, like autoimmune disease and cancer. This is precisely why healthy phase I and phase II detoxification is so important for many of the body's other systems.

Testing: Cholesterol, LDL, and triglycerides can be important indicators of both sugar metabolism and hypothyroidism.

If these are high and your HDL is low and you are eating a "perfect diet," then there could be a couple of causes. The diet could be not so perfect when it comes to sugar or the cause could be hypothyroidism. Or, of course, it could be both.

LIVER ENZYMES: AST, ALT, GGT

High or low liver enzymes can both be problems. Elevations mean inflammation of the liver, while low enzymes may mean deficiencies in important vitamins, such as vitamin B6.

2. P = Prioritize and Plan

Not everything has the same level of importance. This is what 80/20 teaches us. Some things have more of an impact than others. Figure out what they are (the positive feedback loops) and make a plan to fix them.

The liver's importance in many metabolic functions and in the conversion of thyroid hormone makes it a priority for virtually everyone. There really is no downside to improving liver health and function.

3. A = Act and Adapt

Act and put your plan into motion. Then observe the results. Double down on what works and change what doesn't. Results should be apparent relatively quickly. If they aren't, you need to make changes.

An excellent time to work on detoxifying the liver is during the elimination phase of the autoimmune paleo diet. This provides the perfect opportunity to give your liver a break from sugar, processed foods, and other toxins that enter the diet via our food supply.

FOODS

- **Foods that stimulate the liver and relieve stagnation:** watercress, all members of the onion family, mustard greens, turmeric, basil, bay leaf, cardamom, marjoram, cumin, fennel, dill, ginger, black pepper, horseradish, rosemary, various mints, beets, taro root, sweet rice, amasake, strawberry, peach, cherry, chestnut, pine nut, cabbage, turnip root, kohlrabi, cauliflower, broccoli, brussels sprouts.

- **Raw and sprouted foods that are cooling and cleansing:** sprouted grains, beans, seeds, fresh vegetables and fruits. (Not recommended during the elimination phase of the auotimmune paleo diet.)

- **Foods that harmonize the liver:** honey, honey mixed with apple cider, licorice root. (We've discussed the many problems that sugar can cause, so be cautious with sugar of any kind.)

- **Bitter and sour foods that reduce excess heat and inflammation in the liver and surrounding organs:** vinegar (apple cider, brown rice, rice wine varieties), lemon, lime, grapefruit, rye, romaine lettuce, asparagus, amaranth, quinoa, alfalfa, radish leaves, citrus peel.

- **Foods that detoxify and cool the liver:** mung beans and their sprouts, celery, seaweed, lettuce, cucumber, watercress, tofu, millet, plum, chlorophyll-rich foods.

- **Foods that reduce toxicity resulting from overconsumption of meat:** mushrooms, rhubarb root or stem, radish, daikon radish.

- **Foods that nourish liver blood:** spirulina, chlorophyll-rich foods, dark grapes, blackberries, huckleberries, raspberries, blackstrap molasses.

- **Foods that accelerate liver rejuvenation:** spirulina, wild blue-green algae, chlorella, parsley, kale, watercress, alfalfa, collard greens.

- **Foods that cleanse the gallbladder:** parsnip, seaweed, lemon, lime, turmeric, radish (removes deposits and stones from the gallbladder), lemon juice, olive oil.

COMMON LIVER/GALLBLADDER ISSUES

Premenstrual Syndrome (PMS): In Chinese medicine this is seen as a disorder of the blood—stagnant blood, too little blood (anemia), or heat in the blood—and stagnation of liver energy.

Foods to relieve PMS: At least one week prior to onset of symptoms, eat ginger, green onions, fennel, orange peel, spinach, walnuts, hawthorn berries, cinnamon, black pepper, Chinese dates, Dang gui.

Gallstones: cornsilk, water chestnuts, seaweed, beet tops, watermelon and watermelon rind, celery, watercress, winter melon and winter melon rind, green tea powder, distilled water.

One of the most important things to do to prevent gallstones is to ensure that you maintain proper stomach acid levels. Including apple cider vinegar with your meals or supplementing with betaine HCL can help in cases of too little stomach acid.

HERBS FOR LIVER/GALLBLADDER

- **To stimulate the liver out of stagnancy:** lemon balm, angelica root, prickly ash bark.

- **Bitter herbs to clear heat and relieve stagnation:** dandelion root, bupleurum, milk thistle seeds, Oregon grape root, chamomile flowers.

- **For building yin in blood:** flax oil, extracted oils of borage, evening primrose, black current seeds, aloe vera gel.

- **For deficient liver blood:** Dang gui root, prepared rehmannia root, peony root, yellow dock root.

- **To cleanse the gallbladder:** cleavers, chamomile tea.

OTHER HERBS THAT ARE HELPFUL FOR THE LIVER

Ginger: This common spice contains chemicals that have been shown to increase bile secretion and to reduce cholesterol levels by upregulating an enzyme responsible for bile acid production (cholesterol 7 alpha-hydroxylase).

Dandelion: The root of this common weed promotes the production of bile and its delivery to the gallbladder. It causes the gallbladder to contract and release bile.

Milk thistle: This herb increases the solubility of bile and has been shown to significantly lower cholesterol concentrations in the gallbladder. It has potent antioxidant activity that supports detoxification, and it prevents depletion of glutathione in the liver, which often occurs in people with Hashimoto's. It also has anti-inflammatory properties and promotes protein synthesis to replace damaged liver cells.

Panax ginseng: This herb has been shown in several studies to have numerous positive impacts on liver function.[74] It has been shown to reverse fatty liver in animals and can be really helpful in cleaning toxins out of the liver. It also has important benefits for the immune system, like promoting Kupffer cells (specialized immune cells located in the liver), and can be beneficial in balancing the immune system by increasing key proteins like IL-8.

Herba sargassi and Laminaria Kun Bu: These seaweeds have important detoxification properties and can be used to treat metabolic toxicosis that occurs with arthritis,

---

74　*Chinese medical herbology and pharmacology*, by J. K. Chen and T. T. Chen.

rheumatism, dermatitis, and psoriasis. They are quite mild and have very few, if any, side effects. In addition, they are rich in trace minerals and are helpful in reducing swelling, particularly in the lymphatic glands. (A word of caution with seaweeds: They contain iodine, which can be problematic for some people with Hashimoto's.)

Fructus Gardeniae: This herb is the seedpod of the gardenia plant. It has potent antibacterial and antiviral properties and can be used to reduce liver and gallbladder congestion and infections.

Caution: Liver infections can be quite serious, so consult a trained physician if you suspect that you have any form of hepatitis or liver disease.

Rhubarb root: This herb is a potent laxative that can be used to treat acute gallbladder and pancreatic infections. It has potent antibacterial, antifungal, and antiviral properties.

Dosage is *critical* with rhubarb root; too much can cause gastric pain and diarrhea. Never use during pregnancy or lactation or with gout, hemorrhoids, or oxalic acid stones. Consult a trained professional before using this herb.

QI GONG FOR THE WOOD ELEMENT

TWIST AND RELEASE

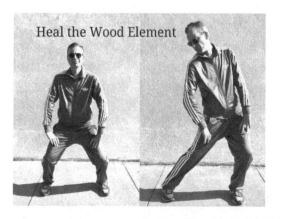

This exercise is beneficial for the whole body. It's effective in relieving tension and lowering blood pressure. In traditional Chinese medicine, twisting the waist helps balance the yin and yang energies in the body; it's soothing to the heart and it increases breathing capacity.

Because this is focused on the wood element, it can also be effective in releasing pent-up anger and aggression.

Begin in a natural standing position, feet shoulder-width apart, weight evenly distributed, and knees slightly bent. To make the exercise more of a challenge, bend the knees more deeply and widen the stance slightly. It's more important that you relax in the posture. So, only go as far as you can and stay relaxed.

Place your hands over your thighs with your fingers pointing inward and your thumbs grasping the outside of the leg.

Put the focus of your mind down to the bottom of your feet. Relax your hips and wrists.

Next, inhale and rotate your torso to the left, leading with the left shoulder. Then turn your head over the right shoulder, looking down toward the right foot. If you need to, you can lower the right shoulder a bit, but try not to hunch forward or pull backward.

As you shift your focus to the right and back, imagine a string pulling your head up and slightly back.

Arch your upper back to get an additional stretch. It is okay to lift the heel of your right foot off the ground, but remember to keep both knees bent the whole time. And keep your hands on your thighs the whole time.

At the end of the movement hold the pose for a second or two.

At first, this movement may seem a bit awkward, but try to keep the movement smooth and do it in one flowing sequence. Stay relaxed and flexible; avoid tightening the hips and waist. As you exhale, bend the right knee and turn back to the starting position.

Repeat the whole movement on the opposite side.

Repeat the exercise three times on each side one or two times per day.

4. R = Reassess and Readjust

Retest, reassess, and ask all over again. Figure out what worked and what didn't. Double down on what worked and either eliminate or re-create a plan for what didn't.

The liver and wood element is constantly under assault in today's world. Revisiting the liver and periodically supporting and cleansing it is an excellent general principle.

Springtime is the best time to do this. Doing a gentle liver cleanse each spring is a great way to "clean house" in your body.

5. T = Try and Try Again

Keep doing it, keep refining, keep building on the positive results, and keep looking for the remaining positive feedback loops that are causing vicious cycles.

Remember that the positive attributes of the wood element are kindness and compassion. As you travel on this journey of healing, always remember to be kind and have compassion for everyone, *including yourself.*

Chapter 25

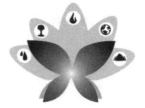

The Fire Element

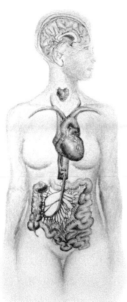

This is a really interesting pairing in Chinese medicine. We saw with the metal element that two apparently unrelated systems actually had a lot of connections (in that case via the lymphatic system).

With the heart and small intestine, the connection is clearly via the cardiovascular system.

Look at the anatomical drawing that we've used for this chapter. See all the vascular activity? The greatest number of arterial vessels supplies the small intestine. Why is there so much?

Well, as every grade school child knows, the heart's job is to pump blood to all the organs, tissues, and cells in your body through blood vessels (arteries and veins). This is really important, because blood delivers the oxygen and nutrients that every cell needs and removes dangerous wastes.

Where do those nutrients come from? Most of them come from the small intestine.

The small intestine is where 90 percent of the digestion and absorption of food occurs; the other 10 percent takes place in the stomach and large intestine. The main function of the small intestine is absorption of nutrients and minerals from food.

THE HEART

The heart circulates those nutrients by pumping blood throughout the body. When blood is pumped through your body, it puts pressure against the walls of your blood vessels.

Right? This is your blood pressure.

When doctors describe blood pressure, they use two numbers, like "120 over 70." These numbers describe the pressure when your heart pumps blood into your blood vessels (the high number) and the pressure when your heart relaxes (the low number).

Imagine squeezing a ketchup bottle. When you squeeze it to "pump" ketchup onto your plate, the pressure is high. When you stop squeezing, the pressure is low.

Blood pressure can change a lot during the day. It is usually lower while you are relaxing and higher when you are active. Other things like pregnancy, smoking, medication, being stressed, and thyroid hormone levels can change your blood pressure.

HYPOTHYROID, BUT HIGH BLOOD PRESSURE?

Usually with hypothyroid conditions, your blood pressure is low and with hyperthyroid conditions, it tends to be high. But there are many reasons why this is not always the case. In fact, many Hashimoto's people actually have high blood pressure.

This is because even though many thyroid patients, or those being treated with T4 meds like Synthroid, can start out with low blood pressure, factors related to having functional hypothyroidism can actually create hypertension and high blood pressure over time.

For example, as we learned when we looked at the water element, hypothyroidism leads to a host of issues physiologically that cause kidney and cardiovascular problems.

For example, there's less blood flow to the kidneys, which causes the kidneys to not filter waste products like creatinine from your body properly.

In addition, when your blood pressure is low, angiotensin is produced to raise it.

When you are hypothyroid, blood is taken from the extremities into the body, which tends to raise pressure by forcing the same volume of blood into a smaller network of vessels.

This process is brought about by a constriction of peripheral vessels. Hypothyroid patients produce an excess of noradrenalin from the adrenal gland, which constricts blood vessels all over the body (another effort by the body to deal with low blood pressure).

This, in turn, is partly related to the effort by the body to raise blood sugar levels when they're low. We've already discussed this as well.

These problems may or may not be caused by overmedication. Anxiety, tachycardia (fast heart rate), and high blood pressure that people with Hashimoto's experience is not always from being hyperthyroid or overmedicated; it may be from noradrenaline that the body is secreting for energy to compensate for the lack of thyroid hormone.

Unfortunately, what often happens is that people are prescribed blood pressure medications (such as beta blockers) and/or antianxiety medications (such as benzodiazepines).

Neither of these drugs corrects the underlying functional hypothyroidism (low thyroid condition) that caused the symptoms in the first place, and both have side effects. In one study, noradrenaline was three times higher in hypothyroid subjects than normal controls when they were lying down.

So what was once low blood pressure now takes a nasty turn toward hypertension (high blood pressure).

It's just another . . . you guessed it, *vicious cycle.*

Obviously, having too-high blood pressure can be dangerous. It means that there is too much stress on your blood vessels. This makes the vessels weak and can damage them. Imagine squeezing a ketchup bottle really hard and fast until it breaks. High blood pressure is a major cause of heart disease.

HOW THE THYROID IMPACTS CARDIOVASCULAR FUNCTION

Okay, so let's look at other ways in which the thyroid impacts cardiovascular function. First, thyroid hormone has a direct impact on cholesterol; with hypothyroidism, serum cholesterol increases.

Thyroid hormone stimulates an enzyme called HMG-CoA reductase, the same enzyme that statin drugs inhibit. This speeds up the synthesis and utilization of cholesterol by the body.

Thyroid hormone stimulates the removal of cholesterol by the liver using LDL receptors. In a hypothyroid state, this whole process is slowed and the result is that cholesterol builds up and isn't cleared as quickly.

Hypothyroidism can also cause homocysteine levels to rise. High homocysteine can lead to inflammation of the arteries and make you more prone to blood clots, heart attacks, and strokes.

We talked about that in the last chapter, too, because nourishing certain pathways in the liver can really help bring down high homocysteine.

C-reactive protein (CRP) is another marker for inflammation in the arteries and is also often high with hypothyroidism.

Another odd thing that too little thyroid hormone can cause is low plasma volume. This is caused by capillaries becoming more permeable; when this happens, albumin and water leak into the interstitial spaces.

> Albumin and water leaking into these spaces causes swelling from edema and water retention, often in your ankles or lower legs.

So here again we have the makings of a particularly dangerous vicious cycle. In the section on the earth element, we spoke about how blood sugar problems like metabolic syndrome can create a lot of conditions that make you more likely to develop heart disease.

Well, when you combine that with hypothyroidism, you have a very potent combination that can put you at risk for heart attack and stroke.

THYROID HORMONE AND THE HEART

Another area that does not get the attention it deserves is the impact of thyroid hormone on the heart and cardiac tissue. One of the things that research is starting to reveal is that thyroid hormone is absorbed differently by different tissues of the body.

In other words, not every part of your body is affected the same way by T4 and T3. For example, the pituitary is different than every cell in the body with different deiodinase enzymes, and it is more sensitive to thyroid hormone receptors.

Many physicians assume, incorrectly, that thyroid hormone is simply absorbed via diffusion (which is basically like the cell sucking the hormone in through a biochemical straw). However, the reality is that the process (called active transport) is energy dependent, which means it requires the body to use energy to push it into the cells.

In addition, different parts of the body respond differently to T3 and T4. Ninety percent of T3 is absorbed by the stomach, while T4 is much less efficient (50–90 percent) and T4 requires much more energy to get absorbed.

T3 affects cardiac muscle cells (myocytes) and contraction of the heart; it also impacts the performance of sodium, potassium, and calcium channels in the heart. What this means is that just throwing more thyroid hormone at the problem may not be the answer and can have unintended consequences.

Something else the research has identified is that thyroid autoimmunity can affect the valves of the heart.[75] So if you have Hashimoto's and have been diagnosed with a heart murmur, an echocardiogram might be a really good idea.

Again, this shows how important it is to deal with this problem from multiple directions. (Jeez, I feel like a broken record sometimes!)

---

75   *"Thyroid hormone and the cardiovascular system,"* by I. Klein and K. Ojamaa, 2001, *The New England Journal of Medicine* 344, pp. 501–509.

CASE STUDY: HEALING THE HEART

Here's a perfect example of how the fire element can be healed.

Edith is a 75-year-old woman with Hashimoto's whose symptoms included palpitations and red, itchy eyes in the morning, an irregular heartbeat, constipation, and sensitivity on her scalp and the back of her head.

Laboratory testing revealed an elevated TSH, low T4, low T3 and free T3, high cholesterol, high homocysteine, and hypertension. Her cardiologist also had done a workup, which revealed atrial fibrillation.

She had recently undergone chelation therapy due to her practitioner finding high levels of lead and pesticides in her body.

We worked to heal her gut and support her liver detoxification pathways. We gave Edith plenty of anti-inflammatories and glutathione, and got her on a strict autoimmune paleo diet.

In addition, we worked to improve thyroid hormone conversion and absorption, and to get her TSH into normal range. We supplemented with B vitamins to bring down her homocysteine levels.

Here is an e-mail Edith sent us six months later:

"I just came home from the cardiologist. Got tested and received a clean bill of health. Yep, he said that everything with my heart is normal and I don't need to come back! This, after continual a-fib and suggestion of beta blockers, blood thinners, and possible ablation [going into the heart to desensitize trigger tissue].

Marc, your course gave me courage to walk your talk. I can't thank you enough for your help in turning my life around.

P.S.: I found a new friend (I'm not kidding). The name is Hashimoto's.

It knows my body better than anything else. It guides me to healthy eating and healthy living. It is always beside me, watching over me. And when I stray, it gently pushes me onto the right path. But if I don't listen, it has a strong voice, for my own good. What a pal. I'm blessed."

Edith S., Maine

Again, we can't promise these results for everyone, but Edith deserves the credit for using our plan, really following through with it, and making the changes she needed to make.

She was also able to change her thinking about this disease and was actually able to see some blessing in it. That's truly inspirational to me, to see that someone could be open to growing and changing—no matter their age.

ANEMIA, NO BUENO

Another area that is of concern with Hashimoto's is anemia. There are a number of theories about why this is.

> One thing that research has revealed is that T4 concentrations are connected to hemoglobin levels.[76]

With less T4, there is less oxygen being carried to the peripheral tissues. We also know that the anemia of hypothyroidism is caused by a decrease in erythropoiesis (production of red blood cells in bone marrow).

There's also iron deficiency anemia, which may be caused by blood loss (during the menstrual cycle) or more often by what we discussed in the chapters on the earth element—low stomach acid levels caused by hypothyroidism.

B12 and folate deficiency are also possible, with absorption being reduced by the same cause. Both T4 and B12 therapy may be helpful.

Another fact, which I mentioned in the chapters on the metal element, is that once you have one autoimmune disease, it's not that hard to develop others, and about 10–12 percent of Hashimoto's patients also have pernicious anemia.

Low B12 levels can be a consequence of Hashimoto's, which can be further complicated by the destruction of gastric parietal cells (and autoantibody inactivation of intrinsic factor). This matters because intrinsic factor is required for B12 absorption.

Thyroid hormone and B12 supplementation are both important here as well.

Bleeding problems can also occur with hypothyroidism. This can lead to bruising easily, prolonged bleeding when injured, or heavy bleeding during the menstrual cycle.

CLINICAL PEARL:

Hypothryoidism can also make bleeding more intense after taking aspirin or other NSAIDs like ibuprofen or acetaminophen. This is another reason to be very careful about NSAID use when you have Hashimoto's.

---

[76] "Effect of thyroid dysfunctions on blood cell count and red blood cell indice," A. Dorgalaleh et al, 2013, *Iranian Journal of Pediatric Hematology Oncology*, 3(2), pp. 73–77.

In particular, it is recommended that you avoid taking NSAIDs while on the elimination diet. These drugs are not that safe to begin with, but when combined with a hypothyroid state, you can have really serious problems.

Okay, that's a lot of heart- and blood-related stuff that we just covered.

RECAP

1. Hypothyroidism can cause high blood pressure. This can be caused by the kidneys and the adrenals, both of which we discussed in the chapters on the water element.

2. Hypothyroidism can impact cholesterol breakdown and utilization and can cause high cholesterol.

3. It can also cause high homocysteine, and high C-reactive protein (CRP). The combined effect of high blood pressure, high cholesterol, high homocysteine, and high CRP is a major risk for heart attack or a stroke. Not good.

4. Hashimoto's can also lead to various anemias: iron deficiency, B12 deficiency, pernicious anemia (another autoimmune disease), and excessive bleeding.

Holy smokes, do you see how this is so much more than a thyroid disorder? And do you see why I wanted to write this book?

I hope so. And I hope you are working with someone and following a similar plan to what we are advocating, because the treatment approach we have shared is one that addresses all of these different areas of the body.

For example, as I've discussed, we recommend limiting the additional causes of high cholesterol by dealing with blood sugar imbalances, reducing inflammation wherever possible, and reducing stress and its corrosive effects.

Here's a little secret: The goal of this book and the process I am advocating is not just to get your Hashimoto's into remission.

Our goal is to help you *keep* it in remission, and to provide you with a blueprint for happiness and longevity, so that you can enjoy life again and be there for your friends and family.

I wish that for you.

Chapter 26

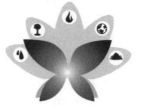

The Small Intestine:
GROUND ZERO

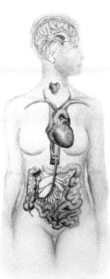

Now let's look a little more closely at the small intestine.

Digestion involves two distinct parts. The first is mechanical digestion: the chewing, grinding, churning, and mixing that takes place in the mouth and stomach. We looked at that in our discussion of the earth element and learned what an important role stomach acid plays.

The second part of digestion is the chemical digestion that uses enzymes and bile acids to break down food material into a form that can be absorbed and then assimilated into the tissues of the body. Chemical digestion occurs mostly in the small intestine.

Enzymes such as trypsin and chymotrypsin are secreted by the pancreas and act upon proteins, peptides, and amino acids. This breaks them down to smaller peptides. Chemical breakdown begins in the stomach and continues until the large intestine.

Enzymes like lipases (also secreted from the pancreas) act on fats and lipids in diet, breaking triglycerides into free fatty acids and monoglycerides.

The process is helped by bile salts secreted by the liver and gallbladder. Lipases are soluble in water, but fatty triglycerides are not.

Bile salts hold triglycerides in the watery environment until the lipases can break them into smaller parts that can enter the villi (intestinal lining) for absorption.

Carbohydrates are broken down to simple sugars and monosaccharides like glucose. Pancreatic amylase breaks down some carbohydrates to oligosaccharides as well.

Some carbohydrates and fibers pass undigested to the large intestine where they may, depending on their type, be broken down by intestinal bacteria. This is where FODMAP comes into play, as we discussed in the section on the earth element.

Once broken down, nutrients are absorbed by the inner walls of the small intestine and ultimately into the bloodstream. Nutrients must be rendered small enough to be transported across the epithelial cells of the gastrointestinal tract and into the blood.

The small intestine is good for absorption, since it has a large inner surface area. This is done by the villi and microvilli. These are damaged with leaky gut.

SMALL INTESTINE IS IMPORTANT FOR ABSORBING EVERYTHING

Approximately 80 percent of water is absorbed by the small intestine, 10 percent by the large intestine; the remaining 10 percent is excreted in feces.

All the important electrolytes are absorbed in the small intestine: chloride, iodine, calcium (these are absorbed with the help of vitamin D), iron, magnesium, and potassium.

Vitamins, including fat-soluble A, D, E, and K, are absorbed together with dietary fats.

Water-soluble vitamins like B and C are absorbed by diffusion. Vitamin B12, combined with glycoprotein, intrinsic factor (from the stomach), is absorbed by active transport.

Of these, iron is absorbed in the duodenum, while most are absorbed in the jejunum; vitamin B12 and bile salts are absorbed in the third portion of the small intestine, the ileum.

HOW DOES THIS RELATE TO HASHIMOTO'S?

Well, if you remember back to the chapters on the metal element, a lot of the lymphatic system is located in and around the small intestine, just as a lot of the arterial blood supply is there.

So when you have leaky gut, a lot of foreign matter can end up in your bloodstream that shouldn't be there. This causes a massive immune response.

THE SMALL INTESTINE IS GROUND ZERO FOR AUTOIMMUNITY

Alessio Fasano, M.D., an expert on the origins of autoimmunity, has found the cause of this intestinal disease. In a paper published in the *Clinical Reviews in Allergy & Immunology*, he writes:

> "Together with the gut-associated lymphoid tissue and the neuroendocrine network, the intestinal epithelial barrier, with its intercellular tight junctions, controls the equilibrium between tolerance and immunity to non-self antigens. Zonulin is the only physiologic modulator of intercellular tight junctions described so far that is involved in trafficking of macromolecules and, therefore, in tolerance/immune response balance. When the zonulin pathway is deregulated in genetically susceptible individuals, autoimmune disorders can occur."[77]

What that means in plain English is that the breakdown of the barrier of the intestines is the pathway to autoimmune disease.

We've already looked at the metal and earth elements and discussed how both are involved in autoimmunity. And we also discussed zonulin, "the zipper" of the intestinal walls.

---

77 "Leaky gut and autoimmune diseases," by A. Fasano, 2012, *Clinical Reviews in Allergy & Immunology, 42*(1), pp. 71–78.

A leaky gut or damaged intestine has been found in every autoimmune disease that has been tested, including rheumatoid arthritis, ankylosing spondylitis, inflammatory bowel disease (Crohn's disease and ulcerative colitis), celiac disease, multiple sclerosis, type 1 diabetes and, yes, Hashimoto's.

In the small intestine this damage leads to immune system stimulation, the wrong types of things in the bloodstream, and, ultimately, a systemic problem that results in the loss of self-tolerance.

This means that the immune system gets so overwhelmed it can't tell the difference between your own tissue and a foreign invader.

SIBO: SMALL INTESTINE BACTERIAL OVERGROWTH

Another serious issue that we touched on earlier in the book is small intestine bacterial overgrowth (SIBO).

Unlike FODMAP, which sounds like a bad corporation, this one sounds like a good charity, doesn't it?

"Please give to SIBO. We understand the plight of the small intestine. We care. Give generously today and save the ecosystem that gives you life."

SIBO could be making your Hashimoto's worse because bacterial gut infections constantly activate the immune system, which can make it difficult to manage the autoimmune part of this party.

WHICH CAME FIRST, LEAKY GUT OR SIBO?

There are many causes of the breakdown of the intestines.

These include NSAID use, alcohol, gluten and other dietary proteins, bacterial overgrowth, environmental toxins, and more.

Once this process breaks down, it alters the whole ecosystem of the gut. It's hard to know which came first.

And at the end of the day, it doesn't really matter.

What matters is what causes it and what we can do to heal it.

SYMPTOMS OF SIBO

SIBO is associated with a number of symptoms, but most often it involves bloating, gas, diarrhea, and constipation.

The hallmark symptom is bloating and discomfort after eating certain foods.

Basically, here's what happens: The wrong type of bacteria end up getting into the small intestine. They migrate from the large intestine and take over.

They feed on certain types of foods like sugars, galactans, fructans, and starches.

In reality, SIBO should be considered if you have abdominal discomfort after eating any of the following:

- Starches
- Sugars/fructose
- Fructans
- Prebiotics
- Probiotics
- Fiber supplements
- Rice or pea powder from protein powders
- Galactans

You may notice that many of the foods listed here can also aggravate candida, which is why candida is sometimes blamed for what is actually SIBO.

FIVE MAIN CAUSES OF SIBO

The causes of SIBO matter, because when we understand the causes, we can figure out how to fix them.

1. Too little stomach acid

Hashimoto's and hypothyroidism leads to lower production of gastrin and stomach acid. This is very common. (We covered this in the section on the earth element.)

Unfortunately, many people develop GERD or acid reflux and are prescribed proton pump inhibitors and antacids that just make everything worse.

2. An immune-suppressed gut

Many factors can lead to immune suppression in the gut. Two important ones are long-term corticosteroid treatment and chronic stress.

In either case, a lot of cortisol or corticosteroids cause the immune system to shut down and can contribute to leaky gut. This results in poor defenses and systemic immune activation.

With Hashimoto's, the body is under a great deal of physiological stress all the time. Therefore, extra emotional stress and abnormally stressful events often result in people getting a lot sicker.

3. Injury to the gut nervous system (known as the enteric nervous system or ENS)

The gut has been called the body's "second brain," because it has its own nervous system and produces many of the neurotransmitters that are also produced in the brain.

Well, just like our other brain, this can degenerate and break down with age and with conditions like scleroderma, IBS, and chronic celiac disease.

And just like neurodegeneration in the brain, this can be permanent. But also just like the brain in our head, this second brain has remarkable plasticity and can relearn things and rewire itself, too.

The gut brain and our main brain are both loaded with thyroid hormone receptors. With Hashimoto's and hypothyroidism, there is often too little thyroid hormone or it's not getting absorbed properly.

This can result in damage to the enteric nervous system (the gut brain).

4. Problems with the vagus nerve

The vagus nerve is a central highway for communication between the brain and the gut. When the vagus nerve stops firing into the gut everything slows down.

This is a major cause of slower motility and constipation.

Thyroid hormone has a direct effect on movement through the entire gastrointestinal tract.

Thyroid hormones increase intestinal neurotransmitters, increase blood flow to the intestines, and support the repair and regeneration of the intestines.

Hypothyroidism can slow movement through the esophagus, can affect muscle function in this area, and can affect the nerves that cause movement. Hypothyroidism also has an effect on the vagus nerve, and this can lead both directly and indirectly to slowing movement through the intestines.

5. Anatomical or structural changes to the small intestine or ileocecal valve

Surgery to the gut (like an appendectomy or resection), diverticulitis, and scarring due to inflammatory bowel disease can all lead to this.

Hypothyroidism can lead to the loss of control of the ileocecal valve that is the doorway between the large and small intestines. When this stops working the way it should, it lets lots of critters from the large intestine into the small intestine.

Later in this chapter, we'll talk about testing and modifying the autoimmune diet for SIBO. Yeah, it's a project.

RECAP

1. The small intestine is a busy place. Lots of nutrient absorption and sharing happens here. Lots of immune cells and immune activity, too.

2. Consequently, it's a place where a lot can happen, both good *and* bad. You can have an overactive immune response and flare-ups. You can have bacterial overgrowth and SIBO.

3. SIBO makes you a gas factory and can lead to lots of other issues, including digestive, skin, and neurological problems.

4. The answer, as always, is diet. Plain and simple.

HASHIMOMENT:
BE PRESENT AND LISTEN TO YOUR HEART

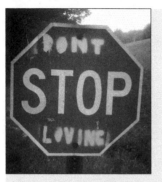

In the West, your heart is associated with emotion. But in the Taoist tradition and in Chinese medicine, that is where your mind lives.

Many psychological disorders are treated as disturbances of shen (the spirit of the heart) using herbs and acupuncture that work on the heart and related channels.

What is also really interesting is that if you have ever known anyone who has had a serious heart attack or open-heart surgery, it is very common for that experience to radically transform their personality—to really change them.

According to Taoist sage Liu Yiming, "When the mind is open, it is aware; the original spirit is in charge of affairs, and illumination is managed properly. One can thereby balance yang.

When the mind is unruly, it wanders: The discriminatory consciousness handles affairs and illumination is not properly directed. This is sufficient to damage yang."

So what does this mean? Well, if you think about it, when we are aligned with our inner self, the heart and the mind function as one.

Following your heart is sometimes really difficult in the short term, but offers the biggest rewards in the long run. So the heart must rule and the mind must follow.

It's easier said than done, I know.

One way to reunite the heart and mind is to aim to be completely present while you are engaged in an activity.

To start, become conscious of all the ways you avoid being present in daily life. Cell phones, tablets, TV, music—all are conspiring to take us out of the present.

Meditation and morning prayer are good rituals to practice to get back in touch with our hearts.

Chapter 27

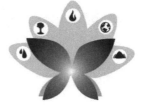

THE CHINESE MEDICINE VIEW OF THE FIRE ELEMENT

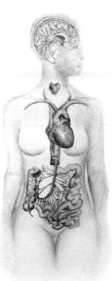

Let's have a look at the Chinese medical take on the fire element.

There are actually four body parts associated with the fire element. The heart and the pericardium represent yin. The heart is the yin organ; the pericardium is the protective membrane that surrounds the heart.

The yang organ is the small intestine, and it represents something unique to Chinese medical thought called *sanjiao*. This is their way of talking about the pleural and peritoneal membranes that surround the lungs and the abdomen in the same way that the pericardium surrounds the heart.

These membranes hold many of the nerves and vessels supplying the organs of the abdomen and the lungs. Though the *sanjiao* is not recognized as an official organ in Western physiology, it does describe actual physiological functions and is important for water transfer and digestive function.

Also interesting in Chinese medicine, the heart is considered the master of the organ systems. It is the emperor.

The *Yellow Emperor's Classic* says, "The heart holds the office of lord and sovereign. The radiance of the spirits stems from it."[78]

Its sphere of influence includes the vessels, the tongue, and controlling speech. Its negative emotion is joy (excessive or over-the-top joy) and its body fluid is sweat.

In Chinese, the heart's spirit is called *shen*. *Shen* is like our soul; it's the spirit within us. It's what makes us unique and is reflected in our mental, emotional, and artistic expressions.

In the chapters on the water element, we discussed the concept of *jing*, which is the water in our well, our DNA, our potential energy. This is the yin aspect of our being.

Shen is *jing*'s yang counterpart. It takes that potential energy and brings it into the world. It brings our latent abilities to life.

When the ancient Chinese spoke of the whole person, they referred to the *shen-jing*, the totality, the union of the spirit, and the tangible parts of our life.

Our *shen* (spirit) rises out of our *jing* (from our kidneys) and fills our hearts. Then this energy radiates out to all other organ systems. This forms a kind of heart-kidney axis.

This yin (*jing*) and yang (*shen*) energy is expressed in all the organ systems of our bodies.

As we discussed, Hashimoto's involves a deficiency of yang, and often our *shen* is tested mightily in this contest. An important manifestation of this energy is reflected in our commitment to things.

Healing Hashimoto's requires a strong sense of commitment. To be successful, we must keep persevering. One thing that breaks my heart is when I see people reach a point of hopelessness.

They know what they should be doing, but because they didn't get the results they hoped for they say "Screw it!" and return to eating whatever they want, ignoring the lifestyle changes that are so important.

---

78   *The yellow emperor's classic of medicine*, M. Ni.

This is another reason why the practices are so beneficial for relieving stress, lowering reverse T3, and strengthening our *shen*. They are not luxuries or optional activities, in my opinion.

They are absolute *necessities*. We must cultivate *shen* energy through meditation, prayer, affirmations, or gratitude lists. Like any part of the body, this can be strengthened.

Another important ingredient to our success, and something that can really help our commitment, is a strong support network. Friends, family, and employers need to know that we're in this for the long haul. And we must learn to communicate what we're going through.

Sometimes we can appear from the outside like we're doing fine, but on the inside we're falling apart. Another reason to cultivate *shen* energy is to give ourselves the strength to ask for help.

We can't do this alone. We need a strong, supportive group of people who understand the magnitude of what we are trying to do.

The endocrine gland associated with the fire element is the pituitary. We've already seen how the pituitary is a master endocrine gland and how the Taoists believed that it's an important energy center.

So we can understand that this is all connected on an energetic level as well. As we consciously work to strengthen these connections—to heal our brains, our kidneys, and our hearts—we can make them begin to work for us and gather momentum in our healing process.

One small victory at a time.

RECAP

So let's sum this up:

Shen, the spirit of the heart, provides the means for us to reconnect to the true self stored in our depths. The heart rules the blood and the constancy of its beat reflects its commitment to fulfilling its role as sovereign ruler.

Hence a person's commitment may be seen as reflecting the quality of the heart's intention. And it comes from our *shen*. We must cultivate this energy with exercises like meditation, qi gong, or yoga.

Chapter 28

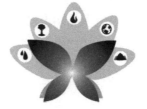

OTHER PARTS OF THE FIRE ELEMENT

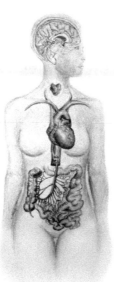

All right, now that your heart and mind have achieved oneness . . .

Let's look at the other parts of the fire element.

If the heart is the emperor or empress, the small intestine is the heart's closest minister and the go-between from the heart to the world and from the world into the heart.

Functionally, the small intestine helps us to clarify how we understand and express the truth and spirit stored within our hearts and the hearts of others.

You don't usually get a private meeting with the emperor; more often it's his minister who first meets you to sort out what is important to convey to the heart.

And the opposite is also true. The top minister must communicate the emperor's decisions to the outside world.

These basic principles are very much aligned with the actual functions of the small intestine.

It has to sort out which vitamins, minerals, and amino acids will be absorbed from food into the blood and delivered to the heart, and it must decide which items are waste and what should be sent downward to the large intestine so it can be eliminated.

An important responsibility of the small intestine is to make sure that communication between the heart and mind, the heart and the outside world, happens in a way that is aligned with virtue or integrity.

If the small intestine is not functioning properly, confusion can result and we can misinterpret others' intentions and second-guess ourselves.

When the heart and mind become separated, the heart can no longer communicate its insight.

Bitterness—the flavor associated with fire—may result from this misunderstanding.

Making unwanted advances or being sarcastic are examples of the small intestine being out of balance and not being able to convey the heart's truth appropriately.

Listening is an important function of both the heart and small intestine. People with small-intestine imbalances may have difficulty listening to what you are saying.

The mind is so disconnected that what is being said and what occurs bear no relation to reality.

Or the person's *interpretation* of what is said is not at all what is being communicated. This can also manifest as a feeling of not being heard by others.

In a way, the small intestine focuses the intention of the heart. Balancing this relationship may be the key to healing, which begins with learning how to listen. Meditation can develop this skill by helping to quiet your mind so that you can be more receptive.

By becoming a better listener, you can better hear others and access your own inner truth.

The pericardium and the *sanjiao* are also part of the fire element. They are unique in that they aren't really organs. They are really more like guards and protectors.

According to the *Neijing*, the pericardium "has the charge of resident as well as envoy. Elation and joy stem from it."[79]

---

79   *The yellow emperor's classic of medicine*, M. Ni.

Just as the emperor lived at the center of the Forbidden City in ancient China, the heart lives at the center of the body surrounded by its own set of guards.

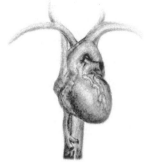

If the small intestine is the minister, the pericardium is like the guard who opens and closes the gate, deciding who to let in and who to keep out.

Like a loyal bodyguard, the pericardium receives the blows intended to strike the heart. Therefore, the pericardium plays a key role in many functional imbalances related to intimacy.

Using acupuncture on points of the pericardium channel can be very effective in helping to heal issues involving betrayal of intimacy.

According to the *Yellow Emperor's Classic*, the *sanjiao* "is responsible for opening up passages and irrigation. The regulation of fluids stems from it."

Physiologically, the membranes of the *sanjiao* help regulate water metabolism in the body. From an emotional point of view, the *sanjiao* is like a customs guard at the border deciding who will be allowed to enter and leave the kingdom of the heart.

Remember the *wei qi* (or defensive *qi*) from the chapters on the metal element? The *sanjiao* contributes to that protection. It creates a barrier that keeps pathogens and emotional attackers outside, preventing them from entering the kingdom of one's heart.

Physiologically, the *sanjiao* is also like the body's thermostat; it maintains balance by regulating fire (yang) and water (yin) throughout our bodies.

To do this, the *sanjiao* has to maintain balance between the internal and external environments. It has to stay connected to our surroundings. In a way, it is responsible for gathering and sharing information that the heart needs in order to rule effectively.

Healthy intimacy involves a balance between the pericardium and the *sanjiao*. The virtue of the fire element is that it empowers maturity.

If the pericardium and *sanjiao* are too strong, one may be overly protective of oneself and not allow intimacy.

If one is too weak and fire gets out of control, one could be promiscuous and act out sexually, not caring about boundaries. Or this person can be an excessive talker who never lets anyone get a word in edgewise.

Treating acupuncture points on the *sanjiao* channel can help regulate boundaries. They are found along the ventral side of the forearm and on the upper back and head.

When the *sanjiao* functions properly, we are not worried about establishing or avoiding connections with others; we simply acknowledge the nature of the connection that is already there.

Only by connecting to our own hearts and the hearts of others can we establish the alignment between heaven internally and externally that leads to fulfillment.

As we work on learning about and healing the fire element, we may be challenged. We may even have a tiny breakdown or two. But sometimes the biggest breakthroughs happen after the biggest breakdowns.

RECAP

1. The fire element of Chinese medicine includes the heart, small intestine, pericardium, and *sanjiao*.

2. We saw how Hashimoto's and hypothyroidism can have a big impact on cardiovascular function and can really make you very vulnerable to heart attack and stroke.

    This makes what we learned earlier about blood sugar imbalances, metabolic syndrome, and diabetes even more important. You do not want to mess around here, people!

3. Emotionally and spiritually we looked at the fire element and the heart as the mind—not the separation we see in the Western medical model, but something more unified.

    A lot of this is about intimacy, and keeping the heart and the mind in alignment. Listening is really an important emotional and spiritual skill. It allows you to hear others and your own heart's direction.

    Ultimately our goal is alignment with our true purpose and with heaven internally and externally.

    The heart is the emperor or empress and lives at the center of the body where it is protected by its loyal ministers and bodyguards.

You can do this. In my heart of hearts, I know you can. All you need is some commitment and support. Together we can find hope, help, and healing by inspiring and supporting one another. At the very least, let's make a commitment to help one another.

Chapter 29

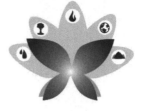

USING the A.P.A.R.T. SYSTEM
TO HEAL
THE FIRE ELEMENT

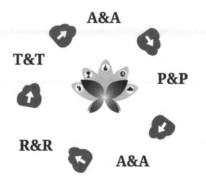

The A.P.A.R.T. System

1. A = Ask and Assess

Your journal should be a book by now! Look for symptoms of problems with the fire element. Note what they are, then create a plan for addressing them. After that, you must act on your plan; follow-through is crucial.

Next, take inventory of what you did. Look at what worked and what didn't. Both will provide valuable information.

Double down on what worked and change what didn't. Summer is a good time to focus on healing fire-related issues. But any time of year is a good time to heal the small intestine.

HEART ISSUES:

Excess conditions: elevated heart rate, chest pain, high homocystein, high cholesterol, LDL, triglycerides, edema, high blood pressure

Deficient conditions: slow heart rate, low blood pressure, anemia (see below for possible kinds)

Small Intestine Issues: constipation from fiber and roughage; pain, tenderness, and soreness on the left side of the body, under the rib cage; undigested, foul smelling, mucus-like, greasy, or poorly formed stool; frequent urination; difficulty losing weight

TESTING: HEART AND SMALL INTESTINE

Okay, we've traveled pretty far down the fire road. Every time I look into something lately it seems to me that an entire universe of discovery awaits.

This is especially true with Hashimoto's. There is so much to learn, so much to explore, so much to discover.

And there are all of these moving parts and connections.

I mean, just look at this chapter: With the small intestine we really can see the convergence of the immune system, the cardiovascular system, and the digestive system.

Everything is affecting everything else. And we are presented with a choice: Either ignore this and allow more vicious cycles to create a downward spiral that compromises our health. Or, see the connections and create a strategy that supports all these systems and allows us to turn things around and build healing momentum.

It's fascinating.

So in this last section, I want to touch on some important things.

First, I'd like to highlight two issues involving the blood that can torpedo your progress.

We covered one of them earlier: blood sugar imbalances. These must be taken seriously and addressed or you may really wind up in a world of hurt.

As we have seen, there are a whole boatload of additional cardiovascular risk factors added on to this equation by just simply being hypothyroid.

We know Hashimoto's and hypothyroidism can have a big impact on the heart and heart function.

And if you don't deal with your blood sugar issues, you can literally become a walking time bomb, having created the perfect recipe for heart attack or stroke.

The second issue involving the blood involves the various anemias. Anemias, like blood sugar imbalances, can torpedo your progress and make all the time and money you are spending absolutely worthless.

Why? Because if you can't get enough oxygen and nutrients to your cells, they won't do you any good and you dramatically reduce your chances of recovering. You are always fighting a losing battle.

A BASIC CBC: COMPLETE BLOOD COUNT

You can get clues regarding anemias from a simple CBC, which costs about 15 bucks. We looked at three anemias:

1. B12

2. Iron deficiency

3. Pernicious anemia

These can be seen in patterns of a basic CBC by looking at red blood cell counts and other related markers.

For example, B12/folic acid deficiency can be identified if you see the following pattern:

Low RBC

Low hematocrit

Low hemoglobin

High MCV

High MCH

High MCHC

You can also simply test serum vitamin B12 and folate (this is the preferred test because it gives you actual levels).

Pernicious anemia can be identified if you see the same pattern as above. If you suspect it may be pernicious anemia, ask your practitioner to order an intrinsic factor blocking antibody (IFBA) test and, possibly, a parietal cell antibody test.

For iron deficiency anemia, the following pattern will be present:

Low RBC

Low hemoglobin

Low hematocrit

Low MCV
Low MCH
Low MCHC
Normal or elevated RDW
and
Low serum iron
Low ferritin
Low iron saturation
High TIBC

MORE ON SIBO

The next thing that you may need to address is SIBO.

We talked about the main issues around SIBO—but wait, there's more!

Many other symptoms of SIBO are a direct effect of nutrient malabsorption. This arises either from the bacteria metabolizing nutrients before we can absorb them or by the bacteria causing enough inflammation in the lining of the gut that it can't work properly anymore.

For example, the bacteria preferentially consume iron and vitamin B12, causing anemia. The bacteria decrease fat absorption by deconjugating bile, leading to deficiencies of vitamins A and D and causing steatorrhea (fatty stools).

As the gut lining becomes increasingly inflamed and leaky, larger and not fully digested food particles enter the body, causing an immune reaction that leads to food allergies and food sensitivities.

Bacteria themselves can enter the bloodstream, causing systemic inflammation and immune reactions that can lead to autoantibody formation and autoimmune diseases.

There really is no end to these vicious cycles.

HOW DO YOU TEST FOR SIBO?

In the conventional medical model there are two methods of testing for SIBO. Both are flawed and not definitive.

1. Direct: endoscopic aspiration and culture

A direct endoscopic aspiration and culture of the small intestine requires a gastroenterologist; the procedure is expensive, and it's invasive (they have to go in and get a sample).

The problem with this is that many of the bacteria removed from the small intestine can't be analyzed, because they don't survive in culture.

Samples must be handled properly for accurate results.

In short, it's expensive, invasive, and sometimes tests don't reveal all the bacteria involved.

2. Indirect: breath testing for hydrogen and methane

This type of testing involves breath testing for hydrogen and methane. Bacteria colonize the large intestine in healthy people and the small intestines in people with conditions that produce hydrogen by fermentation.

Methane is produced by microorganisms from the Archea family that live with bacteria and are thought to be a very ancient species.

This test can be inaccurate if someone has recently taken a course of antibiotics.

It may not be useful in determining all species of bacteria.

The optimal window for collection is different for different people, because transit time is different for different people.

To recap: You may get false negatives due to different transit times or antibiotic use.

Actually, the best test for SIBO is a trial diet and/or a stool test that looks for invasive species.

How Do You Fix SIBO?

TREATMENT DEPENDS ON WHERE YOU ARE IN THE PROGRESSION

One important lesson that I have learned after working with more than 1,000 people with Hashimoto's is that there are two really important things for getting good clinical results:

#1. Figure out the mechanism. In other words, where's the problem? With Hashimoto's it's often in multiple places, not only in the thyroid.

#2. Figure out how advanced it is. Hashimoto's, like all autoimmune disease, is progressive. (Remember in the section on the metal element, where we discussed the three stages of progression?)

In a general sense, the further it has progressed, the more you must do.

HEALING BY SUBTRACTION

Often some of the most effective treatments and solutions come from subtraction.

Many common health problems are problems of excess: too much sugar, too much stress, too much inflammation, too much salt, too many chemicals.

A simple and effective way of treating too much is by taking things away.

If you have insulin resistance or type 2 diabetes, stop eating sugar and refined carbohydrates.

If stress is killing you, stop doing the things that cause you so much stress.

If you have too much inflammation, stop eating and behaving in a way that causes so much inflammation.

If you're sick from too much salt, stop eating salt.

If pollution is killing us and our world, stop using so many chemicals. Such a simple solution that's so hard to actually do.

At first.

The reason is that we are conditioned to be consumers, not subtractors.

However, if you have Hashimoto's, learning the habit of being content with less (sometimes *a lot less*) may just be the key to your healing.

Nowhere is this truer than in the treatment of SIBO.

DIET MUST BE THE FOUNDATION OF TREATMENT

With SIBO, the foundation of treatment is diet, because many bacteria feed on foods that are common in our diets.

And if you're like a lot of people I've worked with you might be asking yourself, "Why not just wipe them out with antibiotics?"

According to *The American Journal of Gastroenterology*, recurrence of small-intestine bacteria after antibiotics is quite high (the most commonly prescribed being rifaximin).[80]

Many people have to keep taking antibiotics over and over again for months with limited results.

And there is a tremendous cost to your immune system and to your future ability to defend yourself.

There is no better way to be defeated by an enemy than to give him repeated opportunities to adapt to your weapons.

The only thing that really works is to use diet as a foundation and then use something to eradicate the bacteria along with it.

There are a number of herbs that are quite effective for this—particularly those in the berberine family (goldenseal, coptis, etc.).

PROBIOTICS CAN ALSO BE BENEFICIAL

A pilot study published in *Acta Gastroenterológica Latinoamericana* in December 2010 found that probiotics may work better than pharmaceutical therapy for patients with chronic abdominal distention and SIBO.

> Based on these pilot study results, we can suggest that the probiotic herein [Lactobacillus casei, Lactobacillus plantarum, Streptococcus faecalis, Bifidobacterium brevis] used has a higher efficacy than metronidazonal in the early clinical response of patients with chronic abdominal distention and SIBO.[81]

In the next section, we'll look into more treatment options for SIBO.

---

80   "Small intestinal bacterial overgrowth recurrence after antibiotic therapy," by E. C. Lauritano et al, 2008, *American Journal of Gastroenterology, 103*(8), pp. 2031–2035.

81   "Comparative clinical efficacy of a probiotic vs. an antibiotic in the treatment of patients with intestinal bacterial overgrowth and chronic abdominal functional distension: A pilot study," by L. O. Soifer et al, *Acta Gastroenterológica Latinoamericana, 40*(4), pp. 323–327.

Recap

The heart is the emperor or empress and lives at the center of the body where it is protected by its loyal ministers and bodyguards.

The fire element is all about relationships and learning to listen to our hearts so that we can become integrated internally and externally.

We looked at SIBO, another potential monkey wrench in the gears of our healing machine. It may take some time to fix this stuff, people, so be aware.

Correcting SIBO can take up to two years. However, you should see improvement in your symptoms fairly quickly, with gradual and continuous improvement.

Stress, poor sleep, infections, and poor diet choices can all create setbacks. It is always difficult to commit to more restrictive forms of a paleo diet (which can be tough enough as it is!).

2. P = Prioritize and Plan

Not everything has the same level of importance. This is what 80/20 teaches us. Some things are having more of an impact than others. Figure out which they are (the positive feedback loops) and then make a plan to fix them.

There's an awful lot here to evaluate. The small intestine, in my opinion, is ground zero for autoimmune disease and Hashimoto's. It could be argued that there is no other place that's more important to focus your treatment.

And because this is also where many important vitamins and minerals that are responsible for healthy thyroid function are absorbed, this ecosystem must be kept healthy.

Finally, this is also where thyroid hormone is converted with the help of good bacteria.

The cardiovascular system is, of course, also important, and if you have many of the risk factors mentioned in this section I recommend focusing on the dietary elements that can heal the heart.

3. A = Act and Adapt

Act and put your plan into motion. Then observe the results. Double down on what works and change what doesn't. Results should be apparent relatively quickly. If they aren't, you need to make changes.

FIRE: HEART AND SMALL INTESTINE

FOODS FOR COMMON ISSUES:

High cholesterol: cholesterol-lowering foods such as apples, bananas, carrots, cold-water fish, garlic, grapefruit, olive oil, and fiber found in gluten-free oats
Stop eating so much sugar! Eliminate all refined sugars and flours.
Iron deficiency: dulse, kelp, rice bran, pumpkin seeds, beans, lentils, parsley, walnuts, apricots, almonds, raisins, Swiss chard, spinach, dates, figs, kale, cucumber, cauliflower, cabbage
B12 deficiency: beef liver, beef kidney, ham, sole, scallops, eggs, oats, pickles, amasake, algae, spirulina and chlorella, brewer's yeast
B6 deficiency: bananas, barley, brewer's yeast, molasses, soybeans, wheat bran, brown rice, liver, beef, cabbage, carrots, potatoes, yams
High homocysteine: Vitamin C, vitamin E, riboflavin, vitamin B6, folate, vitamin B12, and magnesium are all helpful, the B vitamins especially.
Dietary suggestions for calming and focusing the mind: oyster shell, grain, brown rice, oats, mushrooms, silicon foods, oatstraw tea, oat groat tea, cucumber, celery, lettuce, mulberries, lemons, jujube seeds, dill, basil

HERBS/SUPPLEMENTS:

Dietary suggestions for calming and focusing the mind: chamomile, catnip, skullcap, valerian

VITAMINS AND MINERALS:

B vitamins (see food sources in chapter 5 for a complete list), magnesium (found in chlorophyll-containing foods), amino acid L-tryptophan

THE SIBO DIET

The SIBO diet is a terrific exercise in subtraction and should generally be done for a month or so to get the best results.

Since there are many foods that feed these bacteria, there are many foods that must be eliminated from your diet for this initial period of time.

FOODS TO AVOID:

- **Fructose:** sugars, artificial sweeteners, corn syrup
- **Grains:** rice, wheat, quinoa, millet, amaranth, and some non-grains like tapioca
- **Legumes/galactans:** beans, peas, chickpeas, soybeans, lentils
- **Fructan-containing vegetables:** lettuce, onions, artichokes, beets, broccoli, cabbage, brussels sprouts, peas, asparagus, okra, shallots, mushrooms, green peppers, cauliflower
- **High-fructose fruits:** grapes, apples, watermelon, cherries, kiwifruit, bananas, blueberries, mangos
- **Meat products:** Breaded or processed meats such as hot dogs, bologna, potted meats, and most cold cuts (containing added starches). There are some experts who say to also avoid beef, pork, and lamb.

FOODS TO EAT:

- **Nuts:** all nuts, except pistachios
- **Vegetables:** all vegetables, except those listed above
- **Low-fructose fruits:** apricot, avocado, cantaloupe, grapefruit, honeydew melon, nectarine, orange, peach, pineapple, raspberry, strawberry, tomato
- **Meats:** chicken, fish, eggs; beef, lamb, and pork in moderation
- **Fats:** animal fat, oils

STEPS OF TREATMENT

The first step of treatment involves the diet as foundation and something to address the bacteria (like the herbs mentioned above).

Either during or after that Spartan menu, it is important to address the root causes and related issues of SIBO.

These problems include:

1. Too little stomach acid. Here's the exception to the healing by subtraction rule. If you have too little stomach acid, you need more.

A simple treatment is to take things that boost stomach acid levels, such as apple cider vinegar, lemon juice, and ginger root.

Supplementing with betain HCL may also be beneficial (consult your doctor for this).

2. An immune-suppressed gut. Often the cause of this is too much corticosteroid treatment and/or too much cortisol from stress.

Here the subtraction rule works quite well. Stop the corticosteroids (unless you have a condition where you must take them) and do something about stress.

A great daily exercise in doing less? Silent-seated meditation.

3. Injury to the gut nervous system (enteric nervous system)

This type of neurodegeneration is permanent. However, this nervous system also has remarkable plasticity and a capacity to rewire itself.

There are three really important things you can do to improve this damage:

1. **Vigorous gargling.** (I mean *really* vigorous—to the point of tears). Gargle with several glasses of water throughout the day.

    This activates part of the nervous system connected to the vagus nerve, which has a very strong connection to the gut.

2. **Stimulate your gag reflex.** Order some wooden tongue depressors online, and gently stimulate this reflex by pressing down on the tongue.

3. **Coffee enemas.** Make sure the coffee isn't too hot and hold as long as possible. This causes nerve firing in the brain.

    Start with a moderate amount of mild coffee; you can gradually increase both the amount of liquid and the strength of the coffee.

    (Best to do it in the bathtub if you have one, so you are close to the toilet.)

HOW LONG DO YOU NEED TO TREAT SIBO?

Good question. You need to treat it for as long as it takes! And you may have to revisit this periodically. Generally speaking, the more severe it is, the longer and more committed you must be to healing it.

This may take several months.

It's also true that the better you are at really following the diet and not cheating, the better the outcome and the faster your results.

I and others, like Dr. Sarah Ballantyne (The Paleo Mom) and Mickey Trescott, recommend combining one of these diets with an autoimmune paleo diet for the most rapid and effective reversal of SIBO.

QI GONG EXERCISE FOR THE FIRE ELEMENT

THE ARCHER

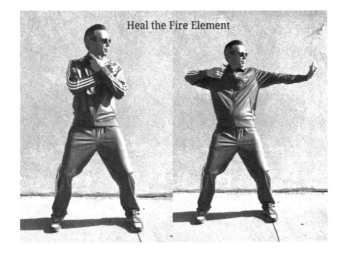

Heal the Fire Element

In this exercise, opening and extending the chest and turning the head increases blood flow in your head, neck, and chest. It also improves heart and lung function. It's a good exercise for improving posture and balance.

How to do it: Start in a natural standing position, feet shoulder-width apart, weight evenly distributed. Bend your knees slightly. Use this same position for the entire exercise.

Inhale and bring your arms in front of your chest in a crossed position about six inches in front of your heart with your palms facing toward your body and your right hand closer to your chest.

As you exhale, bring your gaze to your wrists. Focus on that spot, and in your mind imagine that you are unstoppable. Next, curl the fingers of your right hand as though drawing the string of a bow. Turn your left hand outward, away from your body. Imagine you are drawing the bow with your right hand.

Next, inhale again and turn your head and use your eyes to follow your left arm all the way to your middle finger. Push away from your body with your left hand, extend your arm fully, and point your palm straight up (at 90 degrees).

Imagine that your left hand is pushing against something big like a mountain or a redwood. At the same time, pull in the opposite direction with your right hand until your right fist is even with your right shoulder.

Make sure the whole movement is slow, deliberate, and not rushed.

Also, as you draw the bow, allow your hips to rotate toward your left hand a bit (this opens the lungs even more) and keep the knees bent. As the arms are fully stretched, focus on opening your chest, your lungs, your heart, and your mind.

Finally, exhale and return the hands to the crossed position in front of your body. Repeat the whole exercise in the opposite direction.

Repeat three times in both directions one or two times per day.

4. R= Reassess and Readjust

Retest, reassess, and ask all over again. Figure out what worked and what didn't. Double down on what worked and either eliminate or re-create a plan for what didn't.

With all the challenges that you may have to contend with in treating the fire element, it is very important to reassess and readjust.

Leaky gut, SIBO, and other infections of the small intestine can be long-term projects and it is not unusual for them to recur in the future.

It's very much like growing a garden. A garden requires ongoing care: planting, weeding, adding compost, harvesting, and so on. The same is true of the ecosystem of the small intestine.

And the heart and related issues of the blood, like anemias, high cholesterol, and homocysteine may need to be rechecked periodically. This is particularly important with Hashimoto's because of all the risk factors for heart attack and stroke.

5. T = Try and Try Again

Keep doing it, keep refining, keep building on the positive results, and keep looking for the remaining positive feedback loops that are causing vicious cycles.

As I hope you have seen repeatedly throughout this book, the process of healing requires a long-term commitment and an unwavering willingness to keep at it.

The larger goal of remission is the cumulative result of reaching many smaller goals first. It's important to acknowledge and celebrate these smaller victories as well. They are the building blocks of success.

So pay attention, keep some kind of journal (physical or electronic), keep building on what works, and keeping evaluating and removing what doesn't serve you and your health.

In the final section of the book, I've created an "action plan" that summarizes the most important areas (the 20 percent) that are priorities.

If you focus your attention on these areas, you will find that you get results faster and that you can turn the tide against the downward spirals that can drag your mental, physical, and emotional health downhill.

HASHIMOTO'S HEALING ACTION PLAN

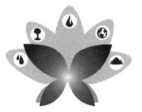

In this final part of the book, I'm going to break it all down for you—everything you need to get started. And we'll look at in two ways: What you need to do and the mind-set you need to have.

You can just jump to this section anytime you feel lost or need a reminder.

As I shared in the introduction to this book, I believe in the 80/20 rule, that 20 percent of things are causing 80 percent of your symptoms.

This Cheat Sheet covers the 20 percent.

Focus on these and chances are you'll see some improvement right away.

As you know, I've worked with an awful lot of people with Hashimoto's (this is all I do) and I've spent years studying and looking at research on how this condition impacts the body.

The most important thing I've learned is that Hashimoto's is much more than a thyroid problem.

It's an autoimmune disease, but it's not just an immune system problem either. It's an all-over-your-body problem.

Your body is not a machine. Like the earth, it's a complex group of ecosystems that all interact. And these ecosystems can all be adversely affected by Hashimoto's.

When this happens you get a downward spiral of vicious cycles all feeding on one another.

POSITIVE FEEDBACK LOOPS

This is caused by positive feedback loops, which is really just another way of saying that things repeat over and over again with time.

These create webs that can lead to problems with virtually all the major systems of the body. These include issues with the brain, adrenals, liver, and gallbladder, and problems with the digestive tract, such as acid reflux, leaky gut, body-wide pain and inflammation, and more.

All of this can result in anxiety, depression, gallstones, poor liver detoxification, poor absorption of vitamins and nutrients, poor conversion of thyroid hormone, blood sugar imbalances, terrible fatigue, and immune responses to various triggers, from foods to environmental toxins and chemicals.

I admit I'm a bit obsessed with this, but there's an argument to make that problems in every system you can imagine are caused by the ripple effect of hypothyroidism and autoimmunity on all the various systems of your body.

I've sometimes heard doctors shame their patients by saying, "People just try to blame everything on this disease." Well, that's because everything *is* being caused by this disease. Thyroid hormone impacts virtually every system of the body.

So, it's not your fault.

However, now that you understand this, it's your responsibility to do something about it. You need to take your health into your own hands.

HOW DO YOU FIGURE OUT WHICH SYSTEMS ARE BREAKING DOWN?

This is half the battle. Once we answer this question, we can start fixing things.

First, you have to be able to see the big picture. Then identify which areas of your body need attention.

Create a plan for healing those areas and then execute that plan.

Next, you need to find the most destructive triggers and eliminate them. (The reality is that both of these things need to be done at the same time to get the best results.)

WHERE THE MAGIC HAPPENS

When you do these two things, something magical happens.

All of those vicious cycles get turned on their heads and start having a positive impact on the other systems.

You start using positive feedback to your advantage. When that happens, you can stop triggering the immune system and start to restore balance.

Then the body can heal itself.

In the beginning, this will give you glimpses of more good days than bad ones, and if you stay the course and work on the big picture you can even get your disease into remission.

(But remember, that's not permission to go back to everything that got you sick in the first place.)

So, break that down into the changes you need to make.

STEP I: START WITH THE DIET

The diet is your foundation for healing. The gut is ground zero for autoimmunity and Hashimoto's. We have discussed this at length in this book.

In my experience, you're just spitting against Niagara Falls if you are trying to heal Hashimoto's without changing your diet.

The first thing you need to do is begin. Don't make excuses or rationalize why you're the exception. In most cases, you aren't the exception. Everyone with autoimmune disease has some degree of breakdown of their gut.

If you've been diagnosed with Hashimoto's, then you do, too. So stop putting it off and stop waiting for the perfect time to get started. Now is the perfect time.

Test this approach first to determine whether it will benefit you. Don't decide before you try it. And understand that this is a long-term project. You might not get miraculous results right away.

If you're already on this diet and aren't getting the results you had hoped for, check out this post in the supplemental section of our website on some of the potential reasons why: www.hashimtoshealing.com/r2rsupplemental

GET YOUR MIND RIGHT:

Something else you need to come to grips with is that this is a long-term project. Like, really long. Basically, the rest of your life.

Face it, accept it, and embrace the idea that from this point on, you're a "gut farmer" and weeding, cultivating, fertilizing, composting, and healing the ecosystem of your gut is your vocation.

Get some cookbooks, start spending some time in the kitchen and the garden, and get into it. It can be fun and incredibly rewarding if you just surrender and go for it.

WHAT DIET IS RIGHT FOR YOU?

I recommend starting with a strict autoimmune paleo diet, which means the elimination phase. You can ease into it and start by eliminating gluten, dairy, and soy 100 percent, or you can just jump into it and cut out everything.

Find a strategy that works for you. Get your family onboard and get some friends onboard and support one another.

Once you get started, think of this diet as home base. Once you've gone through the initial elimination stage and slowly and carefully reintroduced things, you may be able to venture off the farm every once in a while, but don't go too far, and always go back when you have a flare-up of symptoms or start feeling crappy again.

And if you have gone too far, start all over again and go back to the elimination diet 100 percent.

This diet is the foundation and it is home base, but it may not solve all of your problems. And you may need to tweak it for your particular set of circumstances.

Some people do better with a bit more carbohydrates, so adding more resistant starches may be something you need to do.

But first, you need to start, you need to get some data from the experience of doing it, and then you need analyze and reassess (use the A.P.A.R.T. system) and make changes and adjustments as necessary.

STEP 2: START INVESTIGATING THE OTHER SYSTEMS OF YOUR BODY AND START PUTTING TOGETHER YOUR HEALING ACTION PLAN

Let's review those. We'll start at the top and work our way down.

I. THE BRAIN:

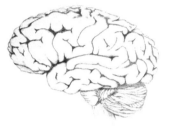

Many of the most common symptoms of Hashimoto's are brain-based.

For example, fatigue, brain fog, memory issues, depression, anxiety, constipation, and more can all come from how the brain is affected by hypothyroidism and autoimmunity.

Here are a few things that a healthy Hashimoto's brain needs (and, as it turns out, all of these things are also beneficial to your thyroid and the rest of your body):

1. Sugar. The brain is the body's biggest consumer of sugar. However, this is not a license to hammer Snickers bars.

The key is to not have too much or too little. There's a "Goldilocks" zone. If you're hypoglycemic, make sure your sugar level doesn't crash. (See below for a more in-depth discussion.)

If you're a sugar addict, admit it, stop living in denial, and get help. Treat your addiction.

2. Oxygen. The brain needs oxygen.

Iron deficiency and other anemia can put a hurt on your brain. Don't do that. Get an iron panel and check your ferritin. Order a CBC and check red blood cell values. Check hemoglobin, RBC, and other red blood cell values.

3. Blood flow. The brain needs blood flow.

Many people with Hashimoto's and hypothyroidism have low/normal blood pressure. That's not always a good thing. Low blood pressure is a major risk factor for Alzheimer's. So get blood flowing to your brain.

If your blood pressure is consistently low, try adding some salt to your diet, especially sea salt or Himalayan salt, as they are high in trace minerals.

Also, anemia is a big problem for the brain. You can't be even a little iron deficient or B12 deficient or any other kind of deficient.

Rule these things out. If you have them, they must be dealt with. Being even "a little anemic" is a big deal. It has major consequences.

4. Less inflammation. Inflammation is the root of all evil.

An inflamed brain is not a good thing. Just ask former NFL players.

Inflammation of any kind in the brain can take a long time to resolve. When you have brain inflammation, the immune system in the brain goes into overdrive and starts destroying brain cells in the process.

No bueno.

Try turmeric and lots of it.

5. Sleep. So important, yet so overlooked.

Turn off the TV. Move it out of the bedroom if you need to. Think of sleep as the most important thing you can do for your health. If you're having trouble sleeping, read on.

6. Get your mind right. Brain inflammation is no joke. This can progress to Alzheimer's or Parkinson's-like symptoms. Hashimoto's can lead to major degeneration of your brain.

It's not your fault, but it is your responsibility to do something about it.

Since the gut and the brain are so closely related, you kind of need to be a brain farmer as well as a gut farmer. The good news is, healthy choices made in one area benefit the other.

II. THE ENDOCRINE GLANDS:

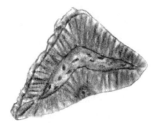

For a lot of people with Hashimoto's, the adrenals are a critical piece of the puzzle.

The warning label on Synthroid and other thyroid replacement hormone warns that if a patient has adrenal insufficiency he or she should not be prescribed the drug.

That's how important the adrenals are.

They can be the difference between you turning this thing around and you treading water and not improving or just continuing to get worse.

In our practice, we do proper testing evaluation and treatment of the adrenals. The best test is the ASI or adrenal salivary index. I also gave you some other tests to consider in the chapters on the water element.

And, of course, it does no good to just test and not do anything about stress. For the vast majority of us Hashimoto's folks, stress can cause major problems.

You don't need testing to understand this.

When you are stressed, you can have more immune flare-ups and this can trigger your Hashimoto's and make it worse.

So, what are you doing about stress?

You need to actually be doing things about it. Meditating, resting, getting massages, doing yoga or qi gong, going for walks in nature, having fun—all of these can have a positive impact.

This is not optional or some luxury that you treat yourself with once a year. This needs to be a daily part of your regimen.

Because here's the tricky thing about adrenal stress: It's almost always caused—at least in part—by something else.

These causes include anemia, blood sugar swings, gut inflammation, food intolerances (especially gluten, dairy, and soy), essential fatty acid deficiencies, environmental toxins, and of course, chronic emotional and psychological stress.

Sound familiar?

These are also all the things that make Hashimoto's worse.

We can't ignore them or pretend like they aren't there. We have to deal with all of them.

We have maxed out our stress cards (like our credit cards for stress). With Hashimoto's your body is under so much physiological stress, all the time, that extra emotional stress will often totally wipe you out.

This happens because we've emptied our accounts and now we have to start putting relaxation and fun back into our "stress savings" accounts.

Seriously, you have to replenish this account. It's not enough to say, "Yeah, I have nothing in that account."

Because just like a bank account, if you aren't putting money back in and you're always just taking money out, what happens?

Eventually you'll go broke, you'll have creditors after you, you'll lose your house and your car, and you'll wind up on the street.

Talked about stressed out!

That's what's happening in your body. You wind up with the functional equivalent of being homeless inside your own body.

So come up with an actual stress strategy. This means real action items, things that you are going to do for yourself on a daily, weekly, and monthly basis to stop stress from preventing you from getting any better.

BLOOD SUGAR PROBLEMS

WELCOME TO THE BLOOD SUGAR VICIOUS CYCLE

Both high blood sugar and low blood sugar levels can make your Hashimoto's worse.

These spikes and crashes of blood sugar add significant stress to the body, cause your adrenals to pump out cortisol (which makes the gut break down), make thyroid hormone not work as well, and push autoimmunity.

You have to deal with sugar like it's one of your top priority issues.

If you are hypoglycemic, you can't let your blood sugar crash; you must be on top of this and make sure you always have something to snack on and that you do not allow yourself to get too irritable, angry, spacey, forgetful, or really hungry.

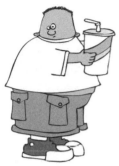

If you reach that point, it's too late.

Instead, start the day with a good protein and fat combination, eat every few hours, and avoid high-sugar foods and refined carbohydrates that will make you spike and crash to the floor like a lead balloon.

If you arc insulin rcsistant and/or you've been diagnosed with metabolic syndrome or type 2 diabetes, chances are you're a sugar addict.

Sugar is more addictive and, arguably, more dangerous than cocaine for people with Hashimoto's. You have to treat it as such.

If you follow an autoimmune paleo diet to the letter, it will help. But you may need to do a sugar detox and really go cold turkey and see just how bad it is.

Sugar is *not* your friend. It's not a good source of energy; it may provide some comfort, but that comfort is short-lived and it comes with a nice helping of increased suffering.

Let go of sugar and set yourself free. Look for other ways to get a rush of dopamine into your life, like exercise, meditation, art, and music. There are so many other ways to feel good.

IT'S ANOTHER VICIOUS CYCLE

If you want to heal your Hashimoto's, you need to deal with blood sugar issues. And that means dealing with your sugar habit.

III. THE GUT

The more I study and learn, the more research I see, and the more people I work with, I am convinced that the gut is ground zero for autoimmunity. It's a place of maximum leverage.

It may be in the top 5 to 10 percent of the 20 percent.

Investing in healing the gut is an investment that can give you a three to ten times return on your investment.

It's worth every bit of time, energy, effort, and money you put into it.

Real gut health begins with what you put in your mouth and then continues on down your digestive tract.

I'm always shocked when patients tell me their doctors say, "Diet doesn't matter."

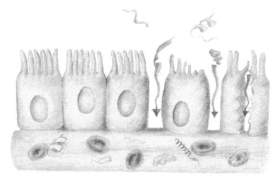

Healing leaky gut should be a priority

This reflects an extraordinary level of ignorance. It's a lie, and ignoring this leads a lot of people to get a lot sicker.

In addition, many doctors say going gluten-free is a fad and isn't such a big deal.

This is also absurd when you look at the research.

Every organ along the way needs to be examined and healed, if necessary.

This begins with the stomach.

Hashimoto's and hypothyroidism can cause too little stomach acid to be secreted, which leads to problems all down the line.

So start there.

Review the earth element section on stomach acid issues.

Once you've addressed the stomach, you need to make sure the pancreas is functioning properly (we have discussed that in detail already).

Balance your blood sugar.

From there it's the liver and gallbladder. These are also hugely important.

Review the chapters on the wood element.

Then we move on to the real home of autoimmune disease, the small intestine.

This is where it all began and where it continues to flourish if you don't do something about it.

One big issue we discussed at length is leaky gut.

Heal the environment of the intestines. Understand that parasites, yeast, and bacterial overgrowth can all be potential problems.

Guess what often helps all of those—cutting out all refined sugars.

Another complication we find is something called SIBO, which stands for small intestinal bacterial overgrowth.

This can be caused by too little stomach acid and can lead to leaky gut. All of these things can make one another worse.

And there you have it.

Here's a quick overview of the most common issues that need fixing.

Get to work on those areas and chances are you'll start to feel a whole lot better.

Get Your Mind Right: Your gut is ground zero. Your health and recovery depends on it getting healed. Invest in gut healing.

Become a gut farmer. Make this your vocation, your passion, your expertise. Heal the earth element. While we're at it, let's heal planet Earth, too.

Finally, here's a reminder of the A.P.A.R.T. System, which is designed to take the guesswork out of this process and is guaranteed to keep you on track and to get results if you use it.

The A.P.A.R.T. System

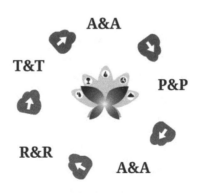

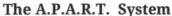

The A.P.A.R.T. System

Apply the A.P.A.R.T. System to all the areas mentioned at the beginning of the Action Plan section.

1. Your brain

2. Your adrenals

3. Blood sugar imbalances

4. Your gut

5. Your stomach

6. Your liver

1. A = Ask and Assess

Data has healing power—if you know what data to collect and analyze and you know what to do with that information. (Both are big ifs.)

You need to ask what the symptoms are and assess the different systems of the body to find out where these symptoms are coming from.

Everything needs to be a suspect. Don't exclude something because you're attached to it or feel like you can't do without it. Everything in your life should be evaluated, and if it isn't working to make you better, it should be eliminated.

This includes people, places, and things, like your favorite foods and drinks.

2. P = Prioritize and Plan

Not everything has the same level of importance. This is what 80/20 teaches us. Some things are having more of an impact than others. Figure out which they are (the positive feedback loops), focus on those first, and then make a plan to fix them.

Use the Cheat Sheet to identify the top suspects that are causing 80 percent of your problems.

3. A = Act and Adapt

Act and put a plan into motion.

Incorporate the foods and qi gong exercises from this book into your everyday life.

Then observe the results. Double down on what works and change what doesn't. Results should be apparent relatively quickly. If they aren't, you need to make changes.

The common practice of prescribing something and then telling the patient to come back in 3 to 6 months is ridiculous, in my opinion. That's way too long, especially if it isn't working.

4. R = Reassess and Readjust

Retest, reassess, and ask all over again. Figure out what worked and what didn't. Double down on what worked and either eliminate or re-create a plan for what didn't.

It sounds obvious, but it is often overlooked or forgotten. Testing and reevaluating what you have done to see the result of your treatment is essential for good care.

Quick side note here: What I have learned over many years of practice is that you need to trust what the data is telling you. In most cases, when you make the right choice you start feeling better.

Things like a "healing crisis," a "die-off," or a "detox reaction" sometimes occur, but they can also be a cover for incompetence. The right decision should yield a positive result relatively quickly.

If you are doing something and you aren't getting better or you continue to feel worse or it causes more discomfort, pain, and adverse symptoms, then you need to question whether or not that is the best course of action.

Eliminate it, reduce variables, and find out which part of what you are doing is causing that reaction or set of symptoms.

And all of this should not be done on the basis of lab tests alone. With Hashimoto's, the process must include a thorough examination of the signs and symptoms as well.

Remember, what you feel is diagnostically important and clinically relevant.

5. T = Try and Try Again

Keep doing it, keep refining, keep building on the positive results, and keep looking for the remaining positive feedback loops that are causing vicious cycles.

People sometimes give up before giving a certain approach a chance. Or they get some good results and then slide back to their old ways of doing things. When you find something that works, keep doing it. Don't quit and don't give up.

Success is defined by the transformation of a vicious cycle into positive healing momentum. This means you start to feel better and then exponentially better.

Lab work and symptoms should all confirm that this has taken place. You can do this!

YOU AREN'T ALONE

Remember, you aren't alone in this.

And you aren't going to fix everything in a day or two. The first step is to identify where the problems are.

The next step is to figure out which systems are in the worst shape and start with healing those.

Then you need to keep moving on to the other systems and periodically circle back to the big ones and reevaluate.

It's not as hard as it seems.

It just takes a little commitment and focus. And it really helps to have a plan.

If you want help, I'm here for you.

If you want to talk to me and learn more, you can contact me at marc@hashimotos healing.com or set up a 30-minute Hashimoto's Healing Discovery Session.

In it you can share where you are and where you want to be, I can make some recommendations right away, and we can discuss how working together can get you better faster.

Yours in Remission,
Marc Ryan, L.Ac.

Resources

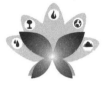

Marc Ryan, L.Ac.

1825 West 153rd Street
Gardena, CA 90249
Telephone: 310-831-2202
Fax: 310-831-2203
E-mail: marc@hashimotoshealing.com

The author of this book, Marc Ryan, L.Ac., is available for appointments virtually via phone or Skype and in his Gardena office. His website and blog also include a great deal of useful information.

ADDITIONAL RESOURCES

Blog: www.hashimotoshealing.com /life-with-hashimotos/

Facebook: www.facebook.com /hashimotoshealing

Twitter: @hashimotohealer

YouTube: https://www.youtube.com /channel/UCneuu5yMTHtfy5DJikTBJqg

Marc also offers professional training for doctors, naturopaths, chiropractors, and acupuncturists.

He is currently working with Bastyr University to create an online version of this professional training, which will be available in 2017. For more information contact him at marc@hashimotoshealing.com.

BOOKS

Dao of Chinese Medicine: Understanding an Ancient Healing Art, by Donald E. Kendall

The Web That Has No Weaver: Understanding Chinese Medicine, by Ted J. Kaptchuk, O.M.D.

Between Heaven and Earth, by Harriet Beinfield, L.Ac., and Efrem Korngold, L.Ac., O.M.D.

Tao: The Subtle Universal Law & the Integral Way of Life, by Hua-Ching Ni

The Tao Te Ching, by Lao Tzu

The Autoimmune Paleo Cookbook, by Mickey Trescott, N.T.P.

The Paleo Approach, by Sarah Ballantyne, Ph.D.

Why Do I Still Have Thyroid Symptoms? When My Lab Tests Are Normal, by Datis Kharrazian, D.H.Sc., D.C., M.S.

Hashimoto's Thyroiditis: Lifestyle Interventions for Finding and Treating the Root Cause, by Izabella Wentz, Pharm.D., F.A.S.C.P., with Marta Nowosadzka, M.D.

Nourishing Destiny: The Inner Tradition of Chinese Medicine, by Lonny S. Jarrett

Your Healthy Pregnancy with Thyroid Disease, by Dana Trentini and Mary Shomon

The Autoimmune Solution, by Amy Myers, M.D.

Grain Brain, by David Perlmutter, M.D.

Why Meditate? by Matthieu Ricard

Chinese Medical Herbology and Pharmacology, by John K. Chen and Tina T. Chen

Healing with Whole Foods, by Paul Pitchford

SKIN CARE

Oessencials Organics
www.oessencials.com

Handmade, organic skin care. Phenomenally effective!

FOOD

Autoimmune Paleo Resources

Autoimmune Paleo
Great recipes and wellness tips
www.autoimmune-paleo.com

Fresh Bites Daily
www.freshbitesdaily.com

The Paleo Mom
Great recipes and research analysis
www.paleomom.com

Simple & Merry
www.simpleandmerry.com

The Weston A. Price Foundation
www.westonprice.org

Coconut Products

Coconut Aminos (soy sauce alternative)
https://www.coconutsecret.com/aminos2
.html

Edward & Sons
This online grocer carries Native Forest brand coconut milks: BPA-free cans of organic, non-GMO coconut milk.

http://www.edwardandsons.com/native
_shop_coconut.itml

Virgin coconut oil and coconut flour
www.tropicaltraditions.com

Fermented Foods

Immunitrition
www.immunitrition.com

Wise Choice Market
www.wisechoicemarket.com/organic-raw
-fermented-vegetables

Kombucha

Health benefits and how to make it
www.foodrenegade.com/how-to-brew
-kombucha-double-fermentation-menthod/

Water Kefir

www.wellnessmama.com/2237/water-kefir
-variations/

Gnowfglins (Traditional Cooking School)

www.gnowfglins.com

Food Organizations/Nonprofits

Center for Food Safety
www.centerforfoodsafety.org

Community Supported Agriculture (CSA)
www.localharvest.org/csa/

Eat Well Guide
www.eatwellguide.org

Environmental Working Group
This site features an excellent, downloadable guide to the fruits and vegetables with pesticide levels (high and low) and lots of other valuable information on environmental toxins
www.ewg.org

Farmers' Markets

This is a national listing of farmers' markets.
https://www.ams.usda.gov/services/local-regional/food-directories

Local Harvest

Use this website to find farmers' markets, family farms, and other sources of sustainably grown food in your area.
www.localharvest.org

Non-GMO Shopping Guide

www.nongmoshoppingguide.com

Organic Consumers Association

www.organicconsumers.org

Seafood Watch

Learn what environmental toxins are found in which type of seafood and which seafood is sustainably harvested
www.seafoodwatch.org

Gluten-Free Food Sources and Information

(These gluten-free products are not recommended during the elimination phase of the Autoimmune Paleo Diet)

Bob's Red Mill
www.bobsredmill.com

Cappello's Pasta
https://cappellosglutenfree.com

GlutenFree.com
www.glutenfree.com

Nuts.com
nuts.com/cookingbaking/gluten-free-flour/

Gluten-Free Flours

On the Go Paleo
www.puretraditionsfoods.com

Top Six Gluten-Free Pastas
www.bewell.com/blog/top-6-gluten-free-pastas/

Grass-Fed Meats and Poultry

Eat Wild
www.eatwild.com

U.S. Wellness Meats
www.grasslandbeef.com

Vital Choice
www.vitalchoice.com

Wise Choice Market
You can buy bone broth here if you don't want to make your own.
www.wisechoicemarket.com/bone-broth

Wild and Organic Fish

Vital Choice
www.vitalchoice.com

Wild Planet
www.wildplanetfoods.com

Online Herb & Grocery Stores

Green Pasture
www.greenpasture.org

Mountain Rose Herbs
www.mountainroseherbs.com

Thrive Market
www.thrivemarket.com

Wild Mountain Paleo Market
www.wildmountainpaleo.com

Teas and Coffee Alternatives

Breakaway Matcha
www.breakawaymatcha.com

Dandy Blend
www.dandyblend.com/

Green Tea
www.traditionalmedicinals.com/product_categories/green-teas/

Guyakí Yerba Mate
guayaki.com/product/47/Traditional-Yerba
-Mate-Tea-Bags.html

Teeccino
www.teechino.com

MEDITATION

Insight Timer
www.insighttimer.com

Buddhify
www.Buddhify.com

Calm
www.calm.com

Headspace
www.headspace.com

RECIPES

Against All Grain
www.againstallgrain.com

Candice Kumai
www.candicekumai.com

Deliciously Organic
www.deliciouslyorganic.net

Elana's Pantry
www.elanaspantry.com

Guilty Kitchen
www.guiltykitchen.com

The Healthy Apple
www.thehealthyapple.com

My New Roots
www.mynewroots.org/site/

Nourished Kitchen
nourishedkitchen.com

Rubies & Radishes
www.rubiesandradishes.com

The Spunky Coconut
www.thespunkycoconut.com

ENVIRONMENTAL SUPPORT AND INFORMATION

Air Filters

AllerAir
www.allerair.com

IQAir
www.iqair.com

Moso Natural
www.mosonatural.com

Cleaning Products

EWG's Guide to Healthy Cleaning
www.ewg.org/guides/cleaners

Gimme the Good Stuff
gimmethegoodstuff.org/safe-product
-guides

Home Products

Allergy Buyers Club
www.allergybuyersclub.com

Baby Earth
www.babyearth.com

EcoChoices Natural Living Store
www.ecochoices.com

Green Home
www.greenhome.com

Lifekind
www.lifekind.com

THYROID

American Association of Clinical Endo-crinologists
www.aace.com

American Thyroid Association
www.thyroid.org

Hashimoto's Awareness
www.hashimotosawareness.org

Hashimoto's 411
Patient-led support
www.hashimotos411.com

HypothyroidMom
Founded by Dana Trentini, a great site with lots of resources
www.hypothyroidmom.com

DrKNews
Dr. Kharrazian's blog, full of lots of great information
drknews.com

National Academy of Hypothyroidism
Led by Dr. Ken Holtorf, great research and information on thyroid disease
www.nahypothyroidism.org

Stop the Thyroid Madness
Patient advocates with great information
www.stopthethyroidmadness.com

Thyroid Change
Working to bring about change in the way thyroid patients are treated; sign the petition so your voice is heard.
www.thyroidchange.org

NONPROFITS

Environmental Working Group
www.ewg.org

Healthy Child Healthy World
www.healthychild.org

Institute for Responsible Technology
www.responsibletechnology.org

Just Label It!
www.justlabelit.org

Non-GMO Project
www.nongmoproject.org

WATER FILTERS

Aquasana
www.aquasana.com

Berkey Filters
www.berkeyfilters.com

PUR
www.pur.com

Additional References
and Commentary

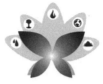

Preface

After creating the A.P.A.R.T. System, I discovered "biohacking" and noticed some similarities. The main point is that we need an approach that is adaptable to change and provides us with a blueprint for long-term improvement.

The current Western medical model doesn't empower the patient with tools for adaptation and progressive improvement. The A.P.A.R.T. System provides an easy-to-repeat program that is both adaptable and designed to create long-term healing momentum.

Introduction

(2014). *Synthroid sales data*. Retrieved from:
https://www.drugs.com/stats/synthroid

According to this data, the hypothyroid medication levothyroxine (Synthroid, AbbVie) continues to be the nation's most prescribed drug.

Holtorf Medical Group. (n.d.). *The best clinical guidelines money can buy: A look at guidelines bias and thyroid treatment*. Retrieved from https://www.holtorfmed.com/best-clinical-guidelines-money-can-buy-look-bias-guidelines-impact-thyroid-patients.

This article cites evidence of clear conflicts of interest in The American Association of Clinical Endocrinologists (AACE) and the American Thyroid Association (ATA) task force on adult hypothyroidism, and their "Clinical Practice Guidelines for Hypothyroidism in Adults" (The "Guidelines") in 2012.

The authors included Jeffrey R. Garber, Rhoda H. Cobin, Hossein Gharib, James V. Hennessey, Irwin Klein, Jeffrey I. Mechanick, Rachel Pessah-Pollack, Peter A. Singer, and Kenneth A. Woeber. In the published guidelines' reference to financial disclosures, only Jeffrey Mechanick was listed as having any financial ties, in this case to Abbott, parent company of AbbVie, which manufactures Synthroid.

While the other guidelines committee members claimed they had "no relevant financial relationships with any commercial interests," this is not true. A search of the ProPublica "Dollars for Doctors" database shows that committee member Rhoda Cobin has financial ties to drug companies.

Peter Singer has disclosed in other venues that he is a consultant for Abbvie Pharmaceuticals, maker of Synthroid. Hossein Gharib and James Hennessey have also been speakers at AbbVie-financed symposia.

At the time of writing this book, I have had 2,325 consultations with Hashimoto's patients. I had 1,093 free consultations and 432 clients. I have tallied more detailed data on the clients, but we are still studying this data.

I surveyed 904 individuals who were diagnosed with Hashimoto's. These took place from April 2013 to June 2015. The average patient age was 46: 870 were female and 34 were male. Five hundred two were on thyroid replacement hormone; 402 were not. The most commonly prescribed drug was Synthroid, followed by Levothyroxine, Armour, and Naturethroid. The most common symptoms included fatigue, brain fog, weight gain, depression, anxiety, hair loss/thinning hair, constipation, and insomnia.

Ho, T. W. T., Shaheen, A. A., Dixon, E., & Harvey, A. (2011). Utilization of thyroidectomy for benign disease in the United States: A 15-year population based study. *American Journal of Surgery, 201*(5), 570–4.

"The authors found that the percentage of patients having total thyroidectomy increased from 17.6 percent (from 1993–1997) to 39.4 percent (from 2003–2007) for benign, non-cancerous, thyroid disease.

While there was very little variation across different regions of the United States, patients were most likely to undergo total thyroidectomy at an urban teaching hospital than in urban non-teaching or rural hospitals.

The authors also found that the length of time spent in the hospital and the hospital charges were significantly more for total thyroidectomy. The data also demonstrated a higher rate of post-operative complications with total thyroidectomy, such as low calcium levels, bleeding, and hoarseness due to vocal cord problems.

Hospitals that performed a higher number of thyroid operations were found to have lower complication rates."

Azad, Kalid. (2007). *Understanding the pareto principle (the 80/20 rule)*. Retrieved from https://betterexplained.com/articles/understanding-the-pareto-principle-the-8020-rule

Chapter 1: Functional Medicine and the 5 Elements of Thyroid Health

Descotes J., & Vial, T. (1994). Immunetoxic effects of xenobiotics in humans: A review of current evidence. *Toxicology in Vitro, 8*(5), 963–966.

Steventon, G. B., Heafield, M. T., Sturman, S., Waring, R. H., Williams, A. C. (1990). Xenobiotic metabolism in Alzheimer's disease. *Neurology, 40*(7), 1095–1098.

Rigden, S., Barrager, E., Bland, J. S. (1998). Evaluation of the effect of a modified entero-hepatic resuscitation program in chronic fatigue syndrome patients. *Journal of Advancement in Medicine, 11*(4), 247–262.

Mckinnon, R. A., & Nebert, D. W. (1994). Possible role of cytochromes P450 in lupus erythematosus and related disorders. *Lupus, 3*(6), 473–478.

Braverman, L. E., & Utiger, R. D. (2005). *Werner and Ingbar's the thyroid: A fundamental and clinical text.* (9th ed., pp. 769–850). Philadelphia: Lippincott Williams & Wilkins.

Chapters 2–5 (Thyroid):

Gibson, P. R., & Shepherd, S. J. (2010). Evidence-based dietary management of functional gastrointestinal symptoms: The FODMAP approach. *Journal of Gastroenterology and Hepatology, 25*(2), 252–258.

Kharrazian, D. (2012). *Mastering functional blood chemistry*. Seminar.

Lord, R. S., & Bralley, J. A. (2008). *Laboratory evaluations for integrative and functional medicine* (2nd ed.) Duluth: Metametrix Institute.

Kharrazian, D. (2011). *Mastering the thyroid*. Seminar.

Braverman, L. E., & Utiger, R. D. (2005). Part II laboratory assessment of thyroid function, Section B causes of hypothyroidism. *Werner & Ingbar's the thyroid: A fundamental and clinical text* (9th ed., pp. 309–373, 701–714). Philadelphia: Lippincott Williams & Wilkins.

Flaws, B., & Sionneau, P. (2001). *The treatment of modern western medical diseases with Chinese medicine: A textbook and clinical manual* (pp. 241–246). Boulder: Blue Poppy Press.

Lakatos, P. (2003). Thyroid hormones: beneficial or deleterious for bone? *Calcified Tissue International, 73*(3), 205–209.

Muller, M. J., Burger, A. C., Ferrannini, E., Jequier, E., & Acheson, K. J. (1989). Glucoregulatory function of thyroid hormones: Role of pancreatic hormones. *American Journal of Physiology, 256*(1), E101–E110.

Calzà, L., Aloe, L., & Giardino, L. (1997). Thyroid hormone-induced plasticity in the adult rat brain. *Brain Research Bulletin, 44*(4), 549–557.

Lima, F. R. S., Gervais, A., Colin, C., Izembart, M., Neto, V. M., & Mallat, M. (2001). Regulation of microglial development: A novel role for thyroid hormones. *The Journal of Neuroscience, 21*(6), 2028–2038.

Oge, A., Sozmen, E., & Karaoglu, A. O. (2004). Effect of thyroid function on LDL oxidation in hypothyroidism and hyperthyroidism. *Endocrine Research, 30*(3), 481–489.

Laukkarinen, J., Kiudelis, G., Lempinen, M., Räty, S., Pelli, H., Sand, J., . . . Nordback, I. (2007). Increased prevalence of subclinical hypothyroidism in common bile duct stone patients. *The Journal of Clinical Endocrinology & Metabolism, 92*(11), 4260–4264.

Inkinen, J., Sand, J., & Nordback, I. (2000). Association between common bile duct stones and treated hypothyroidism. *Hepato-Gastroenterology, 47*(34), 919–921.

Napoli R., Guardasole, V., Angelini, V., Zarra, E., Terraciano, D., D'Anna, C., . . . Saccà, L. (2007). Acute effects of triiodothyronine on endothelial function in human subjects. *The Journal of Clinical Endocrinology & Metabolism, 92*(1), 250–254.

Taddei S., Caraccio, N., Virdis, A., Dardano, A., Versari, D., Ghiadoni, L., . . . Monzani, F. (2003). Impaired endothelium-dependent vasodilation in subclinical hypothyroidism: beneficial effect of levothyroxine therapy. *The Journal of Clinical Endocrinology & Metabolism, 88*(8), 3731–3737.

Pustorino S., Foti, M., Calipari, G., Pustorino, E., Ferraro, R., Guerrisi, O., & Germanotta, G. (2004). Thyroid-intestinal motility interactions summary. *Minerva Gastroenterologica e Dietologica, 50*(4), 305–315.

Green, J. R. (1979). Diminished TSH repines to TRH stimulation in patients with hepatic cirrhosis dispute subnormal T3 levels. Z. *Gastroenterology, 17*(7), 447–451.

Saha, B., & Maity, C. (2002). Alteration of serum enzymes in primary hypothyroidism. *Clinical Chemistry and Laboratory Medicine, 40*(6), 609–611.

Purandare, A., Co Ng, L., Godil, M., Ahnn, S. H., & Wilson, T. A. (2003). Effect of hypothyroidism and its treatment on IGF system in infants and children. *Journal of Pediatric Endocrinology and Metabolism, 16*(1), 35–42.

Jarrett, L. S. (1998). *Nourishing destiny: The inner tradition of Chinese medicine.* (pp. 121–136). Stockbridge, MA: Spirit Path Press.

van den Beld, A. W. (2005). Thyroid hormone concentrations, disease, physical function and mortality in elderly men. *The Journal of Clinical Endocrinology & Metabolism, 90*(12), 6403–6409.

Scobbo, R. R., VonDohlen, T. W., Hassan, M., & Islam, S. (2004). Serum TSH variability in normal individuals: The influence of time of sample collection. *West Virginia Medical Journal, 100*(4), 138–142.

Brown, J. (n.d.) *Food sources of vitamins and minerals.* Retrieved from http://www.epl.umn.edu/let/pubs/img/adol_appendix.pdf

Virion, A., Deme, D., Pommier, J., & Nunez, J. (1980). Opposite effects of thiocyanate on tyrosine iodination and thyroid hormone synthesis. *European Journal of Biochemistry, 112*(1), 1–7.

Yuan, G. F., Sun, B., Yuan, J., & Wang, Q. M. (2009). Effects of different cooking methods on health-promoting compounds of broccoli. *Journal of Zhejiang University SCIENCE B, 10*(8), 580–588.

Zimmermann, M. B., & Kohrle, J. (2004). The impact of iron and selenium deficiencies on iodine and thyroid metabolism: Biochemistry and relevance to public health. *Thyroid, 12*(10), 867–878.

Lee, J. H., Kim, Y., Choi, J. W., & Kim, Y. S. (2013). The association between papillary thyroid carcinoma and histologically proven Hashimoto's thyroiditis: A meta-analysis. *European Society of Endocrinology, 168*(3), 343–349. doi: 10.1530/EJE-12-0903

Trentini, D. (2012, November 26). *Top 5 reasons doctors fail to diagnose hypothyroidism.* Retrieved from http://hypothyroidmom.com/top-5-reasons-doctors-fail-to-diagnose-hypothyroidism

Bowthorpe, J. A. (n.d.). *Rt3-ratio.* Retrieved from www.stopthethroidmadness.com

Holthorf, K. (2012, January 27). *Thyroid hormone transport.* Retrieved from https://www.nahypothyroidism.org/thyroid-hormone-transport/

Ballantyne, S. (2013). *The paleo approach: Reverse autoimmune disease and heal your body.* (pp. 209–210). Las Vegas, NV: Victory Belt Publishing, Inc.

Lotus Institute of Integrative Medicine. (2006). *Clinical manual of Oriental medicine: An integrative approach* (2nd ed., pp. 713–716). City of Industry, CA: Lotus Institute of Integrative Medicine.

Chapters 6–8 (The Metal Element):

Kern, S., & Ziemssen, T. (2007). Psychoneuroimmunology–cross-talk between the immune and nervous systems. *Journal of Neurology, 254*(Suppl 2), II8–II11.

Yaghini, N., Mahmoodi, M., Asadikaram, Gh. R., Hassanshahi, Gh. H., Khoramdelazad, H., & Kazemi Arababadi, M. (2011). Serum levels of interleukin 10 (IL-10) in patients with type 2 diabetes. *Iranian Red Crescent Medical Journal, 13*(10), 752.

Chen, J. K., & Chen, T. T. (2001). *Chinese medical herbology and pharmacology.* (pp. 864–865). City of Industry, CA: Art of Medicine Press, Inc.

Corthay, A. (2009). How do regulatory T cells work? *Scandinavian Journal of Immunology 70*(4), 326–336.

Kendall, D. E. (2002). *Dao of Chinese medicine: Understanding an ancient healing art.* (pp. 124–125). Oxford: Oxford University Press.

Kidd, P. (2003). Th1/Th2 balance: The hypothesis, its limitations, and implications for health and disease. *Alternative Medicine Review, 8*(3), 223–246.

Kharrazian, D. (2011). *Mastering the thyroid.* Seminar.

Van Benschoten, M. M. (2003). *Autoimmune disease and Chinese herbal medicine.* Santa Monica, CA: Emperor's College of Oriental Medicine.

Van Benschoten, M. M. (2009). *Autoimmune disease, multiple chemical disorders, and Chinese medicine.* City of Industry, CA: Lotus Institute of Integrative Medicine.

Mak, T. W., & Saunders, M. E. (2005). *The immune response: Basic and clinical principles.* (pp. 451–453). Burlington, MA: Elsevier Academic Press.

American Autoimmune Related Diseases Association, Inc. (2014). *Autoimmune statistics.* Retrieved from https://www.aarda.org/autoimmune-information/autoimmune-statistics

Trentini, D. (2012). *Hashimoto's: Your body is not supposed to destroy itself right?* Retrieved from http://hypothyroidmom.com/hashimotos-your-body-is-not-supposed-to-destroy-itself-right

Aksoy, D. Y., Kerimoglu, U., Okur, H., Canpinar, H., Karaağaoğlu, E., Yetgin, S., . . . Gedik, O. (2005). Effects of prophylactic thyroid hormone replacement in euthyroid Hashimoto's thyroiditis. *Endocrine Journal, 52*(3), 337–343.

Kresser, C. (2010, August 30). *Basics of immune balancing for Hashimoto's.* Retrieved from https://chriskresser.com

Kharrazian, D. (2012, March 13). *Nitric oxide modulation for autoimmune disease.* Retrieved from https://drknews.com

Drugarin, D., Negru, S., Koreck, A., Zosin, I., & Cristea, C. (2000). The pattern of Th1 cytokine in autoimmune thyroiditis. *Immunology Letters, 71*(2), 73–77.

McGrogan, A., Seaman, H. E., Wright, J. W., & de Vries, C. S. (2008). The incidence of autoimmune thyroid disease: A systematic review of the literature. *Clinical Endocrinology, 69*(5), 687–696.

Boelaert, K., Newby, P. R., Simmonds, M. J., Holder, R. L., Carr-Smith, J. D., Heward, J. M., . . . Franklyn, J. A. (2010). Prevalence and relative risk of other autoimmune diseases in subjects with autoimmune thyroid disease. *The American Journal of Medicine, 123*(2), 183.e1–183.e9.

Ch'ng, C. L., Keston Jones, M., & Kingham, J. G. C. (2007). Celiac disease and autoimmune thyroid disease. *Clinical Medicine & Research, 5*(3), 184–192.

Spadaccino, A. C., Basso, D., & Chiarelli, S. (2008). Celiac disease in north Italian patients with autoimmune thyroid diseases. *Autoimmunity, 41*(1), 116–121.

Kumar, V., Wortsman, J., & Rajadhyaksha, M. (2001). Celiac disease–associated autoimmune endocrinopathies. *Clinical and Vaccine Immunology, 8*(4), 678–685.

Collin, P., Salmi, J., Hällström, O., Reunala, T., & Pasternack, A. (1994). Autoimmune thyroid disorders and coeliac disease. *Digestive Diseases and Sciences, 44*(7), 1428–1433.

Akcay, M. N., & Akcay, G. (2003). The presence of the antigliadin antibodies in autoimmune thyroid diseases. *Hepato-Gastroenterology, 50*(Suppl. 2), cclxxix-cclxxx.

Sategna-Guidetti, C., Bruno, M., Mazza, E., Carlino, A., Predebon, S., Tagliabue, M., & Brossa, C. (1998). Autoimmune thyroid diseases and coeliac disease. *European Journal of Gastroenterology & Hepatology, 10*(11), 927–932.

Yao, C., Shang, J., Wang, L., Guo, Y., & Tian, Z. (2007). Inhibitory effects of thyroxine on cytokine production by T cells in mice. *International Immunopharmacology, 7*(13), 1747–1754.

Strieder, T. G., Prummel, M. F., Tijssen, J. G., Endert, E., & Wiersinga, W. M. (2003). Risk factors for and prevalence of thyroid disorders in a cross-sectional study among healthy female relatives of patients with autoimmune thyroid disease. *Clinical Endocrinology, 59*(3), 396–401.

Hakanen, M., Luotola, K., Salmi, J., Laippala, P., Kaukinen, K., & Collin, P. (2001). Clinical and subclinical autoimmune thyroid disease in adult celiac disease. *Digestive Diseases and Sciences, 46*(12), 2631–2635.

Kresser, C. (2010). *The gluten-thyroid connection.* Retrieved from https://chriskresser.com

Denham, J. M., & Hill, I. D. (2013). Celiac disease and autoimmunity: Review and controversies. *Current Allergy and Asthma Reports, 13*(4), 347–353.

Hodkinson, C. F., Simpson, E. E. A., Beattie, J. H., O'Connor, J. M., Campbell, D. J., Strain, J. J., & Wallace, J. M. W. (2009). Preliminary evidence of immune function modulation by thyroid hormones in healthy men and women aged 55–70 years. *Journal of Endocrinology, 202*(1), 55–63.

Fasano, A. (2006). Systemic autoimmune disorders in celiac disease. *Current Opinion in Gastroenterology, 22*(6), 674–679.

Anti-transglutaminase antibodies. (n.d.). Retrieved from https://en.wikipedia.org/wiki/Anti-transglutaminase_antibodies

Collins, Dan et al. (2012) Celiac Disease and Hypothyroidsism. *The American Journal of Medicine, 125*(3), 278–282

Caja, S., Mäki, M., Kaukinen, K., & Lindfors, K. (2011). Antibodies in celiac disease: Implications beyond diagnostics. *Cellular & Molecular Immunology, 8*, 103–109.

Hadithi, M., de Boer, H., Meijer, J. W. R., Willekens, F., Kerckhaert, J. A., Heijmans, R., . . . Mulder, C. J. J. (2007). Coeliac disease in Dutch patients with Hashimoto's thyroiditis and vice versa. *World Journal of Gastroenterology, 13*(11), 1715–1722.

Dach, J. (2014, January 22). Hashimoto's thyroid disease and molecular mimicry. Retrieved from http://jeffreydachmd.com/2014/01/hashimotos-thyroid-disease-molecular-mimicry

Harris, C., & Kaplan, G. (2010). Two of a kind—Research connects celiac and thyroid diseases and suggests a gluten-free diet benefits both. *Today's Dietitian, 12*(11), 52.

Kučera, P., Nováková, D., Běhanová, M., Novák, J., Tlaskalová-Hogenová, H., & Anděl, M. (2003). Gliadin, endomysial and thyroid antibodies in patients with latent autoimmune diabetes of adults (LADA). *Clinical & Experimental Immunology, 133*(1), 139–143.

Fine, K. (2003). *Early diagnosis of gluten sensitivity: Before the villi are gone.* Transcript of talk by Kenneth Fine, M.D. to the Greater Louisville Celiac Sprue Support Group. Retrieved from https://www.enterolab.com/staticpages/earlydiagnosis.aspx

Human leukocyte antigen. (n.d.) Retrieved from Wikipedia: https://en.wikipedia.org/wiki/Human_leukocyte_antigen

Kharrazian, D. (2012, January 19). *Eating gluten increases the need for thyroid hormones.* Retrieved from http://thyroidbook.com

Martin, A., De Vivo, G., & Gentile, V. (2011). Possible role of the transglutaminases in the pathogenesis of Alzheimer's disease and other neurodegenerative diseases. *International Journal of Alzheimer's Disease, 2011*, Article ID 865432. doi: 10.4061/2011/865432

Nakagawa, H., Yoneda, M., Fujii, A., Kinomoto, K., & Kuriyama, M. (2007). Hashimoto's encephalopathy presenting with progressive cerebellar ataxia. *Journal of Neurology, Neurosurgery & Psychiatry, 78*(2), 196–197.

Hadjivassiliou, M., Grünewald, R., Sharrack, B., Sanders, D., Lobo, A., Williamson, C., . . . Davies-Jones, A. (2003). Gluten ataxia in perspective: Epidemiology, genetic susceptibility and clinical characteristics. *Brain, 126*(3), 685–691.

Seneff, S., & Samsel, A. (2013). Glyphosate, pathways to modern diseases II: Celiac sprue and gluten intolerance. *Interdisciplinary Toxicology, 6*(4), 159–184.

Gerenova, J., Manolova, I., & Gadjeva, V. (2012). Hashimoto's disease—Involvement of cytokine network and role of oxidative stress in the severity of Hashimoto's thyroiditis, A new look at hypothyroidism, Dr. Drahomira Springer (Ed.), Rijeka, Croatia: InTech,

Stojanovich, L., & Marisavljevich, D. (2008). Stress as a trigger of autoimmune disease. *Autoimmunity Reviews, 7*(3), 209–13.

Klein, J. R. (2006). The immune system as a regulator of thyroid hormone activity. *Experimental Biology and Medicine, 231*(3), 229–236.

Galland, L. (n.d.) Leaky gut syndromes: Breaking the vicious cycle. Retrieved from http://www.mdheal.org/leakygut.htm

Fratkin, J. P. (2016, May 10). Leaky gut syndrome: A modern epidemic part I. Retrieved from http://www.ei-resource.org/articles/leaky-gut-syndrome-articles/leaky-gut-syndrome-the-problem/

Brimberg, L., Sadiq, A., Gregersen, P. K., & Diamond, B. (2013). Brain-reactive IgG correlates with autoimmunity in mothers of a child with an autism spectrum disorder. *Molecular Psychiatry, 18*(11), 1171–1177. doi: 10.1038/mp.2013.101

Sapone, A., Bai, J. C., Ciacci, C., Dolinsek, J., Green, P. H. R., Hadjivassiliou, M., . . . Fasano, A. (2012). Spectrum of gluten-related disorders: consensus on new nomenclature and classification. *BMC Medicine, 10* (13).

Trescott, M. (2013, January 24). How do you balance TH1 and TH2 in autoimmune disease? Retrieved from http://autoimmune-paleo.com/how-do-you-balance-th1-and-th2-in-autoimmune-disease/

Ni, M. (1995). *The yellow emperor's classic of medicine.* Boston, MA: Shambhala Publications.

Kharrazian, D. (2011). Autoimmune thyroid. *Mastering the thyroid.* Seminar, 251.

Pitchford, P. (1993). Metal element. In *Healing with whole foods: Oriental traditions and modern nutrition* (revised ed.) (pp. 306–314). Berkeley, CA: North Atlantic Books.

Del Prete, G., De Carli, M., Almerigogna, F., Giudizi, M. G., Biagiotti, R., & Romagnani, S. (1993). Human IL-10 is produced by both type 1 helper (Th1) and type 2 helper (Th2) T cell clones and inhibits their antigen-specific proliferation and cytokine production. *The Journal of Immunology, 150*(2), 353–360.

Corthay, A. (2009). How do regulatory T cells work? *Scandinavian Journal of Immunology, 70* (4), 326–336.

Schmidt, C. W. (2011). Questions persist: environmental factors in autoimmune disease. *Environmental Health Perspectives, 119,* a248–a253.

Parvathaneni, A., Fischman, D., & Cheriyath, P. (2012). Hashimoto's thyroiditis. In D. Springer (Ed.), *A new look at hypothyroidism.* doi: 10.5772/30288

Counsell, C. E., Taha, A., & Ruddell, W. S. (1994). Coeliac disease and autoimmune thyroid disease. *Gut, 35,* 844–846.

Velluzzi, F., Caradonna, A., Boy, M. F., Pinna, M.A., Cabula, R., Lai, M. A., . . . Mariotti, S. (1998). Thyroid and celiac disease: clinical, serological, and echographic study. *American Journal of Gastroenterology, 93,* 976–979.

Kapur, V. K., Koepsell, T. D., Demaine, J., Hert, R., Sandblom, R. E., & Psaty, B. M., (1998). Association of hypothyroidism and obstructive sleep apnea. *American Journal of Respiratory and Critical Care Medicine, 158*(5), 1379–1383.

Chapters 9–12: (Earth Element)

Maclean, W., & Lyttleton, J. (2002). *Clinical handbook of internal medicine: The treatment of disease with traditional Chinese medicine.* Vol. 2: Spleen and Stomach (p. xvii). University of Western Sydney Macarthur.

Jones, M. P., Dilley, J. B., Drossman, D., & Crowell, M. D. (2006.) Brain-gut connections in functional GI disorders: anatomic and physiologic relationships. *Neurogastroenterology & Motility 18*(2), 91–103. doi: 10.1111/j.1365-2982.2005.00730.x

Guinane, C. M., Tadrous, A., Fouhy, F., Ryan, C. A., Dempsey, E. M., Murphy, B., . . . Ross, R. P. (2013). Microbial composition of human appendices from patients following appendectomy. *mBio, 4*(1), e00366–12. doi: 10.1128/mBio.00366-12

Sachmechi, I., Reich, D., Aninyei, M., Wibowo, F., Gupta, G., & Kim, P. (2007). Effect of proton pump inhibitors on serum thyroid-stimulating hormone level in euthyroid patients treated with levothyroxine for hypothyroidism. *Endocrine Practice, 13*(4), 345–349.

Chen, J. K., & Chen, T. T. (2001). *Chinese medical herbology and pharmacology.* City of Industry, CA: Art of Medicine Press, Inc.

Kendall, D. E. (2002). *Dao of Chinese medicine: Understanding an ancient healing art.* Oxford: Oxford University Press.

Jarrett, L. S. (1998). Earth-The axis. In *Nourishing destiny: The inner tradition of chinese medicine* (pp. 278–298). Stockbridge, MA: Spirit Path Press.

Kharrazian, D. (2011). *Mastering the thyroid.* Seminar.

Kharrazian, D. (2010). *Why do I still have thyroid symptoms? When my lab tests are normal.* Carlsbad, CA: Elephant Press.

Van Benschoten, M. M. (2003). *Autoimmune disease and Chinese herbal medicine.* Santa Monica, CA: Emperor's College of Oriental Medicine.

Van Benchoten, M. M. (2009). *Autoimmune disease, multiple chemical disorders, and Chinese medicine.* Lotus Institute of integrative Medicine. Seminar.

Braverman, L. E., & Utiger, R. D. (Eds.). (2005). *Werner & Ingbar's the thyroid: A fundamental and clinical text* (9th ed.) (pp. 796–802). Philadelphia, PA: Lippincott Williams & Wilkins.

Kresser, C. (2010, April 1). The hidden causes of heartburn and GERD. Retrieved from https://chriskresser.com/the-hidden-causes-of-heartburn-and-gerd/

Sugerman, H. J. (2007). Increased intra-abdominal pressure and GERD/Barrett's esophagus. *Gastroenterology 133*(6), 2075. doi: http://dx.doi.org/10.1053/j.gastro.2007.10.017

Theisen, J., Nehra, D., Citron, D., Johansson, J., Hagen, J. A., Crookes, P. F., . . . Peters, J.H. (2000). Suppression of gastric acid secretion in patients with gastroesophageal reflux disease results in gastric bacterial overgrowth and deconjugation of bile acids. *Journal of Gastrointestinal Surgery, 4*(1), 50–54.

Kresser, C. (2010, July 23). Thyroid, blood sugar, and metabolic syndrome. Retrieved from https://chriskresser.com/thyroid-blood-sugar-metabolic-syndrome/

Kadiyala, R., Peter, R., & Okosieme, O. E. (2010). Thyroid dysfunction in patients with diabetes: Clinical implications and screening strategies. *International Journal of Clinical Pratice, 64*(8), 1130–1139.

Ahmad, J., Ahmed, F., Siddiqui, M. A., Hameed, B., & Ahmad, I. (2006). Inflammation, insulin resistance and carotid IMT in first degree relatives of north Indian type 2 diabetic subjects. *Diabetes Research and Clinical Practice, 73*(2), 205–210.

Kresser, C. (2010, July 29). The thyroid-gut connection. Retrieved from https://chriskresser.com/the-thyroid-gut-connection/

Stratakis, C. A., & Chrousos, G. P. (1995). Neuroendocrinology and pathophysiology of the stress system. *Annals of the New York Academy of Sciences 771*, 1–18.

van der Poll, T., Van Zee, K. J., Endert, E., Coyle, S. M., Stiles, D. M., Pribble, J. P., . . . Lowry, S. F. Interleukin-1 receptor blockade does not affect endotoxin-induced changes in plasma thyroid hormone and thyrotropin concentrations in man. *The Journal of Clinical Endocrinology & Metabolism, 80*(4), 1341–1346.

Balkau, B., Shipley, M., Jarret, R. J., Pyörälä, K., Pyörälä, M., Forhan, A., & Eschwège, E. (1998). High blood glucose concentration is a risk factor for mortality in middle-aged nondiabetic men: 20-year follow-up in the Whitehall Study, the Paris Prospective Study, and the Helsinki Policemen Study. *Diabetes Care, 21*(3), 360–367.

De Vegt, F., Dekker, J. M., Ruhé, H. G., Stehouwer, C. D. A., Nijpels, G., Bouter, L. M., & Heine, R. J. (1999). Hyperglycaemia is associated with all-cause and cardiovascular mortality in the Hoorn population: The Hoorn Study. *Diabetologia, 42*(8), 926–931.

Esposito K., Ciotola, M., Carleo, D., Schisano, B., Sardelli, L., Di Tommaso, D., . . . Giugliano, D. (2008). Post-meal glucose peaks at home associate with carotid intima-media thickness in type 2 diabetes. *The Journal of Clinical Endocrinology & Metabolism, 93*(4):1345–1350.

Lenzen, S., Joost, H. G., & Hasselblatt, A. (1976). Thyroid function and insulin secretion from the perfused pancreas in the rat. *Endocrinology, 99*(1), 125–129.

Gullo, L., Pezzilli, R., Bellanova, B., D'Ambrosi, A., Alvisi, V., & Barbara, L. (1991). Influence of the thyroid on exocrine pancreatic function. *Gastroenterology, 100*(5), 1392–1396.

Malaisse, W. J., Malaisse-Lagae, F., & McCraw, E. F. (1967). Effects of thyroid function upon insulin secretion. *Diabetes Journal, 16*(9), 643–646.

Potenza, M., Via, M. A., & Yanagisawa, R. T. (2009). Excess thyroid hormone and carbohydrate metabolism. *Endocrine Practice, 15*(3), 254–262.

Campbell, T. C. (2010, September 28). Low fat diets are grossly misrepresented. *The Huffington Post.* Retrieved from http://www.huffingtonpost.com/t-colin-campbell/low-fat-diets-are-grossly_b_740543.html

Fratkin, J. P. (2016, May 10). Leaky gut syndrome: A modern epidemic part II. Retrieved from http://www.ei-resource.org/articles/leaky-gut-syndrome-articles/leaky-gut-syndrome-the-problem/

Arrieta, M. C., Bistritz, L., & Meddings, J. B. (2006). Alterations in intestinal permeability. *Gut, 55*(10), 1512–1520.

Reardon, S. (2014). Gut–brain link grabs neuroscientists. *Nature, 515*(7526), 175–177.

Granito, A., Muratori, P., Cassani, F., Pappas, G., Muratori, L., Agostinelli, D., . . . Volta, U. (2004). Anti-actin IgA antibodies in severe coeliac disease. *Clinical & Experimental Immunology, 137*(2), 386–392.

Vogelsang H., Wyatt, J., Penner, E., & Lochs, H. (1995). Screening for celiac disease in first-degree relatives of patients with celiac disease by lactulose/mannitol test. *American Journal of Gastroenterology, 90*(10), 1838–1842.

Molodecky, N. A., & Kaplan, G. G. (2010). Environmental risk factors for inflammatory bowel disease. *Gastroenterology & Hepatology, 6*(5), 339–346.

Array 2-Antibody: Intestinal antigenic permeability screen. (2015). Cyrex Tests and Arrays. Retrieved from https://www.cyrexlabs.com/CyrexTestsArrays

Blaser, M. J. (2006). Who are we? Indigenous microbes and the ecology of human diseases. *EMBO Reports, 7*(10), 956–960.

Pitchford, P. (1993). Earth element. In *Healing with whole foods: Oriental traditions and modern nutrition* (Revised ed.) (pp. 302–306, 334). Berkeley, CA: North Atlantic Books.

Ni, M. (1995). *The yellow emperor's classic of medicine.* Boston, MA: Shambhala Publications.

Trescott, M. (2014). *The Autoimmune Paleo Cookbook.* Berkeley, CA: Rockridge Press.

Liu, H. (1997). *The Healing Art of Qi Gong.* New York, NY: Warner Books.

Brooks, M. (2014, January 30). Top 100 selling drugs of 2013. Retrieved from http://www.medscape.com /viewarticle/820011#vp_1

Reimer, C., Søndergaard, B., Hilsted, L., & Bytzer, P. (2009). Proton-pump inhibitor therapy induces acid-related symptoms in healthy volunteers after withdrawal of therapy. *Gastroenterology, 137*(1), 80–87.

Siemińska, L., Wojciechowska, C., Walczak, K., Borowski, A., Marek, B., Nowak, M., . . . Kos-Kudła, B. (2015). Associations between metabolic syndrome, serum thyrotropin, and thyroid antibodies status in postmenopausal women, and the role of interleukin-6. *Endokrynologia Polska, 66*(5), 394–403. doi: 10.5603/EP.2015.0049

Chapters 13–17 (Water Element):

Agmon-Levin, N., Theodor, E., Segal, R. M., & Shoenfeld, Y. (2013). Vitamin D in systemic and organ-specific autoimmune diseases. *Clinical Reviews in Allergy & Immunology, 45*(2), 256–266.

Tzu, L. (1961). *Tao Teh Ching* (10–11). (J. C. H. Wu, Trans.). Boston, MA: Shambhala Publications.

Klein, I., & Danzi, S. (2007). Cardiovascular involvement in general medical conditions: Thyroid disease and the heart. *Circulation, 116*(15), 1725–1735.

Jarrett, L. S. (1998). *Nourishing destiny: The inner tradition of Chinese medicine* (pp. 176–198). Stockbridge, MA: Spirit Path Press.

Braverman, L. E., & Utiger, R. D. (2005). *Werner & Ingbar's the thyroid: A fundamental and clinical text* (9th ed.) (pp. 789–795, 811–816). Philadelphia, PA: Lippincott Williams & Wilkins.

Pitchford, P. (1993). Water element. In *Healing with whole foods: Oriental traditions and modern nutrition* (Revised ed.) (pp. 315–328). Berkeley, CA: North Atlantic Books.

Chen, J. K., & Chen, T. T. (2001). *Chinese medical herbology and pharmacology.* City of Industry, CA: Art of Medicine Press Inc.

Holtorf, K. (n.d.) Understanding the adrenal and thyroid connection. Retrieved from https://www .holtorfmed.com/adrenal-health-understanding-the-adrenal-and-thyroid-connection/

Kresser, C. (2010, August 2). 5 ways that stress causes hypothyroid symptoms. Retrieved from https:// chriskresser.com/5-ways-that-stress-causes-hypothyroid-symptoms/

Mercola, J. (2000). Understanding adrenal function. Retrieved from http://articles.mercola.com/sites /articles/archive/2000/08/27/adrenals.aspx

Rettori, V., Jurcovicova, J., & McCann, S. M. (1987). Central action of Interleukin-1 in altering the release of TSH, growth hormone, and prolactin in the male rat. *Journal of Neuroscience Research, 18*(1), 179–183.

Pang, X. P., Hershman, J. M., Mirell, C. J., & Pekary, A. E. (1989). Impairment of hypothalamic-pituitary -thyroid function in rats treated with human recombinant tumor necrosis factor-alpha (cachectin). *Endocrinology, 125*(1), 76–84.

Kimura, H., & Caturegli, P. (2007). Chemokine orchestration of autoimmune thyroiditis. *Thyroid, 17*(10), 1005–1011.

Baeke, F., Takiishi, T., Korf, H., Gysemans, C., & Mathieu, C. (2010). Vitamin D: modulator of the immune system. *Current Opinion in Pharmacology, 10*(4), 482–496

Kharrazian, D. (2011). *Mastering the thyroid.* Seminar.

Ni, M. (1995). *The yellow emperor's classic of medicine.* Boston, MA: Shambhala Publications.

Janssen, H. C. J. P., Samson, M. M., & Verhaar, H. J. J. (2002). Vitamin D deficiency, muscle function, and falls in elderly people. *The American Journal of Clinical Nutrition, 75*(4), 611–615.

Štefanić, M., Papić, S., Suver, M., Glavaš-Obrovac, L., & Karner, I. (2008). Association of vitamin D receptor gene 3'-variants with Hashimoto's thyroiditis in the Croatian population. *International Journal of Immunogenetics, 35*(2), 125–131. doi: 10.1111/j.1744-313X.2008.00748.x

Panossian, A., Wikman, G., & Wagner, H. (1999). Plant adaptogens. III. Earlier and more recent aspects and concepts on their mode of action. *Phytomedicine, 6*(4), 287–300. doi: 10.1016/S0944-7113(99)80023-3

Streeten D. H., Anderson, G. H., Howland, T., Chiang, R., & Smulyan, H. (1988). Effects of thyroid function on blood pressure. Recognition of hypothyroid hypertension. *Hypertension, 11*(1), 78–83.

Chapters 18–20 (The Brain):

Pert, C. (1999). *Molecules of emotion: Why you feel the way you feel.* New York, NY: Touchstone.

Davidson, R. J., & Begley, S. (2012). *The emotional life of your brain: How its unique patterns affect the way you think, feel, and live—and how you can change them.* New York, NY: Hudson Street Press.

Mallat, M., Lima, F. R. S., Gervais, A., Colin, C., & Neto, V. M. (2002). New insights into the role of thyroid hormone in the CNS: The microglial track. *Molecular Psychiatry, 7*(1), 7–8.

Lima, F. R. S., Gervais, A., Colin, C., Izembart, M., Neto, V. M., & Mallat, M. (2001). Regulation of microglial development: A novel role for thyroid hormone. *The Journal of Neuroscience, 21*(6): 2028–2038.

de La Monte, S. M., & Wands, J. R. (2008). Alzheimer's disease is type 3 diabetes—Evidence reviewed. *Journal of Diabetes Science and Technology, 2*(6), 1101–1113.

Kharrazian, D. (2010, November 12). Thyroid-brain Crosstalk—Part 1: The microglia, neuron and thyroid connection. Retrieved from http://sanjosefuncmed.com/thyroid-brain-crosstalk-part-1 -microglia-neuron-thyroid-connection/

Harry, G. J., & Kraft, A. D. (2012). Microglia in the developing brain: A potential target with lifetime effects. *Neurotoxicology, 33*(2), 191–206. doi:10.1016/j.neuro.2012.01.012

Bonuccelli, U., D'Avino, C., Caraccio, N., Del Guerra, P., Casolaro, A., Pavese, N., . . . Monzani, F. (1999). Thyroid function and autoimmunity in Parkinson's disease: A study of 101 patients. *Parkinsonism & Related Disorders, 5*(1–2), 49–53.

Huang, M. J., & Liaw, Y. F. (1995). Clinical associations between thyroid and liver diseases. *Journal of Gastroenterology & Hepatology, 10*(3), 344–350.

Bowen, R. (2012, February 26). Thyroid Hormones: Pregnancy and Fetal Development. Retrieved from http://arbl.cvmbs.colostate.edu/hbooks/pathphys/endocrine/thyroid/thyroid_preg.html

de Morreale, E. G. (2001). The role of thyroid hormone in fetal neurodevelopment. *Journal of Pediatric Endocrinology and Metabolism, 14* (Suppl 6), 1453–1462.

Patel, J., Landers, K., Li, H., Mortimer, R. H., & Richard, K. (2011). Thyroid hormones and fetal neurological development. *Journal of Endocrinology, 209*(1), 1–8.

Houston Methodist. (2013, August 13). Autism four times likelier when mother's thyroid is weakened. *ScienceDaily*. Retrieved from https://www.sciencedaily.com/releases/2013/08/130813111730.htm

Mittelbronn, M., Schittenhelm, J., Bakos, G., De Vos, R. A., Wehrmann, M., Meyermann, R., & Bürk, K. (2010). CD8+/perforin+/granzyme B+ effector cells infiltrating cerebellum and inferior olives in gluten ataxia. *Neuropathology, 30*(1), 92–96.

Zoeller, T. R., Dowling, A. L. S., Herzig, C. T. A., Iannacone, E. A., Gauger, K. J., & Bansal, R. (2002). Thyroid hormone, brain development, and the environment. *Environmental Health Perspectives, 110*(Suppl 3), 355–361.

Trentini, D. (2013, May 13). Maternal hypothyroidism and fetal brain development. Retrieved from http://hypothyroidmom.com/maternal-hypothyroidism-and-fetal-brain-development/

Bernal, J. (2015, September 2). Thyroid hormones in brain development and function. Retrieved from http://www.thyroidmanager.org/chapter/thyroid-hormones-in-brain-development-and-function/

Ganguli M., Burmeister, L. A., Seaberg, E. C., Belle, S., DeKosky, S. T. (1996). Association between dementia and elevated TSH: A community-based study. *Biological Psychiatry, 40*(8), 714–725.

Schiess, N., & Pardo, C. A. (2008). Hashimoto's encephalopathy. *Annals of the New York Academy of Sciences, 1142*, 254–265.

Wang, J., Zhang, J., Xu, L., Shi, Y., Wu, X., & Guo, Q. (2013). Cognitive impairments in hashimoto's encephalopathy: A case-control study. *PLoS ONE, 8*(2). http://dx.doi.org/10.1371/journal.pone.0055758

Selim, M., & Drachman, D. A. (2001). Ataxia associated with hashimoto's disease: Progressive non-familial adult onset cerebellar degeneration with autoimmune thyroiditis. *Journal of Neurology, Neurosurgery & Psychiatry, 71*(1), 81–87.

Kharrazian, D. (2010, February 17). The effects of hashimoto's and hypothyroidism on brain health. Retrieved from https://drknews.com/hashimotos-hypothyroidism-and-how-to-protect-your-brain/

Braverman, L. E., & Utiger, R. D. (2005). *Werner & Ingbar's the thyroid: A fundamental and clinical text (9th ed.)* (pp. 836–850). Philadelphia, PA: Lippincott Williams & Wilkins.

Hadjivassiliou, M., Grünewald, R., Sharrack, B., Sanders, D., Lobo, A., Williamson, C., . . . Davies-Jones, A. (2003). Gluten ataxia in perspective: Epidemiology, genetic susceptibility and clinical characteristics. *Brain, 126*(Pt 3), 685–691.

de la Monte, S. M., & Wands, J. R. (2008). Alzheimer's disease is type 3 diabetes—Evidence reviewed. *Journal of Diabetes Science and Technology, 2*(6), 1101–1113.

Chapters 21–24 (The Wood Element):

Rigopoulou, E. I., Smyk, D. S., Matthews, C. E., Billinis, C., Burroughs, A. K., Lenzi, M., & Bogdanos, D. P. (2012). Epstein-Barr virus as a trigger of autoimmune liver diseases. *Advances in Virology, 2012*. doi: 10.1155/2012/987471

Oliva, F., Berardi, A. C., Misiti, S., & Maffulli, N. (2013). Thyroid hormones and tendon: Current views and future perspectives. *Muscles, Ligaments and Tendons Journal, 3*(3), 201–203.

Pitchford, P. (1993). Wood element. In *Healing with whole foods: Oriental traditions and modern nutrition* (Revised ed.) (pp. 84–290). Berkeley, CA: North Atlantic Books.

Murrell, G. A. (2002). Understanding tendinopathies. *British Journal of Sports Medicine, 36,* 392–393.

Bensky, D., & Barolet, R. (1990). *Chinese herbal medicine formulas and strategies* (p. 147). Seattle, WA: Eastland Press.

Jarrett, L. S. (1998). *Nourishing destiny: The inner tradition of Chinese medicine* (pp. 234–256). Stockbridge, MA: Spirit Path Press.

Braverman, L. E., & Utiger, R. D. (2005). *Werner & Ingbar's the thyroid: A fundamental and clinical text* (9th ed.) (pp. 796–802). Philadelphia, PA: Lippincott Williams & Wilkins.

Ni, M. (1995). *The yellow emperor's classic of medicine* (pp. 95–97). Boston, MA: Shambhala Publications.

Upadhyay, G., Singh, R., Kumar, A., Kumar, S. Kapoor, A., & Godbole, M. (2004). Severe hyperthyroidism induces mitochondria-mediated apoptosis in rat liver. *Hepatology, 39*(4), 1120–1130. doi:10.1002/hep.20085

Laukkarinen, J., Kiudelis, G., Lempinen, M., Räty, S., Pelli, H., Sand, J., . . . Nordback, I. (2007). Increased prevalence of subclinical hypothyroidism in common bile duct stone patients. *The Journal of Endocrinology & Metabolism, 92*(11), 4260–4264.

Inkinen, J., Sand, J., & Nordback, I. (2000). Association between common bile duct stones and treated hypothyroidism. *Hepatogastroenterology, 47*(34), 919–21.

Liu, H. (1997). *The Healing Art of Qi Gong.* New York, NY: Warner Books.

Hoffmann, M. F., Preissner, S. C., Nickel, J., Dunkel, M., Preissner, R., & Preissner, S. (2014). The Transformer database: Biotransformation of xenobiotics. *Nucleic Acids Research, 42*(Database issue), D1113–D1117.

Huang, M. J., & Liaw, Y. F. (1995). Clinical associations between thyroid and liver diseases. *Journal of Gastroenterology and Hepatology, 10*(3), 344–350.

Tzu, C. (1968). *The complete works of Chuang Tzu* (p. 87). (Watson, B., Trans.) New York, NY: Columbia University Press.

Chapters 25–29 (The Fire Element):

Maclean, W., & Lyttleton, J. (1998). *Clinical handbook of internal medicine: The treatment of disease with traditional Chinese medicine. Vol. 1: Lung kidney liver heart.* University of Western Sydney Macarthur.

Chen, J. K., & Chen, T. T. (2001). *Chinese medical herbology and pharmacology.* City of Industry, CA: Art of Medicine Press, Inc.

Kendall, D. E. (2002). *Dao of Chinese medicine: Understanding an ancient healing art.* Oxford: Oxford University Press.

Jarrett, L. S. (1998). *Nourishing destiny: The inner tradition of Chinese medicine* (pp. 196–232). Stockbridge, MA: Spirit Path Press.

Braverman, L. E., & Utiger, R. D. (2005). *Werner & Ingbar's the thyroid: A fundamental and clinical text* (9th ed.) (pp. 774–781, 790). Philadelphia, PA: Lippincott Williams & Wilkins.

Kharrazian, D. (2010). *Why do I still have thyroid symptoms? When my lab tests are normal.* Carlsbad, CA: Elephant Press.

Jarrett, L. S. (1998). *Nourishing destiny: The inner tradition of Chinese medicine* (pp. 258–276). Stockbridge, MA: Spirit Path Press.

Ni, M. (1995). *The yellow emperor's classic of medicine*. Boston, MA: Shambhala Publications.

Pitchford, P. (1993). Fire element. In *Healing with whole foods: Oriental traditions and modern nutrition* (Revised ed.) (pp. 296–299). Berkeley, CA: North Atlantic Books.

Lauritano, E. C., Bilotta, A. L., Gabrielli, M., Scarpellini, E., Lupascu, A., Laginestra, A., . . . Gasbarrini. A. (2007). Association between hypothyroidism and small intestinal bacterial overgrowth. *The Journal of Clinical Endocrinology & Metabolism, 92*(11), 4180–4184.

Tursi, A., Brandimarte G., & Giorgetti, G. (2003). High prevalence of small intestinal bacterial overgrowth in celiac patients with persistence of gastrointestinal symptoms after gluten withdrawal. *The American Journal of Gastroenterology, 98*(4), 839–843.

Wolfson, A. B, Hendey, G. W., Ling, L. J., Rosen, C., Shaider, J., & Sharieff, G. (Eds.) (2010). *Harwood-Nuss' clinical practice of emergency medicine* (5th ed.). Philadelphia, PA: Lippincott Williams & Wilkins.

Fasano, A. (2012). Leaky gut and autoimmune diseases. *Clinical Reviews in Allergy & Immunology, 42*(1), 71–78.

Fazio, S., Palmieri, E. A., Lombardi, G., & Biondi, B. (2004). Effects of thyroid hormone on the cardiovascular system. *Recent Progress in Hormone Research, 59*, 31–50.

Klein, I., & Ojamaa, K. (2001). Thyroid hormone and the cardiovascular system. *The New England Journal of Medicine, 344*, 501–509.

Urita, Y., Watanabe, T., Maeda, T., Arita, T., Sasaki, Y., Ishii, T., . . . Hike, K. (2008). Extensive atrophic gastritis increases intraduodenal hydrogen gas. *Gastroenterology Research and Practice, 208*(1). http://dx.doi.org/10.1155/2008/584929

Naylor, G., & Axon, A. (2003). Role of bacterial overgrowth in the stomach as an additional risk factor for gastritis. *Canadian Journal of Gastroenterology and Hepatology, 17*(Suppl B), 13B–17B.

Soifer, L. O., Peralta, D., Dima, G., & Besasso, H. (2010). Comparative clinical efficacy of a probiotic vs. an antibiotic in the treatment of patients with intestinal bacterial overgrowth and chronic abdominal functional distension: A pilot study. *Acta Gastroenterológica Latinoamericana, 40*(4), 323–327.

Henriksson, A. E., Blomquist, L., Nord, C. E., Midtvedt, T., & Uribe, A. (1993). Small intestinal bacterial overgrowth in patients with rheumatoid arthritis. *Annals of the Rheumatic Diseases, 52*(7), 503–510.

Davis, P. J., Yoshida, K., & Schoenl, M. (1980). Interaction of thyroid hormone and hemoglobin. I. Nature of the interaction and effect of hemoglobin on thyroid hormone radioimmunoassay. *The Journal of Laboratory and Clinical Medicine, 95*(5), 714–724.

Bures, J., Cyrany, J., Kohoutova, D., Förstl, M., Rejchrt, S., Kvetina, J., . . . Kopacova, M. (2010). Small intestinal bacterial overgrowth syndrome. *World Journal of Gastroenterology, 16*(24), 2978–2990.

Index

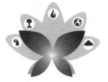

About the Author

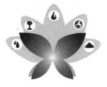

Marc Ryan, L.Ac., is a graduate of Cornell University and a licensed acupuncturist and herbalist in the state of California who practices functional medicine.

After suffering from his own battle with Hashimoto's and discovering an alternative approach to healing it, he decided to devote his life to doing everything he could to help others find hope, help, and healing.

In the last four years, he has spent thousands of hours researching, working with, and talking to over 2,000 Hashimoto's patients.

Website: www.hashimotoshealing.com

HOW TO heal

HASHIMOTO'S

Programs and Services

At Hashimoto's Healing we offer a number of programs and services to support you in healing Hashimoto's and autoimmunity.

These include:

* Consultations and Case Reviews with Marc

* Online membership programs that include access to our Healing Hashimoto's library and private Facebook group

* The How to Heal Hashimoto's Program - Our online program that helps you implement what you learn in *How to Heal Hashimoto's: An Integrative Road Map to Remission*

* Programs that focus on specific problems:

- Save Your Brain: For healing and preventing neurodegeneration caused by Hashimoto's and hypothyroidism

- Abundant Energy: A program designed to help you restore energy, endurance, and strength to mind and body

- Perfect Weight: A program designed to help you lose those stubborn pounds using diet, exercise, and circadian rhythm balance

- 4 Weeks to Healing: A program designed to help you create a lifestyle that supports healing, including: Installing new habits, a diet for reducing inflammation and calming your immune system, healthy stress management, and exercising the right way with Hashimoto's

TO LEARN MORE ABOUT OUR PROGRAMS AND SERVICES:

Visit: www.hashimotoshealing.com
E-mail us at marc@hashimotoshealing.com
Call us at 310-831-2202
Hope, help, and healing for Hashimoto's

We hope you enjoyed this Hay House book. If you'd like to receive our online catalog featuring additional information on Hay House books and products, or if you'd like to find out more about the Hay Foundation, please contact:

Hay House, Inc., P.O. Box 5100, Carlsbad, CA 92018-5100
(760) 431-7695 or (800) 654-5126
(760) 431-6948 (fax) or (800) 650-5115 (fax)
www.hayhouse.com® • www.hayfoundation.org

Published and distributed in Australia by:
Hay House Australia Pty. Ltd., 18/36 Ralph St., Alexandria NSW 2015
Phone: 612-9669-4299 • *Fax:* 612-9669-4144 • www.hayhouse.com.au

Published and distributed in the United Kingdom by:
Hay House UK, Ltd., Astley House, 33 Notting Hill Gate, London W11 3JQ
Phone: 44-20-3675-2450 • *Fax:* 44-20-3675-2451 • www.hayhouse.co.uk

Published and distributed in the Republic of South Africa by:
Hay House SA (Pty), Ltd., P.O. Box 990, Witkoppen 2068
info@hayhouse.co.za • www.hayhouse.co.za

Published in India by: Hay House Publishers India, Muskaan Complex,
Plot No. 3, B-2, Vasant Kunj, New Delhi 110 070 • *Phone:* 91-11-4176-1620
Fax: 91-11-4176-1630 • www.hayhouse.co.in

Distributed in Canada by:
Raincoast Books, 2440 Viking Way, Richmond, B.C. V6V 1N2
Phone: 1-800-663-5714 • *Fax:* 1-800-565-3770 • www.raincoast.com

Take Your Soul on a Vacation

Visit www.HealYourLife.com® to regroup, recharge, and reconnect
with your own magnificence. Featuring blogs, mind-body-spirit news,
and life-changing wisdom from Louise Hay and friends.

Free e-newsletters from Hay House, the Ultimate Resource for Inspiration

Be the first to know about Hay House's dollar deals, free downloads, special offers, affirmation cards, giveaways, contests, and more!

 Get exclusive excerpts from our latest releases and videos from *Hay House Present Moments*.

 Enjoy uplifting personal stories, how-to articles, and healing advice, along with videos and empowering quotes, within *Heal Your Life*.

 Have an inspirational story to tell and a passion for writing? Sharpen your writing skills with insider tips from *Your Writing Life*.

Sign Up Now!

Get inspired, educate yourself, get a complimentary gift, and share the wisdom!

http://www.hayhouse.com/newsletters.php

Visit www.hayhouse.com to sign up today!

 HAY HOUSE

HAYHOUSE RADIO)) *radio for your soul*

HealYourLife.com ♥

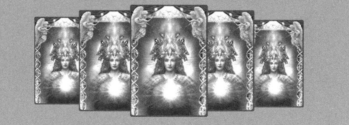